Keith

I could not have realized this book, as much of what is good in it, without your steady, and patient, guidance. Thanks for mentoring me, and most of all for your friendship.

Stephen
7/5/11

THE BLEEDING DISEASE

*Hemophilia and
the Unintended Consequences
of Medical Progress*

STEPHEN PEMBERTON

The Johns Hopkins University Press
Baltimore

The Johns Hopkins University Press
2715 North Charles Street
Baltimore, Maryland 21218-4363
www.press.jhu.edu

Library of Congress Cataloging-in-Publication Data

Pemberton, Stephen Gregory.
    The bleeding disease : hemophilia and the unintended consequences of medical progress / Stephen Pemberton.
        p. ; cm.
    Includes bibliographical references and index.
    ISBN-13: 978-1-4214-0115-7 (hardcover : alk. paper)
    ISBN-10: 1-4214-0115-0 (hardcover : alk. paper)
    1. Hemophilia—United States—History. I. Title.
    [DNLM: 1. Hemophilia A—history—United States. 2. Hemophilia A—therapy—United States. 3. Blood Transfusion—United States. 4. HIV Infections—transmission—United States. 5. History, 20th Century—United States. 6. Liver Transplantation—trends—United States. WH 11 AA1]
    RC642.P46 2011
    616.1'572—dc22   2010049749

A catalog record for this book is available from the British Library.

Special discounts are available for bulk purchases of this book. For more information, please contact Special Sales at 410-516-6936 or specialsales@press.jhu.edu.

The Johns Hopkins University Press uses environmentally friendly book materials, including recycled text paper that is composed of at least 30 percent post-consumer waste, whenever possible. All of our book papers are acid-free, and our jackets and covers are printed on paper with recycled content.

This book is dedicated to the memory of

Dr. Kenneth Brinkhous (1908–2000)

and the many other pioneers of hemophilia management

whose stories, for better or worse, are reflected here.

It is not a book that Dr. Brinkhous would have envisioned me writing,

although I wish I could share it with him, to show him how

I put my time inside and outside his laboratory to use.

One repays a teacher badly if one always remains nothing but a pupil.

—NIETZSCHE, "ON THE GIFT-GIVING VIRTUE,"
IN *THUS SPOKE ZARATHUSTRA*

CONTENTS

For more than six decades, the hereditary bleeding disorder known as hemophilia has spurred parents and doctors to engage in a concerted effort to normalize the experience of patients: to liberate them from the imminent threat of death, to alleviate their pain and debility, and to integrate them fully into society. Crucially, blood transfusions helped physicians render bleeding manageable for patients and families in the middle decades of the twentieth century. Beginning in the 1970s, many Americans with hemophilia could say that their lives were relatively normal and be viewed as normal by others. Yet, the glory of this achievement was short-lived. The therapeutic revolution that delivered this semblance of normalcy soon brought unexpected results in the 1980s: HIV/AIDS, hepatitis C, and the notorious irony of hemophilia patients' contracting virulent diseases borne by the biomedical treatments that they believed had liberated them. In the late twentieth century, the history of hemophilia became a narrative of technological promise and unfolding peril.

While the media have widely publicized stories indicating that many hemophilia patients contracted HIV (human immunodeficiency virus) during the 1980s, the public—in many ways—still does not appreciate the depth of this tragedy. In the United States, among the more than ten thousand patients whom clinicians categorized as "severe hemophiliacs," nearly nine out of ten acquired an HIV infection from the concentrated blood products they infused to control their bleeding disorder. What should we now make of this event? How are we to understand the fact that those hemophilia patients whose conditions were most heavily and expertly managed later proved to be at the highest risk of post-transfusion infections? What does it say about "modern" medicine and society that our most advanced, technology-intensive efforts to manage disease and promote health actually facilitated the opposite—greater debility and premature death?

These questions, as well as the multiple contexts that give rise to them, are the subject of *The Bleeding Disease*.

This history focuses on efforts to manage hemophilia in the United States with the goal of identifying what has been exemplary as well as worrisome about this enterprise. Readers should also know that my decision to write this particular work of history was borne out of circumstances I confronted during the 1990s. I first became interested in hemophilia in the fall of 1993 when Dr. Kenneth Brinkhous (1908–2000) introduced me to the problem. On meeting this vibrant hematologist on my arrival at the University of North Carolina, I could hardly have predicted the path on which it would put me. Then in his eighties, Brinkhous still ran a thriving blood research laboratory at the medical school, one that he had founded nearly five decades earlier.

For three formative years, I worked in the Brinkhous laboratory as an editorial and research assistant. My qualifications for the job were hardly obvious. I was not trained as a scientist, nor did I have a prior interest in medicine or health-related work. In fact, my advanced education at that point was mostly in philosophy. Yet Brinkhous seemed certain that I could play a productive role in his laboratory, and I appreciated the job and encouragement. I soon found myself helping him prepare scientific and historical talks that he was frequently invited to give, assisting him in the revisions of the laboratory's research papers, managing his archive and library, and facilitating his intellectual projects in various ways. Ostensibly, my reason for being in Chapel Hill was to get a graduate degree in history. I took the job with Brinkhous to help pay for my schooling as a historian, but soon found myself spending more time on the medical campus than I had planned. In 1994 I dropped my history classes completely and began working full time for this experimental hematologist. He had a way of making the activities in his laboratory seem all-encompassing.

Dr. Kenneth Brinkhous had a long and distinguished career as a medical scientist, and his many successes as an experimental hematologist paralleled hemophilia's transformation from an intractable disease in the 1930s into the manageable condition it had become by the 1970s. Born and educated in Iowa, Brinkhous began research on blood clotting as a medical student at the University of Iowa. Upon receiving his M.D. in 1932, Brinkhous joined the pathology faculty at Iowa where he made the characterization and correction of bleeding disorders a focus. In 1946, after his World

War II service in the Army Medical Corps, Brinkhous became chair of pathology at the University of North Carolina Medical School, where he immediately took up his hemophilia research to become one of the first hematologists to classify classical hemophilia as a deficiency of clotting factor VIII (then called "antihemophilic factor," or AHF).

Brinkhous's greatest contributions as a hemophilia researcher came in his long tenure at the University of North Carolina where one of the tallest, most imposing buildings on the campus now bears his name. In the late 1950s and early 1960s, Brinkhous and his colleagues were developing methods to produce more potent blood concentrates (aka plasma fractions) to stop hemophilic bleeding. Their major breakthrough in this area came with their 1966 announcement of the first highly potent antihemophilic factor concentrate (factor VIII concentrate). Approved by the Food and Drug Administration in 1968, this concentrate could be stored at room temperature and administered in a few minutes in a physician's office or even by the patient at home. Brinkhous retired as UNC's chair of pathology in 1973 and devoted himself to unsalaried, full-time scientific research until his death in 2000.[1]

My experiences in Brinkhous's laboratory not only initiated my interest in hemophilia, medicine, and their histories but also nourished a prior curiosity that I had about the technological character of our world. On the advice of my friend, the philosopher Todd Newman Davis, I read Bruno Latour and Steve Woolgar's *Laboratory Life* sometime during that first year working for Brinkhous. Todd's recommendation was apt. In the late 1970s, Latour and Woolgar spent time at the Salk Institute in La Jolla, California, to observe the activities of one biomedical research laboratory through an anthropological lens. *Laboratory Life* explained in exquisite detail how lab-based scientists crafted their objects of study and represented them in ways that had transformative power.[2] As Latour later put it, "Give me a laboratory and I will raise the world."[3] That anthropological vision of the laboratory grabbed me, although in different ways from Brinkhous's indigenous perspective. Still, I could not help but read one vision of the experimental laboratory in terms of the other. I was taken by the idea of studying my workplace and focusing my attention on what made Brinkhous's laboratory such a vital enterprise. I chose historian's tools more so than anthropological ones.

Brinkhous's own take on the biomedical enterprise was what you might expect of a productive scientist in the final years of his own distinguished career. In 1995 I told him that I wanted to return to active graduate studies in history, now with a focus on the history of medicine, science, and technology. I shared with him my interest in the history of his laboratory, and he was enthusiastic about my plan to return to my history studies even though it meant spending fewer hours working alongside him. What I then came to realize was that he liked the idea of having someone commemorate his research activities. Indeed, Brinkhous would later tell me that he hoped I might write a biography about him. I declined his invitation to write such a work. Yet, in composing *The Bleeding Disease*, I have communicated what I think is historically significant about the world that Brinkhous rightly wanted to remember. Unquestionably, it would hardly have been possible to render hemophilia manageable in the twentieth century without its being realized in biomedical enterprises such as his.

My efforts to make sense of hemophilia management grew increasingly broad as I learned more about the reach of Brinkhous's work beyond the laboratory and clinic. In 1997 I wrote a master's thesis in history on Brinkhous's use of hemophilic dogs for the study of hemophilia in human patients.[4] That study was rooted in my earliest attempts to provide some historical analysis of the long-standing activities of the Brinkhous laboratory. Yet, when I sought to understand the larger context in which hemophilia became a manageable disease, my research and writing turned beyond an analysis of laboratory life proper; it soon became a study of historical efforts to manage hemophilia in its changing social, cultural, and political milieu. This book is the product of the latter effort; it employs historical sources and methods to narrate and analyze how hemophilia came to be manageable.

My focus is on subjects and arguments that extend far beyond the laboratories and clinics where most hemophilia research occurs. Brinkhous's laboratory was merely my initial vantage point. The goal in studying my workplace was always to connect its activities to the larger world in which hemophilia had become a manageable disease. In the mid-1990s, this meant making sense of the devastating effect of AIDS on almost everything related to hemophilia and its management. I met several people with hemophilia during that time, all of them men who carried HIV and hepatitis C viruses in their bodies. Most had active infections that were killing them. Some of them have since died. These individuals were acquaintances, not friends. But their stories, lives, and work moved me. A couple of these persons were social activists. All of them took precious time out of their lives to impress upon me what mattered to them, what was wrong with the world as they knew it, and how they were trying to change things for the better. My encounters with them were brief; and few as they were, they proved to be a necessary antidote to the hype and self-serving rhetoric that often surrounded the good work that physicians, scientists, and other experts did for the hemophilia community.

This book also addresses some of the chief ironies in the history of hemophilia management—including the high rates of post-transfusion HIV/AIDS experienced by hemophilia patients in the 1980s. A variety of articles and books have appeared over the years that detail the mistakes of pharmaceutical firms, blood banks, the federal government, and even individual physicians in making this iatrogenic tragedy possible. What is missing in this important but occasionally bitter literature is the context for understanding the choices that people often faced. That is not to say that some outrage is not warranted, or to dismiss the incendiary evidence that does exist. Wrongs clearly occurred, and accountability is vitally important. But what is most critical as we move forward is that we understand the conditions that put so many people in difficult, if not compromising circumstances in the first place. Above all, the goal of this book is to promote understanding of efforts to manage hemophilia and other diseases so that such efforts can actually promote health and healing rather than its opposite.

ACKNOWLEDGMENTS

R esearching and writing this book was, at once, a collective enterprise and personal challenge. It took many years to mature as the people who informed my writing compelled me to grow. I am thankful to them all.

The book, and my career as a historian, would not have been possible without the mentorship of Keith Wailoo. He was resolute in helping me realize this project from our very first meeting, through my graduate student and postdoctoral years and, more recently, as a colleague. I benefited most deeply from my extended apprenticeship with Keith but also from the intellectual and material resources he shared with me. Significant funding for my work came directly from the James S. McDonnell Foundation Centennial Fellowship in the History of Science awarded to Keith in 1999, as well as from his Robert Wood Johnson Investigator Award in Health Policy, which facilitated my postdoctoral studies of pain, stigma, and disability issues in chronic disease management. I thank these foundations for investing in Keith's vision of opening new areas of scholarship in the history of science, medicine, and health policy.

My hemophilia research was also funded by a John J. Pisano Grant from the Historical Office at the National Institutes of Health (1998–99), a George E. Mowry Dissertation Research Award from the Department of History at the University of North Carolina, Chapel Hill (2000), a faculty fellowship at the Rutgers Center for Historical Analysis in New Brunswick (2002–3), a Visiting Scholar's Residency at the Institute for Medical Humanities at the University of Texas Medical Branch, Galveston (2004), and a faculty development grant at the New Jersey Institute of Technology (2004–5). My gratitude for these resources extends beyond these institutions to the many individuals who made them possible.

My investments in hemophilia as well as the history of medicine began at the University of North Carolina at Chapel Hill, and there were many people affiliated with UNC in the 1990s who merit special recognition. My

Ph.D. committee included Keith Wailoo, Michael McVaugh, Peter Filene, Peter Redfield (Anthropology), and Duke University's Jeffrey Baker (History/Pediatrics). I thank each of them for their expert guidance but am also thankful for the special assistance of Lloyd Kramer (History), Rosa Haritos (Sociology), and the faculty and graduate students of UNC's Department of History. My scholarly and professional growth was significant during my years as a Research Associate in UNC's Department of Social Medicine. Larry Churchill, Donald Madison, Nancy King, Sue Estroff, Barry Saunders, Jon Oberlander, Gail Henderson, Arlene Davis, Myra Collins, and Desmond Runyon all aided my development as an interdisciplinary scholar of medicine and society. In the Department of Pathology and Laboratory Medicine, my thanks to Dr. Marjorie S. Read and Dr. Timothy Nichols as well as to the professional staff of the Francis Owen Blood Research Laboratory. They each made the Brinkhous laboratory so vibrant in my time there, and greatly facilitated my peculiar interest in hematological science.

Since 2001, I have resided in New Jersey and have benefited enormously from being part of the extended community of scholars affiliated with the New Jersey Institute of Technology and Rutgers University. For all that they have done to improve my productivity and spirits, special thanks are due to my NJIT history colleagues, Richard Sher, Neil Maher, Allison Perlman, Lisa Nocks, John O'Connor, Maureen O'Rourke, Gautham Rao, Doris Sher, and our enlightened dean, Fadi Deek. Thanks as well to my faculty colleagues and students in the Federated History Department of Rutgers, Newark, and to my affiliated colleagues in the Department of History at Rutgers, New Brunswick. My writing was aided by Lisa Troiano, Lucien Patterson, and Katherine Keirns, each one an able research assistant from the Federated History Department's M.A. in History program.

My familiarity with the histories of hematology and the hemophilia community was greatly enhanced by individuals with deep and, sometimes, direct knowledge of events covered in this book. Susan Resnick and Douglas Starr deserve my special thanks. I drew heavily on their books and research along the way. Susan was particularly kind to share her source interviews from *Blood Saga* with me, and Doug was forgiving of me for my failure to give him his full due in my short book review of *Blood*. My own book builds on their path-breaking scholarship. More directly, I benefited from conversations with physicians Jack Alperin, Harvey Alter, Bruce Evatt, Leon Hoyer, Jay Hoofnagle, and Dale Lawrence, and from discussions with filmmaker Marilyn Ness and hemophilia activists Warren Jewett, Craig Epson-Nelms, Bill Horn McGinnis, and Carol Grayson as well as from interactions with several HIV-positive persons with hemophilia (who will remain anonymous).

Oral historians, librarians, and archival specialists were particularly gracious about my requests for help. Laura Gray and Kathryn Hammond Baker facilitated my access to the 2004–5 oral history interviews that Laura Gray and Christine Chamberlain conducted with twenty-one men with hemophilia in the Boston area. Those interviews are now available through the Center for the History of Medicine at Harvard Medical School's Countway Library. Dianne O'Malia ably assisted my use of the Oscar Ratnoff papers at the Stanley Ferguson Archive at University Hospitals Case Medical Center, Cleveland. I also thank the special collections librarians at the National Library of Medicine (for assistance with the U.S. Blood Policy Papers), Harvard University Archives (for access to the Edwin Cohn and Richard Cabot papers), and the Marriott Library at the University of Utah (for use of the Maxwell Wintrobe papers).

Many other individuals in my scholarly and social networks gave constructive feedback or assistance, including Andrew Arnold, Robert Aronowitz, Eric Avery, Allan Brandt, Susan Burch, Susan Carruthers, Ronald Carson, John Chasteen, Thomas R. Cole, Michael L. Dorn, Gary Farney, James Faubion, Gerard Fitzgerald, Gary Frost, Joseph Gabriel, Jeremy Greene, Bert Hansen, Donna Haraway, Victoria Harden, Paul Israel, Will P. Jones, Ann Kakaliouras, Elizabeth Dolan, Carla Keirns, Hannah Landecker, Jackson Lears, Barron Lerner, Susan Lindee, Simi Linton, Julie Livingston, Candida Mannozzi, James Marcum, Harry Marks, Richard Mizelle, Arwen Mohun, Ellen More, Sandra Moss, Khalil Muhummad, Kelly Overton, Randall Packard, Dominique Padurano, Reggie Pearson, Michael Petit, Scott Podowsky, Karen Rader, Edmund Russell, Beryl Satter, David Sartorius, Jessie Saul, Susan Schrepfer, David Serlin, Susan Speaker, Sandra Sufian, John Swann, Karen Kruse Thomas, Moshe Usadi, Helen Valier, William Winslade, and the families of John J. Pisano and Kenneth Brinkhous.

I owe an even greater debt to those individuals who read the whole manuscript or chapters as the book developed and neared completion. This crucial group of readers included Jeffrey Baker, Jacalyn Duffin, Curt Gibson, Gerald Grob, Jennifer Harmsen, Joel Howell, Susan Lederer, Philip

Pauly, Stefani Pfeiffer, Charles Rosenberg, Keith Wailoo, and two anonymous reviewers for the Johns Hopkins University Press. Audra Wolfe became my lifeline to judicious and clear writing in the final months of revisions, and Jacqueline Wehmueller provided the editorial acumen and leadership at the Johns Hopkins University Press. The book is undoubtedly better because of their interventions.

My deepest gratitude is reserved for my wife, Samantha Kelly, and my family and friends, who have supported me throughout this project and carried me through both the best and worst of times. Thank you, Samantha and Hugh, Patsy and John Pemberton, Heather and Juan José Ortiz, Prescott and Pamela Kelly, Judith and Vince McBrien, and the extended Kelly and McBrien clan. Thanks as well to my steadfast gadfly, Todd Davis. "The world of the happy man is a different one from that of an unhappy man." You have all willed only happiness.

Although I have benefited enormously from the help of many giving and talented people in the execution of this work, the way I have posed the problem of hemophilia might be read as peculiar to my own concerns about the biotechnological age in which we live. If the book fails to offer satisfactory answers to the questions it poses, I hope at least that it points readers toward the kinds of questions we should be asking ourselves about the challenges of disease, the promotion of health, and the uncertain terms of biomedical progress.

The Bleeding Disease

Introduction

Hemophilia as Pathology of Progress

K nowledge about hemophilia is not uncommon. In the first half of the twentieth century, this physician's term of art spread into popular usage as journalists reported its effects among the royal families in Great Britain, Germany, Spain, and Russia. Because of hemophilia's colorful reputation among educated laypeople in the 1930s, students of heredity in the United States often mentioned it to familiarize the reading public with the principles of Mendelian genetics and sex-linked traits. Eugenicists likewise found it useful in their promotions of "better breeding" and "fitter families." From the 1940s through the early 1960s, the word gained traction among advocates of hematological science, transfusion medicine, and voluntary blood donation. As the hemophilia patient's demand for blood plasma grew in postwar America, the public learned that this hereditary disorder afflicted many ordinary families, not just aristocratic ones. By the mid-1960s, hemophilia was a focus of the emergent biotechnology industry, and it even had a role in policy and legislative debates about affordable health care in the early 1970s. More recently, Americans witnessed the tragic coupling of hemophilia and AIDS in the tainted blood scandals of the 1980s and 1990s.

The word *hemophilia* has resonated in surprisingly diverse ways in the twentieth century, marking something deeper in modern medicine and society than just its increased visibility. Hemophilia has traveled far in the past century precisely because we, as a modernizing society, have transformed the disease and rendered it manageable. Just as insulin helped transform diabetes (type I) from an acute condition into a chronic, manageable disease, biomedical knowledge and technologies have played a critical role in transmuting how people experience hemophilia.[1] Hemophilia's significance within the developed world has only multiplied as our technology-intensive efforts to manage it have enjoyed success. But it is the paradoxical terms of that success, particularly the new opportunities and dangers that medical management has entailed, that speaks to the enduring relevance of this bleeding disorder and its history. Efforts to manage hemophilia as both a medical and a social problem concern not only the long-standing and deeply felt aspiration to "normalize" the experience of patients with bleeding disorders but also a wide range of issues in modern American medicine and society that have surfaced in conjunction with the rising incidence of heart disease, cancer, stroke, diabetes, kidney failure, and other chronic conditions over the past century.[2] In short, the management of hemophilia is a subject that informs and reflects our increasingly biotechnological way of life, and we ignore it at our own peril.

A Chronicle of Perilous Progress

Although hemophilia is among the oldest hereditary diseases on record, it emerged as a subject of sustained medical attention only in the nineteenth century. Since the 1890s, clinicians have highlighted hemophilia's three cardinal characteristics: frequent and prolonged bleeding into joints and soft tissue, a family history of uncontrollable bleeding among male family members, and a laboratory test that indicates that the patient's blood is slow to clot. Even though the reading public knew hemophilia as little more than a strange malady of European royalty during the 1920s and 1930s, patients, families, and their physicians knew it as a devastating hereditary disease characterized by prolonged bleeding, disabling pain, and social isolation. Whether it was regarded as a curiosity or merited the seriousness befitting its tragic impact on certain families, hemophilia's visibility remained limited before the age of transfusions and mass blood donation.

The widespread use of transfusions for hemophilia that required very public calls for fresh blood and plasma substantially raised the cultural visibility of hemophilia in the United States in the two decades after World

War II. In fact, the need for blood donors prompted families and physicians to work together to provide hemophilic children with the attention and resources they required to treat their condition effectively. Hemophilia communities emerged in the 1950s as the National Hemophilia Foundation (established in 1948) and other family-based advocacy groups aided patients with bleeding disorders.[3] Expectations about hemophilia also changed for the better as physicians and scientists developed increasingly powerful hematological tools for diagnosing and treating bleeding disorders. Postwar physicians were envisioning a life of medical management for their pediatric hemophilia patients and the prospects of healthier lives. Patients along with their families embraced what modern medicine both promised and offered in the late 1940s, and increasingly they spoke of their opportunities to be "normal" beginning by the late 1950s. The media, in their occasional coverage of hemophilia, also began promoting the idea that a "normal life" was possible for "the hemophiliac."[4] As such, the rising visibility of hemophilia in postwar American society was linked to the idea of its medical management and how experts and laypeople could help achieve that goal.

Efforts to render hemophilia manageable were fully realized in the 1970s following the widespread introduction of potent new treatments made from blood plasma. These products—cryoprecipitate and clotting factor concentrates—were rich in the clot-promoting proteins that hemophilia patients lacked. The American hemophilia community emerged as a small but potent political group, one whose significance reflected many factors: dramatic public awareness campaigns and lobbying by the National Hemophilia Foundation; growing recognition by the federal government that the hemophiliac's plight as a blood consumer was a telltale sign of the state of the nation's blood resources; and increased visibility for the medical management of hemophilia, which in turn highlighted discussions of the proper roles of private industry and government in delivering life-promoting technologies to health consumers. Experts were aware that serious complications and risks remained part of hemophilia management even as they witnessed enormous progress. Conditions were hardly ideal. Yet there was widespread consensus by the decade's end that every hemophilia patient in America could expect a "near normal" life-span given the current state of medical management. In fact, by 1980 comprehensive care programs for hemophilia had brought the median life expectancy of American patients in line with that for all U.S. males (67.5 years and 71.1 years, respectively).[5] Such progress was cause for celebration.

The attainment of some normalcy for persons with hemophilia proved tragically brief. In the 1980s, through their now standard transfusions of pooled plasma products, nearly 60 percent of patients with hemophilia contracted the human immunodeficiency virus (HIV) that causes acquired immunodeficiency syndrome (AIDS). The infection rate approached 90 percent among the severe hemophiliacs who routinely used clotting factor concentrates.[6] This turn of events brought the normalizing expectations of physicians and the hemophilia community into question. The intense media attention accorded to AIDS created a new cultural and social context for persons with hemophilia: the "hemophiliac" was now widely portrayed as a victim not only of disease but also of society. The patient's fate was being attributed to diverse sources by the late 1980s: "technology gone awry," biomedical mismanagement, incompetent government, and corporate greed.[7]

In the two decades before AIDS, many persons with hemophilia had the opportunity to experience themselves as members of a distinctive community—an experience that proved critical in the 1990s in lobbying for public, governmental, and biomedical attention to their plight. Concurrently, biomedical scientists, blood bankers, and the pharmaceutical industry sought technical and administrative solutions to the crisis. By fine-tuning public health policies and creating new biomedical technologies, this community of experts helped shield hemophilia patients not already infected with HIV/AIDS from the terror of blood-borne pathogens, proffering anew (albeit in a different environment from that of the 1950s to 1970s) the possibility of a technologically normalized life.

The transfusion-related AIDS crisis is one of the most notorious catastrophes of recent medical history, yet it also suggests why the history of hemophilia management provides fertile ground for examining the intended and unintended consequences of biomedical progress in the twentieth century. There were at least sixteen thousand Americans under intensive treatment for hemophilia in the 1980s; the majority of them contracted HIV during the first few years of the AIDS epidemic. By 1994, more than a quarter of the U.S. hemophilia population had died of causes related to AIDS. Many were children and adolescents.[8] People in the hemophilia community began to wonder what this medical and social catastrophe meant. They were shocked, angry, and disappointed. Many patients felt betrayed by their doctors. Most blamed the corporations that sold them their blood products. Some targeted the federal government for failing to protect them. There was even anger at the National Hemophilia Foundation for downplaying the risks of AIDS when it might have prevented the spread of HIV among hemophilia patients and their families. Blame also spread easily because the doctors, drug industry, government, and hemophilia associations had all failed to deliver on their respective promises of care. And while it remains debatable who was actually responsible for this collective failure, no one had any doubts about the tragic character of it all. AIDS threw into question the considerable progress that medicine and society—comprising essentially the same doctors, drug companies, government agencies, and hemophilia associations—had made in the preceding decades.

While the epidemic of AIDS among hemophilia families was an unwanted effect of the substantial progress made in managing this bleeding disorder in the twentieth century, this disaster is also symptomatic of a technological approach to disease that requires considerable historical and sociological perspective to evaluate. Most people with hemophilia who lived in the 1980s have already died. The few hemophilia patients who survive are now being treated for multiple diseases (e.g., HIV infections, hepatitis C infections) beyond their primary bleeding disorder (factor VIII or factor IX deficiency). The healers who treat these patients carry a different but related sort of burden: the obligation of hemophilia management's past successes and failures. Interpreting the burdens on both healers and patients can be aided by greater knowledge of the ways that medical progress in the management of hemophilia and other diseases has been constituted as a technological enterprise.

The need to understand the burdens of technological success in the treatment of chronic conditions such as hemophilia, diabetes, or cardiovascular disease is one reason why Edward Tenner devoted two chapters of his 1996 book *Why Things Bite Back* to past efforts by physicians to use technology to manage health and disease. As he put it, modern medicine is full of "revenge effects" that strike back on the medical enterprise itself. Robotic surgery and laparoscopy are recent examples. Each procedure entails localized cutting that is less traumatic for the patient than the conventional scalpel. Yet, as Tenner explains, surgeons using these technologies peer at the body through a "television image," unable to "feel organs directly with their fingers." To avoid poorer outcomes for their patients, surgeons using robots or laparoscopy must become proficient at a different skill set from that of surgeons using the spatial-motor abilities of classic surgery. Moreover, the introduction of computer-assisted surgery has not obviated the need for traditional surgical skills, thus requiring more of the doctor, not less. Yet the demands of technological medicine go beyond a greater need for training and professionalism; they call for heightened vigilance as well. Medical care tends to become more intensive where technology is employed, and the risk of medical complications can increase with greater technical savvy. Thus, as suggested by the rise of multidrug-resistant tuberculosis or the onset of graph-versus-host disease following organ transplantation, when complications do occur in contemporary medicine, they are more often serious or fatal.[9] Similar arguments can be made about AIDS and hepatitis among hemophilia patients and other recipients of blood products. Certainly, hemophilia doctors have become all-too-familiar with the revenge effects of technological sophistication.

Although technology has been a double-edged sword for Americans with hemophilia and the physicians who treat them, it also represents a challenge to those writing histories of hemophilia and other diseases. In 1963, for instance, physician Charles Baldwin Kerr reflected back on the life prospects of hemophilia patients in the nineteenth century. His historical essay addressed the period running from 1793 until about 1910 and described various clinical observations and ineffectual treatments of that era. In rendering hemophilia's past, Kerr added his gloss on its future:

> When the final history of haemophilia is written it will be divided into three parts. The first part will describe the era of clinical observation and ineffectual treatment. The second part will deal with an age of increasingly effective medical management and better understanding of the underlying mechanisms of haemophilia. The third and final chapter is yet to come. Not until the disease can be permanently suppressed or, at least, controlled in the manner in which insulin restores the disturbed physiology of a diabetic will the haemophiliac face life on equal terms with his healthy colleagues.[10]

Since Kerr wrote in the early 1960s, historians and other scholars have begun examining the ways that disease not only shapes social relations, politics, cultures, and ideologies but also embodies their diverse qualities and effects. Kerr undoubtedly wrote about hemophilia in a simpler era, at a time (pre-AIDS) that was not perceived to be "out of joint" or "at odds with itself."[11] His conception of the history of hemophilia was not one of confrontation with technology but rather one of congeniality toward it. For him, the management of hemophilia was a benign enterprise: if things were not getting better, they were at least getting no worse. For a time, Kerr's vision of the future seemed assured. Management of hemophilia got dramatically better. By 1973, when clotting factor concentrates for controlling hemophilic bleeding were first becoming widely available in the United States, Donna Boone added, "Progress has been made in the third chapter in the history of hemophilia described by C. B. Kerr, with the temporary normalization of the disturbed coagulation status of the hemophilia patient."[12] Boone was a physical therapist working daily with pediatric hemophilia patients in Los Angeles. Indeed, much of what Kerr projected for the hemophilia patient in 1963 had seemingly come to pass by 1973. Unfortunately, Kerr's melioristic categories do not allow us to make much sense of what has happened since the 1970s. To put it bluntly, the aims of hemophilia management are no longer as self-evident or benign as they once seemed. HIV/AIDS and other events of the past quarter century require us to examine the ends of therapy in ways that Kerr and Boone could not have imagined.

As Kerr and Boone remind us, "normalization" was the goal that hemophilia management set for itself in the post–World War II decades. In researching this history, I have traced how this elusive therapeutic goal came into being, and how it has fared in the midst and wake of the transfusion AIDS tragedy. As such, the story I relate confronts the hold that technology exercises within American medicine and society by examining what the management of disease has actually entailed in its affirmations of both technology and normality.

Entwined with hemophilia's narrative of technological promise and peril is also a story of gender and social identities repeatedly negotiated, challenged, and redefined. In the first half of the twentieth century, scientists and physicians characterized hemophilia as a sex-linked trait transmitted by asymptomatic females to their male offspring. It was, in short, a "male" disease; and many experts of this era believed that symptomatic hemophilia in the female was a practical impossibility. New diagnostic technologies and growing awareness of the variety of existing bleeding disorders led, in the early 1950s, to the first medical discoveries of "female hemophiliacs," followed over the next decade by a medical redefinition of hemophilia that again limited its diagnosis almost exclusively to males. Such long-forgotten events exemplify how social and cultural factors as well as our disease concepts shape the story of biomedical advance, for while hematologists could now detect a more diverse range of bleeding disorders, the interpretation of that evidence, and the delineation of categorical boundaries around it, allowed these experts considerable room for choice in how they defined and diagnosed hemophilia. The decision to limit hemophilia diagnoses almost exclusively to males reflected a complex mix of attitudes in the mid-twentieth century that included commitments to using biological sex as an ordering mechanism and a related preference to reinforce a therapeutic culture that had become visibly gendered over the years.

The gendered aspects of hemophilia culture has had profound ramifications for those afflicted: for females with bleeding disorders whose status within the hemophilia community was often ambiguous, and for males whose treatment-based "normalization" was deeply infused with notions of idealized masculinity. This focus on masculinity included an unspoken hope for transcendence beyond the aspects of disease and disability that both experts and laypersons sometimes characterized as emasculating or "feminizing" influences on the hemophiliac's otherwise male identity.[13] Such patterns of thought took shape in the 1950s and early 1960s, years well known to historians as an era of gender retrenchment and anxiety.[14] Anxieties about gender emerged again in the mid-1980s when the enormous attention directed at the gay community and its affliction with HIV/AIDS brought the hemophilia community—and its long history of embracing mainstream masculine norms—into sudden and close identification with stereotyped perceptions of homosexual men and gay lifestyles.[15]

The histories of hemophilia and the hemophilia community should also be seen in the context of broader American debates about health care, the rights and responsibilities of individuals, the character of civil society, and the boundaries of citizenship. As diverse scholars have highlighted in recent years, normality is itself a powerful means of governance in liberal democratic societies such as the United States.[16] The promise that American society holds out to its citizens and immigrants—of upward social mobility, of economic prosperity, and of opportunities for personal fulfillment—has frequently been predicated upon the individual's conformity to norms such as physical autonomy and productivity. Failures to meet these normative standards all too often become evidence of a person's unfitness for full participation in society.

Social norms profoundly inform the history of hemophilia as well as the histories of other diseases and disabilities.[17] These norms are evident in the varied efforts to transform "hemophiliacs" into autonomous, vigorous, and productive male members of society and in the enthusiasm for their status as health consumers, which in the 1960s and 1970s involved them in a profitable, yet dangerous, blood economy.[18] These norms are at stake in the advocacy efforts that presumed certain rights (of organization as an interest group, of legal recourse for their grievances, of legislative protection from health risks, of economic access to new treatments) belonging to the diseased or disabled. Of course, what constitutes the normal and the pathological is also a continually contested and contestable question.[19] As widely evident in American debates about health care, the recent history of hemophilia has frequently illustrated such disputation in the larger arena of U.S. history where efforts to manage chronic disease have presented social, political, and commercial challenges for Americans and their institutions. Finally, the ambiguous status of the American "hemophiliac"—at once citizen and stigmatized individual, in varying proportions over time—invites comparison with women, African Americans, gays and lesbians, and other groups whose historically ambiguous and challenged status in the American polity are more familiar to students of U.S. history.[20]

Recent efforts to manage hemophilia well illustrate the powers, conflicts, and ironies of living in a "normalizing" society in which science and technology play critical roles. In rendering hemophilia's history as a lens onto normalization in twentieth-century medicine and society, I have identified three themes—technology, gender, and governance—that are critical to any historical analysis of hemophilia management. These themes are visible in the ways that expertise and biomedical technology shape our experiences and aspirations (in the laboratory, the clinic, and home care), the ways gender affects our persistent efforts to sustain ourselves and our communities (as seen through the lens of a sex-linked disorder that is limited almost exclusively to males), and the ways our bodily conceptions figure into recent debates over the rights, responsibilities, and borders of social and political identity (as evidenced by issues of health care access and transfusion-related AIDS).

Running throughout these key themes, and integral to how people with hemophilia interpreted normality, are the problems of stigma and dependency. Hemophilia patients and families have long interpreted advances in medicine as a means to combat stigma and constitute personal autonomy. For this reason, *The Bleeding Disease* situates the problems of stigma and autonomy as critical, yet largely underrecognized dimensions of the hemophilia experience. Thus, when I say that American medicine and society framed hemophilia as a bleeding disorder predominantly found among males, or when I remark that doctors imagined or treated hemophilia as controllable using modern medical technologies, or when I intimate that social organizations and institutions were creating the social forms of life necessary for people with hemophilia to govern their own lives, I am also speaking to the fact that management of hemophilia extends beyond the control of bleeds, the reduction of pain, and the avoidance of crippling. In short, effective healing transcends the technological framing of disease management that often dominates our descriptions of contemporary medicine.

Interpreting Hemophilia's History

How have we—as a modernizing society—treated hemophilia as a manageable problem? Historians have not tackled this question in any depth, though it is essential for our understanding of the disease and the experiences of those who suffer from it. While historians have long been interested in accurately describing the patient's experience of hemophilia, they have usually focused on the scientific understanding of the disease and the medical, economic, and even political revolutions associated with it. While it is fascinating to ponder how hemophilia impacted the course of the Russian Revolution, or the critical role it played in the transformation of blood into a commodity in the past century, this book travels a different path.[21] It lays out a context for interpreting how modernizing people have transformed hemophilia into a manageable experience and have learned to live with it on those terms.

If hemophilia can be seen as having powerful significance for contemporary society, that is because effective disease management only begins with the patient and the physician. Rendering diseases manageable requires social support for both doctors and patients, and such care of the doctor-patient relationship involves individuals and institutions throughout modern society. Thus, patients and families have been as critical to hemophilia management as the work of medical and scientific experts. On another level, the institutions that sustain these human actors are equally crucial to the success or failure of disease management. By *management,* I am therefore referencing a broader enterprise than the services that modern medicine has offered patients and their families. This managerial enterprise has amplified the significance of a relatively rare problem and thereby rendered hemophilia's history into a significant event for sectors of society that have no direct contact with, or little knowledge of, the disease itself. Where this book intimates how hemophilia speaks to issues of technological medicine in the United States and other advanced industrialized nations, it is speaking about some of the key ways that modernizing societies have constituted hemophilia as a manageable problem.

A disease, on one level, is a highly sophisticated way of conceptualizing illness; it is a tool of art, an abstraction created and sustained by physicians in a mostly good-faith effort to promote the health of patients who are facing a debilitating biological event.[22] The fact that physicians use science to realize their disease concepts and improve their healing craft does not make medicine any less of an art. It just makes it "modern." And there is nothing so modern in medicine as the act of transforming an acute condition into a chronic disease that can be managed over the life course of an individual.[23]

The transformation from acute to chronic disease requires social progress as well as advances in science and technology. It matters that hemophilia experts and advocates in the mid-twentieth century conceptualized this disease not only as correctable but also as a predominantly male problem that could be "normalized." Patients and families did not think of advances in transfusion medicine simply as a means to control bleeding; they also interpreted them as a means of lessening physical pain, avoiding crippling, overcoming isolation, combating stigma, constituting autonomy, and maximizing their personal happiness. Postwar technological investments in hemophilia management, the appearance of a recognizable hemophilia community, and this community's long-standing commitment to realizing "normal lives" for predominantly male patients were closely linked. Normality, I therefore argue, became a historically important concept in the 1950s that both experts and laypeople increasingly used to mark progress in their efforts to manage hemophilia.

In postwar America, people with hemophilia learned to embrace the notion that normality was attainable for them and their families with the assistance of modern medicine. Normality became a critical ethic within the American hemophilia community precisely because the advancement of medicine played off the very human inclination that patients and their families had to pursue meaningful lives. Medicine was promising to transform their hereditary condition into something manageable. Disease management thus came to mean more than freedom from bleeding, pain, and crippled joints; it promised healthier, more fulfilled lives.

This book treats normality as an acculturated commitment to modern disease management. As I understand it, the flexible concept of normality signified a critical but understated strategy in postwar America for making people with hemophilia into credibly healthy people. By "credibly healthy people," I simply mean that people with hemophilia could say that their lives were relatively normal and be viewed that way by others. People with hemophilia have long confronted stigma in the unwanted scrutiny or prejudice their hereditary bleeding disorder has often invited in the minds of others.

Normality and stigma are intertwined, and no one seems to have captured this dynamic relationship in post–World War II America quite as well as sociologist Erving Goffman. For this reason, my interpretation of Goffman's 1963 book, *Stigma: Notes on the Management of Spoiled Identity*, played a formative role in how I have presented the story of American society's uneven progress in managing hemophilia. People with hemophilia confronted stigma in the unwanted scrutiny or prejudice their hereditary bleeding disorder often invited in the minds of others. In his analysis of how people manage perception of stigmatizing conditions that are identified with them, Goffman not only explores how postwar Americans differentiated stigmatized individuals from so-called normals but also explains what marks an individual as "discreditable."[24] Goffman's analytical distinction between the normal and the discreditable individual points to the fact that health conditions that are potentially stigmatizing are experienced differently depending on their visibility to others; and, by extension, that these experiences also change over time as the conditions governing the visibility of illness and debility change. This logic also means that any stigmas associated with a disease will themselves evolve as our efforts to manage that malady succeed or fail. The degree to which a sick person can be socially discredited, or cast as discreditable, or portrayed as "normal" or resistant to social discrimination should matter in any historical assessment of medical efforts to manage disease. And, as I have already said, Americans with hemophilia were often as invested in managing stigma as they were in alleviating the physical symptoms of disease. Thus, the hemophilic individual's changing status from a discreditable individual into a normal person in the postwar decades not only marks progress in the history of hemophilia management but also enhances our capacity to understand the cultural and social investments that the American hemophilia community had going into the AIDS-crisis years and beyond.

Hemophilia, for natural and social reasons, has never been as stigmatized as some other diseases. For example, the fact that this hereditary bleeding disorder is far less stigmatized than sexually transmitted diseases played an important role in public understandings of the AIDS epidemic because it allowed Americans in the late 1980s to see in images of hemophilic children with AIDS a less alien, more "normal" disease challenge. But the fact that people with hemophilia might seem more "innocent" or creditable than other kinds of sick people does not mean they have not and do not face serious stigma.

Only by seeing the rise of disease management as a social and cultural project to transform sick individuals into credibly fit individuals does it truly become clear how deeply the recent history of hemophilia is marked by uneven progress and how tenuous such progress is. Thus, as Americans with hemophilia began to experience increasing levels of fitness with twentieth-century advances in the medical and social management of their condition, these individuals entered a world in which others could no longer easily discredit them for their physical vulnerability. The visible symptoms of hemophilia began to disappear in the post–World War II decades with accelerating advances in treating bleeding disorders. Indeed, by 1980 the bodies of people with hemophilia were beginning to look no different from normal bodies before AIDS suddenly challenged that perception. Yet the AIDS years have also signaled for everyone in hemophilia management just how fragile the medical and social progress surrounding disease is.

A Trajectory for Understanding
the Hemophilia Experience

Like every disease, hemophilia generates experiences that are unique to it. When seen in the proper light, those experiences reveal both how we choose to live and how we make sense of our choices. To interpret how small groups of Americans became invested in managing hemophilia, I focus each chapter of this book on a particular dimension of this effort at a specific point in time.

Chapter 1 examines how experts in the United States and Europe conceptualized hemophilia in the years between 1800 and 1940. By highlighting how knowledge of hemophilia circulated for this nearly 150-year period, I treat the emergence of the modern hemophilia concept as a way of introducing the biological and social aspects of a disease that have been a cause of fascination and concern for laypeople as well as experts up to the present day. I argue here that issues of class, race, ethnicity, and gender have long mattered in the history of hemophilia. For instance, the chapter explains that inquisitive physicians and biologists of the early twentieth century sometimes framed hemophilia as a biological marker of social progress and degeneration even as they articulated the modern portrait of hemophilia's clinical and hereditary aspects that they hoped might one day make the condition medically manageable. But the principal argument made in this chapter is that the conceptualization of hemophilia—like any disease—is subject to the social and cultural assumptions of those who seek to understand and transform it.

Chapter 2 turns to the technological ethos that developed among hematological enthusiasts from the 1890s through the 1930s. Laboratory studies of hemophilic blood not only helped clarify the previously obscure pathology responsible for the hemophilia patient's interminable bleeding but also began transforming the care of hemophilia patients in Europe and North America. Here, the book highlights how laboratory studies of blood helped render hemophilia into a "blood disease" proper, and I explain through explicit examination of America's most prominent hemophilia investigators how a technological ethos was a critical factor in the making of a more optimistic, interventionist strategy toward this long-intransigent malady. It is a story not only about dedicated physician-researchers but also of people with hemophilia who made their blood and bodies available for study.

Chapters 3 and 4 examine the critical era after World War II (ca. 1947–64) when modernizing physicians utilized the science of hematology and the practice of transfusion medicine to redefine how the hemophilia patient could be effectively treated. It was an era when diagnostic and therapeutic technologies intersected with social norms regarding gender to shape a growing spectrum of bleeding disorders beyond "classical hemophilia" in the male. I detail how the collective decision by hematologists to limit hemophilia diagnoses almost exclusively to males reflected a complex mix of attitudes in the mid-twentieth century that included commitments to using biological sex as an ordering mechanism and a related preference to reinforce a therapeutic culture that had become rigidly gendered over the years. Yet these chapters also relate an uplifting story about how postwar patients and families emerged as a visible community in America and began to organize with a focus on medical resources mobilized around bleeding disorders. Here, I explicitly examine how affected individuals and families constituted themselves as a distinct lay community that could advocate for its interests, even as it came to rely on experts to help define how more "normal lives" were within its reach.

Chapter 5 turns to the therapeutic innovations of the 1960s that more completely fulfilled hemophilia's transformation into a manageable disease and effectively helped hemophilia patients and families realize their aspirations to be regarded not as sickly and dependent but as "normal" persons who could be more fully integrated into American society. The appearance of potent new plasma treatments—namely, cryoprecipitate and clotting factor concentrates—illustrates how dependent the nascent revolution was on technological innovation. Yet I argue that this revolution was social. The forces driving it were far too complex to be captured by any narrative that focused on medical and technical innovation alone. In fact, the social character of this therapeutic revolution derived from the fact that hemophilia patients in the United States had acquired a new and distinctive identity by virtue of how Americans embraced medical and technical innovation in the two decades after World War II. People with hemophilia now had a visibly "manageable" disease that made their aspirations for normal lives increasingly credible in the eyes of Americans. Indeed, the rising credibility of the claim that people with hemophilia could live normal lives when given access to modern treatment would provide Americans with bleeding disorders greater leverage to stake out their concerns about the nation's delivery system for blood plasma products and healthcare. Thus, this chapter points to a series of overlapping developments in American society that helped patients and their various advocates define what interests were now critical to the "hemophiliac."

Chapter 6 builds on my preceding arguments about the hemophiliac's changing status as a health consumer to address the pivotal 1970s, a decade in which the hemophilia community became more effectively involved in concerns such as how blood and blood banks should be managed as national resources, how the needs and interests of the chronically ill and economically disadvantaged could be met in the United States, and how changing demographics and other large-scale changes in American society were impacting discussions about civic responsibility, social justice, and civil rights. This chapter details further how and why the promises of hemophilia management—especially commercial clotting factor concentrates— must be understood in terms of the larger social and political economy of which this therapeutic enterprise was a part. This point is driven home with discussions of how patients and families sought autonomy for themselves, even as the National Hemophilia Foundation argued to the American public and the U.S. Congress that the plight of the "hemophiliac" was deserving of public support. Theirs was a largely successful argument, one that solidified the medical and social progress of the preceding decades by establishing federally funded hemophilia treatment centers across the United States. Not only did it seem by the late 1970s that that the majority of America's hemophilia patients were leading "normal lives," but there was guarded optimism that the emerging risks and problems that arose from recent successes in treating hemophilia were themselves manageable.

Chapter 7 brings the story of hemophilia management into the tumultuous 1980s by detailing how AIDS unexpectedly transformed the experience of hemophilia for the worse, transmuting what had been a medical success story into what some have called a "natural disaster" and what others have more correctly termed an "iatrogenic catastrophe." Transfusion-related AIDS reoriented how patients and experts experienced efforts to manage hemophilia; it changed how they understood the goals of "normalcy," autonomy, and improved health. This chapter familiarizes readers with the controversies surrounding AIDS, hemophilia, and the nation's blood economy. It not only examines how the AIDS crisis impacted the historical goals of hemophilia management but provides documentation and interpretation that should allow future investigators to explore this medical and social tragedy beyond what I have been able to do at the current time.

The book's conclusion brings the story of hemophilia management's successes and failures into the 1990s and early twenty-first century as it again addresses the significance of modern medicine's and society's efforts to manage this bleeding disorder. The question here is one of governance: namely, how should we interpret the history of hemophilia in light of the paradoxical effects of ongoing efforts to manage this bleeding disorder?

CHAPTER ONE

The Emergence of the
Hemophilia Concept

Hemophilia's unusual visibility in the twentieth century reflected its cultural status as a disease of heredity and blood. As a bodily marker of both identity and kinship, hemophilia has provided experts and laypeople with opportunities to express their thoughts and anxieties about matters of class, race, ethnicity, and gender. Thus, in covering the Second International Congress of Eugenics in 1921, the *New York Times* quoted biologist Charles Davenport as saying of hemophilia and other traits: "Already there is being developed a well-defined conscience in the matters of cousin marriages and matings into families with grossly defective members." By linking hemophilia to eugenic prohibitions against "cousin marriages," Davenport was playing off American anxieties about class and racial difference at a moment when eugenicists also sought to identify what types of hereditary traits should mark immigrants as unfit for participation in American society. As told by the reporter, Davenport and other leading eugenicists sought strict immigration laws to ensure "the healthy racial progress of the American people."[1] Markers of social identity—class, ethnicity, and race—should therefore matter to anyone interested in understanding the history of hemophilia and its management. And because scientists have long regarded hemophilia as a sex-linked hereditary trait, gender plays a particularly important role in this story.

Throughout the history of hemophilia, experts have been no less inclined than laypeople to hold the characteristic class, gender, and racial views of their era. Even in the clinic and laboratory, hemophilia has been signified in ways that reinforced and even performed widely held, if not hegemonic, ideas about class, gender, or racial identity. It is impossible, then, to appreciate the range of social and cultural experiences that have circulated around hemophilia without first understanding the history of the disease concept itself.

This chapter details how the medical community came to share an understanding of the disease concept known as hemophilia and, in doing so, introduces the biological and social aspects of a condition that was a sustained subject of fascination and concern for both experts and laypeople in the past century. Although physicians first articulated our current portrait of hemophilia's clinical and hereditary aspects in the mid-nineteenth century, it would take them another century to begin managing hemophilia in ways that effectively addressed the primary bleeding problems associated with it. Hemophilia's transformation into a manageable disease in the second half of the twentieth century should be seen not only against the backdrop of sustained medical and scientific interest in hemophilia between 1800 and 1940 but also in terms of the range of social and cultural matters that knowledge of the disease raised for experts and laymen alike.

By design, our modern hemophilia concept has provided a way of marking progress in efforts to understand and treat disease; it has circulated as a signifier for a variety of social and cultural phenomena as knowledge of that disease has evolved. Some of these changes in our knowledge of hemophilia (e.g., the recognition of sex-linked inheritance and the growing realization of the functional mechanisms of blood clotting) have had a profound and lasting impact on efforts to manage the disease. Subtler, however, are the ways that particular circumstances have shaped interpretations of hemophilia beyond the treatment of individual patients or families. For instance, what difference did it make that the first medical reports of hemophilia came from the fledgling nation of the United States in the early 1800s? Or that German clinicians operating in urban hospitals standardized our formal conception of the disease in the mid-nineteenth century? What role did hemophilia's early status as a hereditary disease play in the formation of the science of heredity and the notorious eugenics movements of the twentieth century? And what practical effects, if any, did hemophilia's place within the new medical and life sciences of the twentieth century have on efforts to manage the disease?

As with all diseases, physicians have used the hemophilia concept to describe a distinct clinical reality, one that presumably captures the illness experience of the bleeding patient at the same time that it helps everyone comprehend what natural course of events is occurring in the patient's body and/or mind. This means that at any given moment, the concept of hemophilia bears a critical relationship to the illness it seeks to describe in biological terms. But it is also a mistake to confuse hemophilia's biological nature with the disease concept. Hemophilia has a natural history apart from the cultural and social history described in this book

Naturally speaking, hemophilia has always been with us. The natural history of hemophilia began somewhere in the course of mammalian evolution. We know this as a matter of scientific fact, but there is apparently no way to locate the beginning of this history other than to follow the lead of hematologist Isley Ingram, who notes that "hemophilia results from a relatively common mutation in the mammalian genome, and has its origins there."[2] Of course, there are no conventional texts that speak to hemophilia's existence millions of years ago. The "documents" that make Ingram's claim valid are presumably "written" into the genome of various mammalian species, including humans.[3] If one wants to read and interpret them, one must either be literate in contemporary bioscience or accept the authority of those who are. In any case, on this naturalistic model, the history of hemophilia is very, very old.

There are, however, a handful of written sources dating from the ancient and medieval eras that confirm that certain communities and peoples within the Western world knew of hereditary bleeding that disproportionately affected males. The earliest known reference to a condition resembling our modern concept of hemophilia originates from the second century A.D., in the compilation of Jewish law known as the Babylonian Talmud. Drawing on this earliest precedent, rabbinical rulings within Judaism have traditionally exempted male siblings from the circumcision ritual in cases where the child's family has suffered previous deaths from the ritual cutting. Two of the greatest physicians of the medieval period, Albucasis (ca. 936–ca. 1013) and Moses Maimonides (ca. 1138–1204), also had occasion to comment on hereditary bleeding conditions that can in retrospect be described as hemophilia.[4]

While hemophilia has always been present in human populations, its existence did not amount to a continuous body of knowledge about the disease. Before the modern era, there was some recognition of the experience of familial bleeding and its capacity to cause death or suffering (*pathos*), but there was still no formal knowledge (*logos*) of hemophilia within medical circles, still no *pathology*.[5] Assertions that human societies have long recognized hemophilia are relatively commonplace in historical writing about this disease. Such awareness is frequently interesting, sometimes informative; in the case of the Talmudic prohibition on ritual circumcision, it has even become a source of ethnic identity and pride.[6] Yet, if one attends to the cultural as well as social conditions of this knowledge, it is clear that a concept of the disease was absent from Western societies before the modern era. Hemophilia existed among us, but humans did not know it as such.

What follows, then, is the history of the hemophilia concept as modern medicine and society made and remade it before 1940. People's fascination with and worry about the biology of hemophilia has therefore been experienced in a variety of contexts where the social identities of the afflicted have mattered to the experts who took the lead in conceptualizing this terrible disease. And because concepts are always developed in a context, this chapter dwells on the fact that the inquisitive physicians who pioneered our modern concept of hemophilia were often invested in seeing the class, race, ethnicity, and gender of their bleeder patients in ways that impacted the evolution of knowledge about hemophilia.

Made in the USA: The Democratic Constitution of Hemophilia

Hemophilia became an object of continuous medical and scientific concern at the beginning of the nineteenth century. This formal concern with the disease was localized in two ways. On the one hand, the concept of hemophilia began to circulate between 1803 and 1820 among learned physicians on both sides of the Atlantic. On the other hand, a handful of practitioners first articulated this disease concept in relation to a familial illness experience that a small number of Anglo-American communities in the northeastern region of the United States had recognized for at least seventy years.[7] This historical circumstance places the origins of our hemophilia concept in a decidedly democratic context. Popular media in the twentieth century often portrayed hemophilia as a disease of European royalty, yet the Anglo-American physicians who first forged our modern conception of the disease did so out of a concern for hereditary bleeding among ordinary citizens in the wake of the American Revolution.

Our modern concept of hemophilia was effectively born in 1803, the year that Philadelphia physician John Conrad Otto (1774–1844) published "An Account of an Hemorrhagic Disposition Existing in Certain Families" in the New York *Medical Repository*. Otto's account begins with the story of the descendants of a woman named Smith, who settled in Plymouth, New Hampshire, in the late 1720s. Many of Smith's descendants exhibited a condition that Otto called alternately a "hemorrhagic idiosyncrasy" or a "hemorrhagic disposition." "If the least scratch is made on the skin of some of them," Otto wrote, "as mortal a hemorrhage will eventually ensue as if the largest wound is inflicted."[8] The "idiosyncrasy" did not afflict Smith or any of her female descendants.

> It is a surprising circumstance that the males only are subject to this strange affection, and that all of them are not liable to it. Some persons, who are curious, suppose they can distinguish the bleeders (for this is the name given to them) even in infancy; but as yet the characteristic marks are not ascertained sufficiently definite. Although the females are exempt, they are still capable of transmitting it to their male children.[9]

There is good reason to be suspicious of claims that locate twentieth-century concepts, such as, "sex-linked inheritance," in texts that predate that era.[10] However, Otto's account does articulate many of the hereditary and clinical features of our modern concept of hemophilia. It also stands apart from earlier sources on hemophilia for three basic reasons. First, it conceptualized hemophilia as a distinct disease whose distinguishing mark was a familial propensity to bleed (hemorrhage) among males. Second, it initiated a discussion of hemophilia among elite physicians in Europe as well as the United States. Third, it encouraged these medical practitioners to treat hemophilia as an object of continuous scientific concern.

Otto, who had studied with Benjamin Rush at the University of Pennsylvania in the 1790s, was only twenty-nine years old when he wrote and published his account in 1803.[11] Its publication in the New York *Medical Repository*, which was among the first and finest forums for medical communication in the United States, surely raised his reputation as a man of medical science in an era when America was aspiring for respectability among civilized nations. Otto's publication proved to be among the most important scientific contributions of any medical practitioner living in the early American republic, largely because it enjoyed wide readership in Europe throughout the nineteenth century at a time when it was difficult for Americans to keep pace with scientific movements in Europe or have their contributions appreciated there.[12]

More significantly, Otto's description of the "hemorrhagic idiosyncrasy" was characteristically American in its focus on how the patients, rather than the physicians, viewed the malady and its treatment. The medical marketplace in the early American Republic was a laissez-faire economy that required physicians to compete with a wide variety of healers for their patient's trust. Unlike in Great Britain, where royal charter regulated medical practice, in the United States physicians could not rely on special learning, credentials, or government decree to command the trust of their patients (or higher fees). American health consumers decided themselves how much authority and value they would place in the healer's services.[13] Physicians earned trust, and customers, by taking the patient's perspectives on illness and treatment to be major factors in how they dispensed their knowledge and care. Otto's description of the "hemorrhagic idiosyncrasy" bears the marks of this social and economic reality. When compared to subsequent case studies of hemophilia by European investigators, Otto's account reflected this egalitarian flavor of American medical practice.

According to Otto, Mrs. Smith's descendants lived in fear not only of the "idiosyncrasy" but also of medicine itself. At a time when American physicians were inclined to bleed their patients for a variety of ailments, members of the Smith-Shepard family were quite wary of doctors who wished to draw their blood: "So assured are the members of this family of the terrible consequences of the least wound, that they will not suffer themselves to be bled on any consideration, having lost a relation by not being able to stop the discharge occasioned by this operation."[14] Moreover, the family had consulted several physicians of "acknowledged merit" over the years, and these physicians had employed "various remedies . . . to restrain the hemorrhages," including bark, strong styptics, opiates, and astringents used topically or taken internally. Yet all the usual remedies were "tried in vain," according to Otto. The Smith-Shepard family ultimately resorted to a folk remedy of sulfate of soda that it found routinely efficacious. This "family receipt," as Otto called it, was their preferred treatment for bleeding.[15] Otto's account of hemophilia thus narrated the reputed efficacy of this folk remedy in relation to the life-threatening nature of the condition, the need to give the "bleeder" prompt relief, and the Smith-Shepard family's rightful distrust of physicians.

Ironically, Otto never actually saw a case of hemophilia himself. He based his descriptions of the Smith family's illness entirely on the written testimony of three men from New Hampshire: the Honorable Judge Livermore and two physicians, Drs. Rogers and Porter, who resided in the family's "neighborhood." The illness was well known in the community of the Smith family (and their descendants, the Shepards). As Otto noted, people in the community had been calling members of the Smith-Shepard family "bleeders" for at least a generation. Moreover, given Otto's relation to Benjamin Rush, it is notable that the account identifies Rush's long-standing familiarity with the malady, that Rush had himself seen two separate cases of it in different parts of Pennsylvania earlier in his career, and that Rush provided Otto with another, more recent account of the family of "A.B." in Maryland, "four of whom . . . died of a loss of blood from the most trifling scratches or bruises."[16] There is no evidence in the 1803 account or any subsequent source to indicate that Otto ever attended a case of the "idiosyncrasy."

One might wonder why Otto did not seek out the Smith-Shepard family to acquire firsthand clinical knowledge of their condition. While impossible to give a definitive answer, it is helpful to consider the distinctive character of American society in the early 1800s and the self-consciousness with which Americans balanced the rights of individuals against invocations of authority and privilege. Like many American physicians, Otto believed that the patient and his family had every right, as the bearers of a familial affliction, to control how doctors viewed and treated them. He also understood that the Smith-Shepard's distrust of physicians made it difficult, if not impossible, for doctors to conduct proper studies of the condition or its possible cures. When the family did call a physician to aid with a bleeder, Otto noted that it was "with a view of directing him how to proceed" with the family's chosen remedy rather "than of permitting him to make a series of trials and observations which might be at the hazard of the life of the patient." Given its expressed wishes, Otto was content to study the Smith-Shepard family from afar. His notably egalitarian account makes no mention of an effort by himself or any other physician to persuade the family to submit to a formal investigation of its "haemorrhagic disposition" or its "family receipt."[17] Rather, Otto's dutiful promotion of the Smith-Shepard's sulfate-of-soda remedy suggests his desire to represent the truth of the family's condition as members of the family and the community saw it. Otto's preference for authentic representation tempered his pursuit of knowledge, rendering his account both an artifact of democratic spirit and a seminal document in the history of the hemophilia concept.

Otto's peers in the medical community greeted his documentation of the "hemorrhagic idiosyncrasy" with respect, if not enthusiasm. By formalizing extant testimonies of this familial illness and transforming them into a provisional disease concept, Otto prompted interested practitioners to pursue a dual strategy of investigation. First, in saying that "cases shall become more numerous," Otto assumed that physicians would find more families of "bleeders" once they armed themselves with a formal disease concept. Second, the account outlined a definite set of concerns (such as whether "the female sex is not entirely exempt") that future investigators would need to confront as they identified cases.[18] The concept prompted physicians to inquire systematically about the bleeding patient's familial history, which in turn could lead to the discovery and investigation of more cases.

What effectively marks Otto's 1803 account as the beginning of modern knowledge about hemophilia is found, then, in the formal manner of its thinking: the fact that Otto structured the information he collected about an "idiosyncratic" illness experience in a way that allowed subsequent medical thinkers not only to conceptualize hemophilia as a familial disease but to test the concept and think it differently. This was a critical step forward for doctors who had previously attended "bleeders" with little hope of successfully treating or even characterizing the familial problem in a useful way. As Otto emphasized, physicians could now clarify the nature of the idiosyncrasy by examining future "cases" of the disease.

"Love of Bleeding": Hemophilia's Maturation in the German Clinic

The scientific study of hemophilia in the nineteenth century was hardly an American story. In fact, efforts to understand and treat hemophilia since the early 1800s have always been international in character. After a relatively short period (1803–17) in which American physicians and cases played a critical role in shaping medical conceptions of the disease, German physicians proved themselves to be far more interested in documenting cases than doctors from other nations.[19] By 1872 the London physician John Wickham Legg observed in his *Treatise on Haemophilia* that nearly 50 percent of all known cases of hemophilia were "German."[20]

The legacy of German engagements with hemophilia, particularly as they evolved in and around clinical settings, had far-reaching implications for the management of the disease in the twentieth century as well as in the nineteenth. These effects are discernible where the emergence of our modern concept of hemophilia is linked not only to clinical work on hemophilia among Germanic physicians but also to the cultural and social conditions of its production.

Sustained German study of hemophilia began in 1805 when Christian Erhard Kapp (1739–1824) published an unsigned review of Otto's account in the medical journal he edited in Leipzig. The author of that review stated that he knew of several cases of the disease affecting only males from his own medical practice and that two of these patients experienced unusual bleeding after tooth loss.[21] This anonymous report was enough to signal to German clinicians that they had a scientific opportunity at hand. As one physician familiar with the "idiosyncrasy" put it, the disease was "a wonderful circumstance most interesting for physiology and pathology, and one I cannot yet properly explain!"[22]

The fascination that German clinicians expressed for cases of hemophilia has its roots in the decades-long transformation of academic medicine that overtook German universities between 1750 and 1820 and its immediate catalyst in the new form of hospital medicine that physicians throughout Europe began embracing in the first half of the nineteenth century.[23] German physicians were more likely to encounter "bleeders" than their counterparts in the United States and other parts of Europe because they were more frequently engaged in hospital work. The impulse to classify diseases (nosology) and think systematically about their clinical presentation was also characteristic of German academic medicine during the era. Hemophilia was among a broadening array of novel diseases that German physicians elucidated by embracing the hospital as a preferred site for clinical training as well as scientific work.[24]

By the time Legg wrote his *Treatise on Haemophilia* in 1872, German clinicians had already rendered hemophilia into a distinctive clinical entity. Their portrait highlighted the various presentations of the bleeding, the joint involvement and crippling, the evidence of familial inheritance, the preponderance of cases among males, and even the physical and intellectual qualities that physicians witnessed among the afflicted. Among the German clinicians who significantly advanced the concept of hemophilia between 1820 and 1855, Christian Friedrich Nasse (1778–1851) and Johann Lukas Schönlein (1793–1864) were the most influential. Both men used their university faculty appointments and clinical teaching posts to refine thinking about peculiar cases of bleeding among the relatively large patient populations they oversaw in their hospital work. Their hospital-based casework and their faculty chairs within their universities helped them to establish standards for clinical thinking about hemophilia in the German-speaking world.

In 1820 Nasse published the results of a comprehensive investigation on the "hereditary disposition to fatal bleeding" that provided a principle for differentiating between hemophilia and other forms of bleeding.[25] Nasse's characterization of hemophilia differed from all previous writing on the subject in its insistence that cases of familial bleeding limited to males were distinct from those cases in which familial bleeding occurred in both males and females. In their clinical rounds, Nasse and his assistant Krimer observed that the "hereditary disposition to fatal bleeding" occurred only in males, that these males showed no signs of transmitting the disease themselves, and that it was their unaffected female relations—namely, their mothers and sisters—who transmitted the condition through marriages with men who exhibited neither symptoms nor a familial history of bleeding. Physicians began referring to Nasse's nosological principle as "Nasse's law" because he maintained that the observed inheritance pattern was a necessary condition for any diagnosis. For instance, Nasse's study described one family from Bonn whose five sons all bled frequently from their adolescence forward and whose female relatives—including their sister, mother, grandmother, and great-grandmother—had all suffered from profuse menstruation and postpartum bleeding. The grandmother and great-grandmothers even bled to death at their menopause. Tellingly, Nasse excluded this family from a diagnosis of the "hereditary disposition to fatal bleeding" because the bleeding afflicted its female as well as male members.[26]

Nasse's 1820 study also heightened interest in hemophilia among German physicians at a time when the clinical research and teaching of Johann Lukas Schönlein were just beginning to provide German physicians with additional opportunities to advance knowledge of a growing variety of diseases.[27] Schönlein helped revolutionize German medicine in the mid- to late 1820s by embracing the methods of clinical practice and teaching made famous in Parisian hospitals in the wake of the French Revolution.[28] Schönlein's contributions to our modern conception of hemophilia, as with most of his pursuits, are found today not in his own hand but in the notes, dissertations, and personal recollections that his students penned in the course of their own medical work. The word *haemophilie*—which means "love of blood"—first appeared in the medical literature in the 1828 medical thesis of Schönlein's student, Friedrich Hopff.[29] Hopff's thesis described a familial hemorrhagic disposition occurring predominantly in males and credited Schönlein with originating the term *haemophilie* to identify it. From Schönlein's private research records, we know that he initially used the term *haemophilie* to describe cases of bleeding in female as well as male patients, but sometime between 1825 and 1828 he began to use it in the restricted sense of an inherited bleeding disorder found predominantly in males.[30] Yet Schönlein appears to have been less satisfied than Hopff with the term *haemophilie*. Around 1832 he began using the term *haemorrhaphilia*—"love of bleeding"—to designate the condition more accurately. And though Schönlein's students—among them Rudolf Virchow—occasionally used the latter term, the term *haemophilie* emerged as the German medical community's preferred term for the disease by the 1860s.

Schönlein's contributions to knowledge of hemophilia went beyond terminology and spoke to the nature of the disease itself. The words he employed in his clinical research and teaching on pathology reflected his systematic approach to the problem of nosology. The terms *haemophilia* and *haemorrhaphilia* were not meant to evoke "love of blood or bleeding" in some metaphorical or romantic register (though they have that unfortunate air about them). They were actually terms designed to signify an essential symptom of the disease around which a proper classification of the disease could arise. For Schönlein, a symptom became essential wherever it reflected a material change in the deeper recesses of the patient's body that the physician could potentially localize. Thus, a diagnostic term like *haemophilie* not only signified bleeding as an essential symptom of a disease but pointed the clinician to the nature of pathology that precipitated the disease's symptoms in the first place. There was, in other words, a specific organic lesion within the patient's body that correlated to the essential symptom of bleeding, and which the clinician could discern by autopsy upon the death of the patient. The nature of hemophilia was, in Schönlein's view, evident in the organic lesion that the bleeding signaled to the clinician. On the basis of the medical literature as well as his own bedside and morbid experiences with "Bluters," Schönlein observed that the heart muscles of these patients were frequently irregular in size or shape. He therefore characterized hemophilic bleeding as essentially related to cyanosis (a bluish coloring of the skin related to poor circulation) and its underlying cause, malformation of the heart.

Nasse and Schönlein share a great deal of the credit for placing hemophilia on the modern nosological map, but it was Ludwig Grandidier (1810–78) who helped clinicians throughout Europe articulate an increasingly uniform understanding of the disease.[31] Grandidier, who was a spa doctor in Nenndorf, made hemophilia the major scholarly interest of his life. He spent more than forty years compiling observations and statistics on cases of hemophilia from medical literature and correspondence. Grandidier published his first book-length study of hemophilia in 1855 and revised and updated the book for a second edition in 1877. Grandidier provided German-speaking clinicians with a single, comprehensive source about the disease and also helped popularize the term *hemophilia* (*haemophilie*) within the medical profession.[32]

Most importantly, Grandidier was among the first physicians to document the grim prospects for hemophilia patients. More than half of the 197 males with hemophilia he identified died before their eighth year (n = 111), and only 12 percent of those patients who survived past eight years actually lived beyond their twenty-first birthday (n = 23).[33] After 1855, clinicians began using Grandidier's statistics on hemophilia as a measure of the disease's character and scope. By the 1870s some physicians were questioning the value of Grandidier's statistics, but they also had little choice but to use them.[34] Such criticism did not discourage Grandidier. He continued to compile statistics on hemophilia for the second edition of his monograph, and this work continued to influence how nineteenth-century clinicians thought about the disease.

German studies of congenital bleeding in the nineteenth century were crucial to the maturation of our modern hemophilia concept. In fact, the progress that German-speaking clinicians made in understanding hemophilia in the mid-1800s reflected a cultural and social setting whose ethos was rigorously devoted to the production of new medical knowledge. Yet, while German clinicians may have been the uncontested experts on hemophilia during the nineteenth century, the quality of their investments in the disease did not translate into visible benefits for bleeder patients or their families. That is because clinical studies of hemophilia focused almost exclusively on describing the nature of the disease. German clinicians were more likely than their counterparts in other parts of Europe to provide bleeder patients with a clear diagnosis and prognosis. However, their treatments were no different from what doctors throughout the Western world provided for bleeding, bruises, inflammation, or joint pain.

Any benefit that *Bluters* derived from their clinical care was likely the result of factors other than the German clinician's special interest in hemophilia. Grandidier's mortality statistics confirm that the prospects of living with hemophilia were dismal among German-speaking peoples. Unfortunately, nineteenth-century statistics are poor markers of the quality of life experienced by people with hemophilia. We can only imagine, for example, how painful life must have been for the "fortunate" 12 to 15 percent who survived into adulthood. Much of their suffering was undoubtedly due to the natural progression of hemophilia, but the role of physicians and their institutions should not be discounted as a source of grief as well.

On the basis of what is known of the clinics and hospitals where German physicians took a special interest in hemophilia, it also appears unlikely that patients suffering from congenital bleeding utilized these institutions for reasons other than brute necessity. Generally speaking, the patients who populated Europe's urban hospitals and larger clinics came predominantly from the working and poorer classes of society, while the physicians and surgeons who attended them often benefited from a good education, social connections, and a guaranteed salary. Unlike physicians who derived their living from private practice, the salaried doctors in state-run hospitals and clinics had less incentive to cater to the demands of their patients.[35] They were freer, in other words, to practice medicine as they saw fit. The social inequalities inherent to these nineteenth-century clinical settings also made it possible for clinicians such as Nasse and Schönlein to wield considerable power over their patients and, thereby, use them to increase their knowledge of disease. As such, German clinicians who took an interest in cases of congenital bleeding often did so in the interest of advancing medical science. Whenever these "men of science" took charge of a patient's case, it was unlikely to escape the notice of their patients that treatment was not their primary concern. In this setting, it did not bode well for the bleeder patient to be viewed as clinically interesting.

By the 1870s, the very name of the disease reflected the German clinician's cultivated sense of detachment from his patient's lived experience and suffering. After all, *hemophilia* (love of blood) and *hemophiliac* (one who loves blood) were not designations that any person with the disease would have chosen. Legg recognized the incongruity here. He decided to use the word *haemophilia* in the title of his 1872 *Treatise* because the preferred Anglophone names for the disease, "haemorrhagic diathesis or tendency," had "too wide a meaning" for clinical precision. Yet Legg undoubtedly knew he was sacrificing empathy for the sake of utility. In one of the *Treatise*'s most revealing footnotes, Legg explained that he was "unable to say" for certain that "the word haemophilia" was Schönlein's invention before concluding: "The word is so barbarous and senseless that it is not wonderful that no one should be proud of it."[36]

Anglo-Germanic Heritage and the Risks of Intermarriage

From the earliest American and German reports of hemophilia, the hereditary aspects of this congenital bleeding tendency intrigued physicians. The focus of these early nineteenth-century reports was on the patterns of inheritance, the predominance of male cases, and whether heredity should be considered an essential feature of hemophilia because a significant number of patients presented as "*de novo* cases" (i.e., cases identified among patients who clearly lacked a family history of congenital bleeding). By the mid-nineteenth century, clinicians were becoming bolder in their pronouncements about hemophilia. They moved beyond entirely descriptive writing of hemophilia's symptoms and patterns of inheritance to engage in more speculative thinking about the sources of congenital bleeding and its prevalence within some populations.

One popular medical theory attributed *de novo* cases of congenital bleeding to a history of familial intermarriage and thus prompted physicians to think about the prevalence of hemophilia and intermarriage in certain ethnic and social groups. Not surprisingly, this line of thought was examined closely in Great Britain, where it was an open secret among physicians that Prince Leopold (1853–84), Queen Victoria's eighth child and youngest son, suffered from a chronic tendency to bleed.[37] John Wickham Legg, whom I earlier identified as the author of the 1872 *Treatise*, had briefly served with the royal family as Leopold's personal tutor and medical attendant. In his lifetime, Leopold received the best care for his hemophilia that the British medical establishment could provide even though doctors were unable to stop bleeding or prevent its disabling effects. A few British physicians did, however, acquire a detailed clinical understanding of hemophilia between the 1860s and early 1880s, one that increasingly allowed physicians in the Anglophone world to provide patients with a clearer diagnosis and prognosis. Then, upon Leopold's untimely death in 1884, the editors of the *British Medical Journal* published a short piece on the "haemorrhagic diathesis," also known as "haemophilia," adding the note: "The recent bereavement in the Royal Family will naturally turn the attention of the medical public towards the constitutional affection to which the illustrious deceased was subject."[38] Certainly, the hereditary nature of Leopold's fatal illness helped ensure that physicians would continue to study hemophilia for decades to come. As the eminent clinician Sir William Osler noted in 1885, "Much interest was excited in the disease in England from the fact that the late Prince Leopold was a sufferer."[39]

Over the course of 1856–57, Leopold's physicians concluded he had a constitutional bleeding tendency. British physicians thought that hemophilia was a peculiarly German malady in the 1850s, which may be one reason why many months passed before Sir James Clark, the queen's ordinary physician, treated Leopold's illness as a hereditary bleeding tendency. Given that British physicians relied on German clinical sources for information about Leopold's bleeding tendency, there is evidence suggesting that Queen Victoria expected her family's physicians to be fluent in German.[40] While it is uncertain when Leopold actually received a definitive hemophilia diagnosis, the royal physicians undoubtedly provided the queen and her family some information about hemophilia in Leopold's early years. The family's communications about Leopold from 1856–57 indicate a rudimentary awareness of the medical concept of a constitutional bleeding tendency. It appears unlikely, however, that family members used the word *hemophilia* or stressed its hereditary nature as suggested by the more common medical term of that era, the *hereditary haemorrhagic diathesis*. In the 1850s British physicians knew that the tendency could pass through symptomless mothers to their sons. At least one historian has suggested that the royal physicians kept the hereditary nature of Leopold's condition to themselves in the early years or told only Prince Albert about it.[41] Certainly, the hereditary nature of hemophilia would have been one of the most troubling features of the disease for the royal family.

The capricious nature of hemophilia may have also confused Victoria's family. Hemophilic bleeding is episodic and unpredictable. In his lifetime, Leopold had periods of obvious health in which his bleeding tendency seemed to disappear. In his early twenties, Leopold had two teeth pulled with no prolonged bleeding, and he even fell from a horse and walked away without any ill effects. These periods of relative health provided the royal family with reasons to doubt its physicians or to maintain hope that Leopold's bleeding problems were not deeply ingrained. For the most part, however, the royal family seemed to embrace what the physicians did tell them of Leopold's condition. In his 1872 *Treatise*, Legg maintained that hemophilic bleeding resulted from an "alteration of the blood vessels" due to an "imperfect development of the entire vascular system." This theory had been circulating around medical discussions of hemophilia for some time. As early as 1861, the queen, Prince Albert, and other family members were describing Leopold's bleeding tendency within court circles as "weak" veins.[42]

From 1873 forward, however, the British royal family was wholly conscious that the health of its bloodline was in question. This was the year that the queen's hemophilic grandson, Prince Friedrich Wilhelm (1870–73), died from a brain hemorrhage after a tragic fall from a window. Queen Victoria's writings show that she worried about the quality of the family's bloodlines, but her statements on the royal "bloodlines" were consistent with very common notions about heredity and health circulating in Western societies in the mid-nineteenth century. Using the old language of humoralism, the queen thought of the royal bloodline as too "lymphatic" in character and advised at least one of her pale, fair-haired, blue-eyed daughters of the need to infuse "darker" blood into the family. In fact, Victoria was consistent in maintaining that Leopold's ailments were a constitutional weakness that bore no relation to the royal bloodline. She had various ways of rationalizing this idea. When explicitly confronted with the hereditary argument, for instance, Victoria protested that it did not come from "her" side (that is, the "royal" Hanoverian side) of the family. In other words, if Leopold's illness was to be labeled hereditary, the queen insisted that it be attributed to some deficiency in the Saxe-Coburg bloodline (which it may have been). There was even talk in court circles of a "Coburg Curse." In any case, the matter was never discussed given the stigmas involved. Official royal policy in the Victorian era was to silence talk of hereditary maladies.[43] The high stakes within aristocratic circles of having "unmarriageable" sons and daughters made it virtually impossible for the British royals to deal openly with the issue of hemophilia.

By the early 1870s, the physicians treating Leopold and the royal family had considerable knowledge of hemophilia that they could relate to the royal family, and this knowledge included definitive evidence that the malady could be prevented in future generations. In his *Treatise*, for example, John Legg sought the family health histories of his bleeder patients in order to document the patterns of familial transmission and to determine if there was intermarriage among the patients' families. Legg was interested in knowing if intermarriage was a precursor to hemophilia because the German clinical literature highlighted that marriage between cousins was common in the families of bleeders.[44]

Some physicians did debate possible prohibitions against marriage for bleeders and their family members in Victorian England. Legg raised the issue in 1872.

> Should a bleeder, or one of a bleeder family, be allowed to marry? I think that if the person himself be a bleeder, the question of marriage ought not to be entertained. His sons may possibly escape the disease, but it is almost sure to reappear in his daughters' sons. The prospect of the certainty of so dreadful an entail of disease must repel every right thinking person from such a step, even at so great a sacrifice to himself; and it seems only necessary for the fact to be known to prevent such marriages among the better classes.[45]

Legg added in a footnote: "I say in the better classes: for the artizan class are so ruled by their passions, that no moral restraints would ever be allowed to interfere with the gratification of a lust: the law must stop such contracts." While this footnote signals Legg's own prejudice against the lower, artisan classes from which most of his clinical patients originated, his opinions on the necessity of his prohibition were so strong that he did not exempt the "better classes." As suggested by the recommendation to render such marriages illegal, Legg's prohibition extended to all family members of a male bleeder, and most especially to the sisters of bleeders.[46]

Despite his insistence that hereditary hemophilia was a preventable malady, Legg stressed that cases of *de novo* hemophilia remained a source of uncertainty. Legg found little satisfaction in the various theories that clinicians had offered for *de novo* cases. First, he dismissed contemporary reports of the age-old maternal impression theory that stressed that hemophilia manifested *de novo* in children whose mothers witnessed trauma or bleeding in the course of their pregnancy. He also thought it "extremely unlikely" that "the disease can be produced in a healthy child by food or external agencies." Legg ultimately endorsed no particular view on the generation of *de novo* cases, but his *Treatise* did identify the intermarriage idea as the only hypothesis with any confirming evidence. He found support for the view in the "greater prevalence of the disease in Germany where the marriage of cousins is so little discouraged" as well as "among the Jews who are obliged to intermarry." Like most physicians in the 1860s and 1870s, Legg saw the prevalence of hemophilia in certain populations as a way to clarify the essential nature of the disease.[47]

The royal family's situation oddly constrained knowledge of hemophilia from the Victorian era well into the twentieth century, making it difficult for British experts to speak too forcefully of prevention (fig. 1.1). During Queen Victoria's reign, many in the court and learned medical community knew about Leopold's bleeding tendency, and most probably thought of it as hereditary. But no one could do much to deter Prince Leopold, his sisters, or nieces from marriage or parenthood. In fact, in the 1880s and later, British eugenicists were unable to advance formal prohibitions against marriages involving people with hemophilia.[48] The nation's hereditary monarchy and the open secret of royal hemophilia made that politically improbable. Of this climate, British geneticist and Marxist J. B. S. Haldane later wrote: "The blood royal has actually been corrupted by snobbery, which puts 'high' birth before health." Haldane was writing in favor

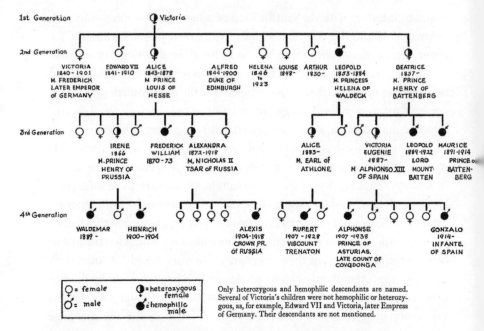

FIGURE 1.1. "Royal Hemophilia" as Illustrated by J. B. S. Haldane, 1939.
Source: J. B. S. Haldane, "Blood Royal: The Dramatic Story of How Hemophilia Has Affected the Recent History of the World," *Living Age* 356 (March 1939): 29.

of a more egalitarian form of eugenics, and he cited his own 1938 study of "royal hemophilia" as evidence "that it is not only among the 'lower' classes that eugenic principles might be applied."[49]

In the absence of concerted efforts in Great Britain to curb procreation among carriers of hemophilia, what one can find in British writing on hemophilia from the Victorian era forward is a dutiful effort to clarify for the medical profession the best treatments and social regimens for managing hereditary bleeding. Indeed, Legg's published work with hemophilia patients at St. Bartholomew's Hospital in the 1870s suggests links between his earlier experience with Leopold (which is nowhere mentioned in his *Treatise*) and the charity patients he so dutifully studied and treated in London. There is no clear evidence that British physicians were more interested in hemophilia in the late nineteenth century than American or even German investigators. But given the "open secret" of royal hemophilia, they certainly had a unique motivation to develop strategies for therapeutic management of a disease that they routinely saw as a malady of the Anglo-Germanic races.

Controlling Transmission in an Age of Eugenics

As case reports of hemophilia multiplied in the second half of the nineteenth century, clinicians increasingly began to speak of it in terms of its hereditary transmission. Questions of race and gender were critical to this discourse. The racial cast of hemophilia in nineteenth-century medical talk was partly an artifact of the successes of German clinical medicine and academic scholarship. By the 1860s, many physicians had concluded that hemophilia was a "special inheritance of the Teutonic race." Not only did Legg dismiss this idea as a consequence of the special interest that German physicians exhibited in the disease, but he also insisted that the prevalence of hemophilia among Jews residing in German territories was "opposed to the idea that haemophilia is confined to the Indo-Germanic race." Still, Legg ultimately could not say if the malady was the inheritance of a particular race because he thought it remained an open question "whether haemophilia be more frequent in one country than another."[50]

After the publication of Legg's *Treatise* in 1872, hemophilia was often regarded as an Anglo-Saxon as well as an Indo-Germanic disease. Basel's Hermann Immermann commented on the rise of reported hemophilia cases in Great Britain and correlated it with the early American cases among Anglo-Saxon stock. In his 1876 study of hemophilia, Immermann concluded, "the frequency of the disease appears to be largely influenced by the *nationality* of the population, the *Anglo-Germanic* race exhibiting a special disposition to the affection." A "similar disposition," he added, "seems to exist in the widespread Jewish race." Immermann proved no more willing than Legg to draw a definitive conclusion about the relationship between race and hemophilia. The "scantiness" of evidence from "non-European countries makes it impossible," he said, "to decide whether race really exerts a predisposing influence or not."[51] Even though Legg and Immermann both exhibited a desire to employ race as a tool for understanding the national incidence of hemophilia, they expressed greater doubt about the evidence than most physicians did.

Hemophilia's status as an Anglo-Germanic inheritance did not mark it as unusual. Physicians routinely employed race as a marker of a disease's identity in the late nineteenth century, and as might be expected, they used racial characterizations to help them identify and treat their patients. This idea did, however, have clear effects on the evolution of the twentieth-century disease concept.

A telling example of the racial climate that surrounded hemophilia in the United States was the small but significant medical literature that sought to explain "hemophilia in the negro" in the first half of the twentieth century. The literature emphasized that most of the hemophilia cases identified in "the negro" were found in people with some mixed-race ancestry.[52] Writing in 1949, Chicago physicians Robert Nesbit and Julius Richmond reviewed the medical literature in order to determine whether hemophilia occurred in "racially pure Negro individuals." They found more cases in the literature of hemophilia among "Negro patients" of "both mixed" and "pure" blood than had African American pathologist Julian Herman Lewis in his magisterial *The Biology of the Negro* (1942), but they concluded that further studies of West African and African American populations would be necessary for any definitive conclusions on the matter.[53] Later studies would find that hemophilia occurred in African and African American populations at relatively equivalent rates to the Caucasian populations of Europe and North America. That is why hemophilia is widely characterized today as a pan-ethnic disease. But for the most part, hemophilia's transformation from an "Anglo-Germanic" malady into a pan-ethnic disease did not occur until the late 1960s and 1970s, when American physicians began paying as much attention to the cases of hereditary bleeding in "colored" and "nonwhite" patients as they had traditionally done with their ethnically white patients.

But race was always a marginal issue to hemophilia experts when compared to the pressing matter of sexual identity. Since the beginning of the nineteenth century, leading physicians had formulated their concept of hemophilia in relation to the occurrence of most cases of hereditary bleeding in male patients. As previously noted, Otto was among the first to mark out the concept of hemophilia in relation to sex, and Nasse elevated sex characteristics into a principle for deciding what constituted a legitimate hemophilia diagnosis and what did not.[54] After Nasse, one might think that a hemophilia diagnosis was reserved exclusively for male bleeders with a family history of the disease. However, judging from uses of the word *hae-mophilia* across the nineteenth century, the disease concept was occasionally employed with cases of bleeding among females.[55] There was disagreement, in other words, on the importance of the patient's sex as a defining characteristic of the disease.

By the 1870s, Legg and others were openly wondering how to interpret the statistical findings of Grandidier that approximated the proportion of male to female hemophilia cases as high as fourteen to one. Legg also noted that the female bleeders in the medical literature rarely presented the disease in terms of its typical symptoms. It "affects women with a lower degree of intensity than men," he said; "they do not bleed more than is usual when wounded, and the disposition may limit itself to the occurrence of spontaneous haemorrhages, or to early, abundant, and prolonged menstruation of the disease." Childbirth, he added, was also a common time for "floodings."[56] Some American physicians interpreted Legg's *Treatise* as evidence that one cannot assume that "females were exempt from haemophilia . . . although women are far less disposed to the disease than men."[57] In 1898, however, Legg clarified his stance on the issue: "I have never seen a case of true haemophilia in a woman, and I am inclined to think that the diagnosis of cases of haemophilia in women is founded on mistaken assumptions."[58] Still, Legg did not rule out the possibility of a classical form of hemophilia in females.

Consensus on the issue of sex in hemophilia was effectively achieved in the 1910s after British physicians William Bulloch and Paul Fildes published their path-breaking study of hemophilia. Bulloch and Fildes defined hemophilia quite simply as "an *inherited* tendency in *males* to *bleed*." This definition emphasized what they described as the disease's three cardinal characteristics and reinforced their "opinion" that hemophilia should be known as a "chronic liability to immoderate haemorrhage" that was essentially "hereditary" and "confined to the male sex." Although Bulloch and Fildes recognized that the "question of the immunity of the female sex from haemophilia" was one in which experts had always disagreed, they found little evidence in their extensive study of the medical literature to support the idea that females were afflicted by bleeding with comparative frequency to males.[59]

The positive evidence that Bulloch and Fildes compiled in support of their view was, by all accounts, "monumental."[60] They based their findings on an annotated literature review of 949 known sources extending from 1911 back to 1519. They thereby identified more than six hundred cases of

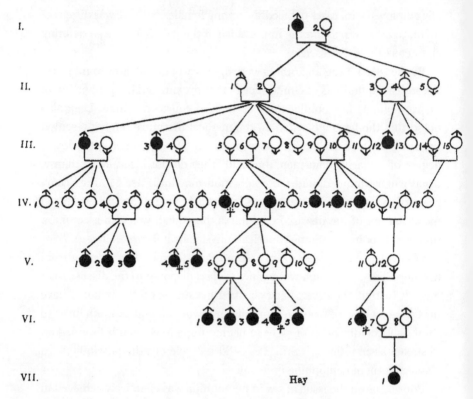

FIGURE 1.2. John Hay's 1813 Study of the Appleton Family with Hemophilia. The family of Oliver Appleton, studied in the early nineteenth century by American physician John Hay, is here illustrated in pedigree form by eugenic scientists William Bulloch and Paul Fildes in their 1911 contribution to Karl Pearson's *Treasury of Human Inheritance*. *Source*: William Bulloch and Paul Fildes, "Haemophilia," in Karl Pearson, ed., *Treasury of Human Inheritance*, vol. 1 (London: Cambridge University Press, 1912), pedigree 408, following reference 24 on p. 198.

abnormal bleeding involving dozens of families. After an extensive analysis in which they authored 607 pedigrees of individuals with histories of abnormal bleeding, Bulloch and Fildes determined that only forty-four families in the literature exhibited indisputable histories of hemophilia (fig. 1.2). Ten of these forty-four families claimed to have female bleeders among them, for a total of nineteen individual cases. Bulloch and Fildes then expressed reasonable doubts about the authenticity of these nineteen confirmed cases of hemophilia in females. They determined that the available evidence in each case was too limited, too circumstantial, or too easily explained by other, more prevalent disorders.[61]

The idea that only males got hemophilia rose to the level of orthodoxy following the rise of Mendelian thinking among eugenicists and geneticists in the 1910s. When the mid-nineteenth-century breeding experiments of Gregor Mendel were "rediscovered" in 1900, Mendel's laws of segregation and independent assortment soon became the preferred way among Anglophone biologists to explain the transmission of hereditary defects such as hemophilia.[62] While Bulloch and Fildes did not employ a Mendelian perspective in their hemophilia studies, many of their readers found confirmation of Mendel's relevance there. Famously, in 1910 Thomas Hunt Morgan utilized fruit flies in his laboratory at Columbia University to demonstrate that certain heritable traits are linked to sex characteristics and transmitted in accordance with Mendelian principles. Geneticists soon deduced that the well-documented hereditary defect for hemophilia was located on the X chromosome and conformed perfectly to a Mendelian understanding of sex-linked recessive inheritance. Hemophilia thus emerged as a model sex-linked disorder in this way of thinking. By the 1930s, hemophilia was understood to be not only "an *inherited* tendency in *males* to *bleed*" but also a sex-linked genetic defect of the first order (fig. 1.3).

In keeping with its peculiar inheritance pattern, the role of sex in hemophilia was not limited to talk about its higher incidence or possible exclusivity in males but extended to discussions of its transmission. Such discussions emerged decades before modern genetics confirmed hemophilia's sex-linked nature. As soon as it was widely reported in the medical literature that asymptomatic women could transmit the condition to their sons, discussions of the role of females in transmitting the disease became commonplace among physicians. Such females were identified by a variety of names—most commonly in English, as "carriers," "transmitters," or "conductors." The dominant question was whether the reproduction of such otherwise healthy women should be prohibited or otherwise controlled.

Already as early as the 1870s, Legg and Immermann were discussing the matter of female and male transmission in detail. Legg recommended a prohibition on marriage of any "bleeder" and members of his family, adding: "The physician, whose advice is asked on this subject, should be on his guard not to be deceived by any appearance of freedom from haemophilia

"SEX-LINKED" INHERITANCE

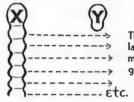

The "X" chromosome is many times larger than the "Y."

The "Y" chromosome lacks duplicates of almost all the "X" genes.

If a recessive "black-X" gene is circulating in a family,
(A) for COLOR-BLINDNESS

DAUGHTER
Receiving one "color-blindness" gene usually has in her second "X" a normal gene to block it.

SON
Receiving a "color-blindness" gene in his single "X" has no normal gene to block it.

Result: Perfectly NORMAL (but a carrier)

Result: COLOR-BLIND

(B) "CRISS-CROSS" TRANSMISSION
As in Hemophilia

(1) WOMAN
Normal, but a carrier

"Bleeding" gene covered by normal one.

(2) ONE-IN-TWO SONS A BLEEDER

All his sons receiving only his "Y" are normal.

(3) Every one of "b l e e d e r' s" daughters is carrier, like grandmother.

PROCESS repeated as from No. 1.

FIGURE 1.3. Sex-Linked Inheritance, as Illustrated for the American Public in 1939. *Source*: Amram Scheinfeld, *You and Heredity* (New York: Frederick A. Stokes, 1939), p. 132.

in the women: they may seem perfectly well and free from any trace of the complaint, and yet the disease will certainly reappear in their sons." As he saw it, a "sadder heritage of disease could scarcely be entailed . . . [and any] person entering upon marriage with a knowledge of all these facts would indeed be open to great blame."[63] Immermann was more forceful but only for female family members. He invoked both familial and scientific experience that suggested that male members of bleeder families demonstrated no evidence of transmission if they were free from the disease. But the prohibition was absolute when it came to the females in such families: he recommended that "marriage should be forbidden to all the females of a bleeder family without exception." Strikingly, Immermann saw no compelling moral reason to prohibit the marriage of male bleeders unless there was evidence of father-to-son transmission in the man's health history. As he and many other physicians concluded, the absolute prohibition to marriage should be applied only to the females from hemophilia families.[64]

With the rise and popularization of eugenics in the Anglophone world (ca. 1905–35), it became increasingly common for American physicians to speak in moral terms about the necessity of controlling the reproduction of families afflicted by any hereditary disease. In the case of hemophilia, physicians and many eugenicists were less inclined to speak of outright prohibitions on marriage for individuals. The disease was just not considered a prevalent problem in the population at large. However, as was true of hemophilia in the 1870s, physicians did make the reproductive capabilities of females in bleeder families a focus. Thus, for instance, Charles Davenport, the reputed dean of the American eugenics movement, insisted that however healthy they might seem, the sisters of hemophiliacs should be barred from having children.[65]

It remains unknown to what extent, if at all, physicians and public health advocates targeted female members of hemophilia families for sterilization and other forms of reproductive control in the heyday of eugenics. Short of combing through case histories of sterilization cases in the United States—and there were at least sixty-four thousand Americans who were involuntary sterilized on health grounds between 1907 and 1965—it is impossible to determine if American authorities really translated such medical and eugenic moralizing about hemophilia into actual social practice. It is clear that male bleeders were not targeted for either voluntary or involuntary sterilization in the United States or Great Britain because, as

J. B. S. Haldane put it in the late 1930s, "the operation [vasectomy] would probably kill them, and nature sterilizes them already to a considerable extent by killing them off as children."[66] But the female "carriers," given their health and the reigning medical opinion, were readily portrayed in the medical literature as potential candidates for eugenic measures (including involuntary sterilization). We can say definitively—in light of hemophilia's rising profile as a sex-linked disorder in the first half of the twentieth century—that the female members of hemophilia families have long faced moral scrutiny on account of their sons or brothers having hemophilia. The mothers, sisters, and daughters of male hemophilia patients were frequently the target of medical and health prescriptions that could severely impact their life choices. In effect, the fitness of these females for marriage and parenthood was always in question.

"The Most Hereditary of All Diseases"

Hemophilia's status as a symbol of social progress (or degeneration) hinged in the first half of the twentieth century on its reputation as an archetypal hereditary disease. Along with its prevalence in European royalty, hemophilia's rendering as a hereditary disease played a critical role in making it more visible to the American public in the 1920s and 1930s. Echoing Grandidier's 1855 characterization of hemophilia as "the most hereditary of all diseases," many Americans—laypeople and experts alike—increasingly framed hemophilia as an exemplary instance of poor heredity.[67] Hemophilia's inheritance could be readily illustrated using pedigrees—for example, the paper tools of lineages and family trees—that were familiar to educated people in Europe and North America (figs. 1.1–1.3). Such pedigrees of hemophilia families helped the public grasp the relevance of both genetics and Mendelianism to their lives, and it often inclined Americans to presumptuous statements about who should or should not intermarry or breed.

Thus, in the 1930s hemophilia could be invoked as an example for understanding various aspects of eugenics as well as genetics. Consider *You and Heredity*, a popular science book authored by American journalist Amram Scheinfeld in 1939. Calling hemophilia a "black gene" (by which he meant a gene that produced a detrimental abnormality or disease), Scheinfeld used the now familiar "royal" hemophilia to explain not only sex-linked inheritance (in a chapter titled "For Men Only") but also the importance of mutation in life processes and the shortcomings of sterilization as a means for eradicating undesirable traits in human populations.[68] Specifically, Scheinfeld saw in hemophilia a troublesome problem for those who wanted to sterilize the "carriers" of hereditary disease: "How are we to identify these women when they are themselves perfectly normal? Remember in Queen Victoria's case that only until hemophilia appeared among her descendants was it known that she was a 'carrier.' (It might be interesting to speculate what would have happened to history had Queen Victoria been forced to undergo sterilization!)"[69] Even as Scheinfeld and other thoughtful eugenicists hoped to curb the incidence of hemophilia, they were beginning to question the practicality of doing so.

In the 1930s, genetic studies of hemophilia had seriously undermined the notion advanced by most eugenicists that hemophilia could be eradicated by merely preventing hemophilic carriers from reproducing. By the time Scheinfeld published his book, geneticists J. B. S. Haldane and Lionel Penrose had already demonstrated that the high mutation rate in hemophilia undercut such simplistic eugenic proposals, and Haldane reminded the public of this fact in his popular essay "Blood Royal" (published the same year as *You and Heredity*). Haldane and Penrose argued that roughly a third of all hemophilia cases were *de novo* cases attributable to spontaneous gene mutation (a fact that has been subsequently confirmed). Following this line, Haldane infamously concluded in 1938 that hemophilia among Queen Victoria's progeny most probably originated from a gene mutation "in the nucleus of a cell in one of the testicles of Edward, Duke of Kent, Victoria's father, in the year 1818." In light of this refined understanding of the genetic basis of hemophilia, Haldane continued to advocate for eugenic control of hemophilia carriers, but he did so merely out of the social need to reduce incidence of a harmful disease, rather than the impractical hope of completely eradicating it. That said, Haldane was a Marxist who likely would have been sympathetic to government actions that required the mothers, sisters, and daughters of hemophilic patients to avoid reproduction. He certainly encouraged the prohibition.[70]

Like Haldane, Scheinfeld was interested not only in educating the public about genetics and eugenics as war loomed in Europe but also in stressing that science could be corrupted by politics and prejudice. In fact, Scheinfeld's *You and Heredity* and Haldane's "Blood Royal" each used hemophilia as an exemplar for arguing for a more rational, democratic, and therefore just form of eugenics than had hitherto been promoted in the United States, Great Britain, and other nations. Thinking explicitly of the "Aryanism" of Hitler and the Nazis, Scheinfeld concluded: "All that we have learned [of heredity] proves that one section of mankind cannot long maintain a corner on 'superior' genes, biologic or 'social,' or rid itself and keep free of the 'inferior' genes in circulation."[71] Moreover, as Haldane did in *Heredity and Politics* (1938), Scheinfeld attacked the validity of "race" as a useful category for the politically progressive thinker:

> If the advancement of mankind has come through the efforts of a
> handful, civilization has again and again been hurled back by a few
> individuals, who, like cancers, have corrupted the rest. We have no
> more right, therefore, even in these questionable times, to condemn all
> civilization as hopeless because of some evil specimens than we have to
> consider that all persons are diseased because a few have hemophilia or
> Huntington's chorea.[72]

Hemophilia—from this reformed eugenics perspective—offered society sufficient cause to limit the private liberty of a few individuals while promoting health and autonomy for the population as a whole. For Scheinfeld, this was eugenics for the social good. But the existence of a few "black genes" in any given group or population was not sufficient cause to pathologize everyone belonging to it. Scheinfeld saw no place in eugenics for most contemporary talk of races, and he even argued against universal bans on inbreeding because he saw little evidence that cousin marriages were inherently harmful to society (except where they clearly raised the risk of reproducing an undesirable hereditary disease such as hemophilia or "congenital deaf-mutism"). "Only by improving others . . . can we improve ourselves, and only by promoting progress on a broad front, throughout mankind, can we give our own advancement significance and permanency," opined Scheinfeld.[73] Unfortunately, in calling hemophilia a "black gene," *You and Heredity* did symbolically for people with hemophilia and their families what Scheinfeld said Hitler was actually doing to Europe's Jews: for many of his readers, Scheinfeld's rhetoric undoubtedly stigmatized families with hemophilia as an impediment to "civilization" and the "advancement of mankind."[74]

As signaled by eugenicists as far removed from one another as Charles Davenport and J. B. S. Haldane, hemophilia's status as an archetypal hereditary disorder has long made it a source of fascination and interest for people whose primary concern is not merely the medical treatment of individual patients or the social support of their families. From the inception of the hemophilia concept in the nineteenth century to its popularization in the first half of the twentieth century, our modern concept of hemophilia long reflected the cultural, social, and political sensibilities of the physicians and biologists who made patients with hemophilia and their family members a subject of scrutiny. Without question, then, various hereditary bleeding disorders are manageable today by virtue of medical and scientific endeavors that wielded the hemophilia concept over the past two centuries. Physicians and biologists—even before the era of effective treatments—undoubtedly served the interests of biomedical progress by advancing their conceptions of hemophilia. Yet this disease concept has held complex meanings beyond the immediate challenge of treating congenital bleeding in certain patients and families. The diverse ways that eugenicists wielded the hemophilia concept in the first half of the twentieth century are merely the most prominent example of how talk of hemophilia could be used beyond the clinic to serve a variety of social agendas.

Our modern conception of hemophilia has at various times, and in diverse ways, reflected how physicians in particular treat people who not only happen to be ill but also happen to have a particular social identity. The hemophilia concept has been repeatedly used, for instance, to recommend certain relationships between bleeder patients and their physicians that are ostensibly (but not always) in the service of patients, their families, and society. People have also used the concept to reinforce their particular preferences for certain configurations of modern society along recognizable lines of class, race, ethnicity, and particularly gender. And the hemophilia concept has understandably been used to promote the usefulness and value of scientific and medical knowledge to the public at large. Thus, when I say that hemophilia has long resonated as a measure of progress or decline or as a bodily marker of identity and kinship in the modern world, I am alluding directly to the diverse ways that the concept of the disease has been deployed for better and for worse over the years. Hemophilia's characterization as a blood disease effectively marked it in the second half of the twentieth century as a malady whose management was not only feasible but also capable of producing both beneficial and troubling effects throughout modern society.

CHAPTER TWO

The Scientist, the Bleeder, and the Laboratory

In 1893 British bacteriologist and immunologist Almroth Edward Wright (1861–1947) made an important hematological discovery, one far less celebrated than the turn-of-the-century vaccine discoveries for which he is typically remembered.[1] The blood of Wright's patient, an eleven-year-old hemophiliac known in the literature as S.W., clotted very slowly when compared to his own "normal" blood. S.W.'s clotting time was "9 to 10 minutes" on average, which was significantly longer than the "2.5 to 5, or rarely 6 minutes" that it took Wright's blood to clot. This result compelled Wright to put S.W.'s "subnormal" blood to work as a research tool. Wright imagined that he might shorten the clotting time of S.W.'s hemophilic blood by adding substances to it. His intuition paid off when he witnessed "an increase of coagulability" after the addition of calcium chloride to samples of S.W.'s blood. Excited by this promising result, he immediately turned his attention from bench to bedside. Wright fed calcium chloride (lime salts) to S.W. to see whether ingesting the substance would reduce the patient's blood clotting time. The experiment, however, was cut short before it produced any conclusive results; "my observations," as Wright put it, "were unfortunately broken off by the departure of my patient."[2]

Wright's application of the whole blood clotting time to hemophilia proved to be the most enduring contribution to hematology, for it effectively demonstrated that hemophilic blood was marked as different from normal blood by its delayed ability to clot.[3] After seeing that clotting times in hemophilic blood were measurable, others soon improved upon Wright's technique.[4] Unfortunately, whole blood clotting times proved to be too blunt a tool for determining whether readily available substances such as calcium chloride might be used to effectively treat hemophilia. Yet Wright's clotting experiments embodied two fundamental features of subsequent efforts to manage hemophilia. First, it was early confirmation that laboratory assays that could measure blood clotting activity would play a critical role in subsequent efforts to understand and treat hemophilia and other bleeding disorders. Second, it affirmed that advancing a medical and scientific understanding of hemophilia would require a ready supply of hemophilic blood and bodies. To early twentieth-century hematologists, laboratory-based tools and knowledge held real promise for understanding and treating the root of the hemophiliac's affliction.

But before a laboratory perspective could transform hemophilia into a clinically manageable disease, researchers first had to reach a consensus that hemophilia was, in fact, a blood disease. The practices and perspectives of hematological enthusiasts like Wright were critical in orchestrating this shift because, paradoxically, investigators before the 1890s had been unable to demonstrate that there was anything demonstrably wrong with hemophilic blood. Understanding the making of modern hemophilia management therefore hinges on seeing how medical scientists employed laboratory perspectives and technologies to transform the prospects for treating the disease.

This chapter explores the pivotal role that the laboratory would play in twentieth-century efforts to manage hemophilia by showing how inquisitive physicians conceptualized congenital bleeding in hemophilic patients as a treatable blood disease. These experimentalists did so by introducing laboratory-based instruments and perspectives that not only solidified hemophilia's reputation into the archetypal bleeding disorder it is today but also shaped how the emergent practice of blood transfusion would help transform hemophilia from the intractable, invariably fatal malady that it was in the first quarter of the twentieth century into the chronic but manageable disease it became in the second half of the century. The rapid advances in hemophilia management that were so characteristic of the four decades after World War II grew out of a technological ethos that already pervaded experimental medicine by the 1930s. That ethos, I argue, bound scientist, bleeder, and the laboratory into a productive and ostensibly progressive-minded enterprise.

The Elusive Promise of Being a Blood Disease

Today, it is hard to imagine that inquisitive physicians ever doubted that hemophilia was a blood disease (i.e., as due to a defect in the blood) or that transfusing normal blood into the hemophilic patient would be an obviously beneficial thing to do. But neither idea was easily demonstrated in the nineteenth century. While physicians were virtually unanimous in grouping hemophilia as a constitutional disease with hereditary features before the twentieth century, there was great diversity of opinion when it came to explaining its pathology and causes. In the 1830s, for instance, the prominent British surgeon James Wardrop (1782–1860) suspected that there might be a defect in blood clotting when he noted the similarity between cases of hemophilia and those of typhus fever and scurvy; the latter patients also demonstrated a diminished capacity to clot firmly. However, the blood-clotting hypothesis advanced by Wardrop was merely one theory among others that doctors proposed in the nineteenth century, and hardly a very popular one.[5]

By the 1870s, decades of observation at bedside and autopsy led many medical investigators to conclude that the congenital bleeding tendency in hemophilia patients was due to vulnerabilities in the blood vessels and, possibly, the heart. Recall Schönlein's influential observation that heart malformation was often seen in hemophilic patients and that British physicians told the royal family that Prince Leopold had weak veins.[6] There was also general agreement that this consensus was an unsatisfactory explanation. In the 1850s, for instance, the preeminent German pathologist Rudolf Virchow (1821–1902) proposed that hemophilia might be due to a splenic abnormality. Autopsies had occasionally revealed large spleens in some hemophilic patients, and the spleen was particularly appealing as an organ of concern because physiologists and pathologists associated it with the formation of the blood. By the early 1870s, however, Virchow had abandoned his spleen hypothesis after several of his German contemporaries used microscopic and chemical analysis to demonstrate that hemophilic blood was visibly normal in its color, cell composition, and ability to clot.[7]

Nor was there any definitive evidence in the 1870s or 1880s to suggest that hemophilia should be characterized principally as a blood disease. Thus, while endorsing aspects of both the abnormal vasculature and the malformed heart theories, Hermann Immermann's influential hemophilia entry for the *Cyclopedia of the Practice of Medicine* (1876) stressed the diversity of pathological findings among patients by noting that "there is in all probability no absolutely single pathology for all cases of haemophilia." Moreover, by 1885 explanations of hemophilia's pathology were so full of unwarranted speculation that William Osler (1849–1919) cautioned that any discussion of them would be a "profitless" exercise for the physician who focused on practical medicine.[8] Seen in this light, Almroth Wright's 1893 demonstration of prolonged clotting times in hemophilic blood was a critical breakthrough. Claims that hemophilia was a blood disorder now had legitimate support.

To contemporary minds, the leap from thinking of hemophilia as a blood disease to considering blood transfusion as a therapeutic strategy would seem to be obvious. Before 1900, however, blood transfusions were considered extremely dangerous as well as impractical. Physicians and surgeons had argued about the advisability of the practice since the infamous animal-to-human blood transfusions of 1667 conducted in France by Jean-Baptiste Denis and in England by Richard Lower. These cross-species experiments captured the imagination as well as scrutiny of many Europeans in the late seventeenth century. Initially, a variety of healers emulated the practice, using blood from humans, sheep, cows, dogs, and other creatures; some made extraordinary claims about the curative effects of transfusion for a host of mental and physical maladies. Learned physicians and surgeons were more guarded in their interest (if not openly hostile to the procedure). There was talk of violent and sometimes fatal reactions to the transfusions. Some patients died following such transfusions, including one of Denis's subjects, the "madman" Antoine Mauroy. In 1668 Denis's practice came under attack from many quarters. A murder trial followed. Denis won his case, but the victory was Pyrrhic. The judge also declared transfusion in need of regulation by the medical profession, which allowed Denis's enemies to bring his experimentation to an end. Soon thereafter, authorities in France, England, and Italy banned the practice of human blood transfusions outright. Such prohibitions were favored by the Catholic Church after the Pope characterized blood transfusion as a mortal sin.[9]

Blood transfusions remained a disreputable practice for more than 150 years until 1818, when the English physiologist and obstetrician James Blundell conducted a relatively promising series of blood transfusion experiments on dogs and a few patients in an effort to determine the procedure's potential as a corrective for severe blood loss.[10] On the basis of his physiological experiments, Blundell insisted on the exclusive use of human blood for transfusions to patients, and he recommended against the use of the practice as a remedy for anything other than a life-threatening bleed. Although Blundell publicly urged caution with transfusions in the 1820s, he also invoked controversy by introducing it into obstetric practice at Guy's and St. Thomas Hospitals in London. Most of his early transfusion recipients died. Blundell's supporters—who were predominantly obstetricians—praised the practice as a heroic, last-chance effort to save the lives of women "exhausted" by postpartum bleeding. Even where transfusionists observed Blundell's guidelines, the treatment was unpredictable for all parties, painful for donor as well as recipient, and quite dangerous for the patient receiving the blood. Understandably, the practice of transfusion received heated criticism throughout the nineteenth century, but its few proponents were often fervent about its potential to save lives (especially where all other efforts to staunch bleeding had failed).[11]

During this extended period of agitation for Blundell's transfusions, English physician Samuel Lane successfully transfused blood into a hemophilic boy at St. George's Hospital in London. As far as we know, the intervention was the first of its kind. Lane consulted Blundell before performing his blood transfusion and noted in his 1840 report to the *Lancet* that Blundell had "kindly, and with great perspicuity," explained to him how to conduct "the steps of the operation."[12]

The circumstances of Lane's 1840 hemophilia transfusion case demonstrate both the difficulty of the procedure and the fact that the intervention was conducted only because his patient seemed likely to die without it. Lane's patient was an eleven-year-old named George Firmin. The boy's father brought him to St. George's one morning so that Lane could perform a surgery to correct a "deformity of squinting." The operation proceeded successfully, and Lane noticed nothing unusual about it except that "the boy became faint, and there was more bleeding than usual." Lane even allowed the young Firmin to walk home after the bleeding stopped. Unfortunately, Lane was called later that evening to attend the boy again.

Firmin's eye had begun bleeding about fifteen minutes after he returned home, sometime around noon. Lane figured that his patient had been bleeding continuously for six or seven hours before he inquired about the boy's health history. Only then did Lane learn that Firmin often experienced serious bleeds following slight injury. Lane soon discovered that St. George's Hospital had admitted Firmin on three previous occasions: twice around 1836 for prolonged bleeding following tooth extractions and once in 1839 for a swollen knee joint. On that last occasion, doctors bled Firmin's knee with leeches and then encountered great difficulty stopping the bleeds they had induced. Lane's questioning led him to the conclusion that the boy had a "hemorrhagic diathesis" and that he had caused young Firmin's life-threatening bleed by subjecting the boy to what initially seemed like a routine eye operation.

Although Lane did not say so, he likely felt a special burden to save George Firmin. Over the next five days, he attempted a series of increasingly desperate attempts to stop the boy's bleeding. Nothing seemed to help. On the sixth day, he decided that a blood transfusion might be necessary to restore Firmin's strength. Despite a little improvement the preceding day, Lane now found Firmin "in a more deplorable condition than ever." For readers of the *Lancet*, Lane portrayed Firmin's state as desperate, as "the bleeding had returned during the night; the features were shrunk; the skin was of the paleness, and almost coldness, of death; the pulse could not be felt at the wrist; the arms, and even the head, remained wherever they were placed, so utterly was he deprived of all muscular power." Thus, at seven that evening, with the aid of colleagues and a blood donor, Lane performed a transfusion on Firmin utilizing a custom-made apparatus containing a funnel that could pipe fluid into a large syringe. Blood was drawn from an open vein of the donor (a "stout, healthy young woman") and allowed to flow into the funnel of Lane's apparatus. After inspecting the donated blood for air bubbles, Lane "carefully depressed the syringe" and "the blood was thus propelled into the boy's system." The operation was interrupted four times, and the apparatus repeatedly rinsed in warm water because "of the tendency of the blood to coagulate."

Lane halted the transfusion for good when the donor's blood began to flow too slowly to continue. He estimated that Firmin had received ten to twelve ounces of the young woman's blood and hoped it was sufficient. Firmin's pulse soon returned, but the beneficial effects of the operation were "not instantaneous." Two hours later (and much to Lane's relief), Firmin sat up in bed and drank a glass filled with wine and water. Firmin's eye had ceased to bleed. After ten days, the wound in Firmin's arm had healed. Once the boy regained his strength and appetite, he was treated to three weeks in the country air. When Lane next saw him, Firmin's previously swollen eye was "restored to a straight position." There were no complications from the transfusion as far as Lane or anyone else could tell.

In retrospect, the success of Lane's transfusion operation seems improbable given all that might have gone wrong. When reporting his "successful transfusion" case to the readers of the *Lancet* in October 1840, Lane used his report as an occasion to recount Blundell's principles, to insist that at least twelve lives had been saved by Blundell's own transfusion experiments, and to advertise his personal belief "that many of the fatal cases from haemorrhagic tendency [that are recorded in the medical literature] . . . might have terminated favourably by the timely performance of this operation."[13] Lane was fortunate that his patient endured the procedure without complication. Even without solutions to the problems of air bubbles, premature clotting, and blood incompatibility, it is remarkable that a whole blood transfusion of only ten to twelve ounces was able to stop Firmin's bleed.

Apart from the obvious danger of the procedure, it is hard to know why physicians treating hemophilia patients did not follow Lane's transfusion success with experiments of their own. There is no available record suggesting that any nineteenth-century physician ever tried another transfusion to a hemophiliac or even that Lane attempted to promote or perfect the procedure beyond the publication of his life-saving treatment of George Firmin. If practiced after 1840, blood transfusions for hemophilia were a hidden activity until the early twentieth century. Those physicians who believed that it might be possible to treat hemophilic bleeding increasingly looked to laboratory-based studies of blood in the closing decades of the nineteenth century. There were many attempts to determine what was wrong with hemophilic blood but little insight until Wright's breakthrough.

The successful efforts in the 1890s by Wright and others to measure the clotting time of blood facilitated a rising tide of enthusiasm for the idea that hemophilia was a measurable blood defect capable of being controlled. But this tide also came in gradually. In 1901, for example, William Osler's influential *Principles and Practice of Medicine* still categorized hemophilia as a constitutional disease, not a blood disorder. Here, hemophilia was grouped with diabetes, rheumatism, arthritis, gout, rickets, scurvy, and purpura rather than being placed alongside the anemias and leukemia.[14] Many medical and surgical textbooks did the same around 1900. However, the emergence of whole blood clotting-time techniques combined with growing interest in hematological practice at the turn of the century to elevate the idea that hemophilia was best categorized as a blood disease. By 1914 there was little doubt about it. In criticizing Bulloch and Fildes's recent characterization of hemophilia as "an inherited tendency in males to bleed," one of America's eminent hematologists noted that this "unsatisfactory" definition overstressed the hereditary features of the malady and downplayed the primary pathology. He then enforced the new consensus: "All recent workers agree" that "this delayed or deficient coagulability" is "the characteristic feature of hemophilia" and that "attempts to explain the proximate or ultimate cause of the condition [should] start from this point."[15]

Hemophilia and the Science of Clotting

Scientific interest in hemophilia blossomed during the first two decades of the twentieth century as physicians witnessed investments in experimental laboratories, techniques, and materials that made blood's hitherto opaque nature seem increasingly accessible to human understanding and control. Just as many geneticists had seized on hemophilia in the 1910s to investigate and to popularize the principles of heredity, hematologists would increasingly embrace laboratory-based investigations of hemophilia for their promise to advance greater technological sophistication in clinical medicine as well as the life sciences. By the 1930s, the conventional wisdom among hematologists was that knowledge of hemophilia promised to illuminate the interlocking mysteries of both heredity and blood.

The work of Thomas Addis (1881–1949), a young Scotsman who devoted sustained attention to the study of blood clotting between 1908 and 1910, well illustrates the promise of hemophilia research in the early twentieth century.[16] In 1906 or 1907, Addis met surgeon Ernest W. Hey Groves of the Medical Faculty in Bristol, England, who introduced him to the Webb-Curtis family. Groves had recently published on the surgical aspects of hemophilia and thought he might recruit Addis to Bristol by introducing the idea that Addis might also study this long-suffering family of hemophiliacs.[17] Addis decided instead to go to Edinburgh to obtain his M.D. in the physiology department, but he was apparently inspired enough by the prospects of doing research on hemophilia that he took up the study of normal blood clotting for his medical thesis in his native Scotland.

Addis's thesis research for his medical degree was quite remarkable. In 1908 he devised a cumbersome but reliable apparatus for measuring the clotting time of whole blood. When compared to other clotting-time techniques of the day, Addis found that his achieved a higher degree of control on four key criteria: the means of drawing blood, regulating temperature, avoiding contamination, and providing clear end points for consistent measurement. Addis's apparatus allowed him to evaluate the effects of temperature on clotting (a critical variable), to determine whether the clotting time of normal blood varied significantly over the course of each day (it did not), and to test standing claims that oral administrations of calcium chloride or citric acid impacted clotting (they did not). This research earned Addis a prestigious Carnegie Fellowship in 1909 and encouraged him to expand his hematology studies immediately into the arena of abnormal coagulation.[18]

After earning his medical degree, Addis traveled to Heidelberg, Germany, in 1909 to visit the prominent clotting expert Paul Morawitz. By 1909, and largely because of Morawitz's recent synthesis of existing theories of blood coagulation, clotting researchers had generated some tenuous agreement around the idea that the prolonged clotting of hemophilic blood was due to the insufficient release of tissue thromboplastin into the plasma by damaged cellular matter (fig. 2.1).[19] A reigning experimental question at this time was whether low levels of tissue thromboplastin were due to an abnormality in the vascular tissue, blood platelets, or possibly even the blood's red or white cells. Addis was interested in learning more about hemophilia in its relation to contemporary clotting theory, and Heidelberg was the premiere place to study.

While in Germany, Addis worked with several hemophilic patients that Morawitz and other German investigators had long studied.[20] Thus, when he returned to Edinburgh, Addis immediately sought out more opportunities to study patients with hemophilia and other diseases. Having recently qualified (as a member of the Royal College of Physicians) to treat patients

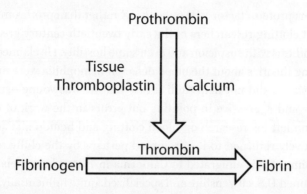

Prothrombin

Tissue
Thromboplastin   Calcium

Thrombin
Fibrinogen ⟶ Fibrin

FIGURE 2.1. The Classic Theory of Blood Clotting, circa 1905–40. According to Paul Morawitz's "classic" theory of blood coagulation, clotting took place in two steps. Tissue thromboplastin initiated the conversion of prothrombin to thrombin in the first step; then the evolving thrombin converted fibrinogen to a fibrin clot. Tissue thromboplastin is a substance liberated into the bloodstream by disintegrating cellular matter (typically as the result of trauma). Today, tissue thromboplastin is known as *tissue factor*, which initiates the extrinsic pathway of blood clotting. Morawitz's own term for it was *thrombokinase*. Over the years, other synonyms for tissue factor have included *platelet tissue factor* and *factor III*. *Source*: Stephen Pemberton, illustration based on Oscar D. Ratnoff, "Why Do People Bleed?" in Maxwell Wintrobe, ed., *Blood, Pure and Eloquent: A Story of Discovery, of People, and of Ideas* (New York: McGraw-Hill, 1980), p. 609.

who came to Edinburgh's Royal Infirmary, he planned to locate and study English and Scottish hemophilia patients to complete his earlier research on German patients. He also reconnected with members of the Webb-Curtis family he had met earlier through Dr. Groves and even secretly transfused one patient, William Webb, in the course of his research. By July 1910 Addis had studied twelve subjects with hemophilia and presented his preliminary findings to a meeting of the Pathology Section of the British Medical Association. Addis stunned the knowledgeable audience with his controversial claim that the defect in hemophilic blood lay not in the mechanisms of a tissue thromboplastin deficiency but rather in a qualitative abnormality in the blood plasma (specifically, in the prothrombin).[21]

Ironically, even though hematologists now recognize Thomas Addis's coagulation studies as prescient of the later discovery (ca. 1937–47) that the prolonged clotting of hemophilic blood results from a qualitative deficiency in a plasma protein (factor VIII or factor IX rather than prothrombin), the dominant clotting researchers of the early twentieth century greeted Addis's hypothesis with suspicion and even some hostility. He claimed that all the leading theories about the blood defect in hemophilia were mistaken; and it certainly did not help Addis's case that he was young—still in his twenties—and aggressive in pointing out errors in the work of others.[22] Addis soon left his research on blood clotting and hemophilia aside and never actively returned to it—prompted perhaps by the chilly reception to his claims. Addis emigrated to California in 1911, where he later married, obtained U.S. citizenship, and specialized, quite influentially, in renal medicine for three decades as Stanford Medical School. His hemophilia studies were, however, an inspiration to researchers in later years. By the early 1930s, a new generation of hematological researchers actively embraced Addis's clotting studies as a seminal influence. Many of these investigators would prove to be pivotal actors in what became known as the "golden age of blood coagulation research" in the two decades after World War II.[23]

In 1910 there were several theories in circulation regarding the source of the prolonged clotting of hemophilic blood, but the leading hypothesis (promoted with some variation by Morawitz and others) held that a defect in the cellular matter of blood—probably the platelets—led to deficiency of tissue thromboplastin in the plasma, which then delayed clot formation. Another prominent theory proposed by French investigator Paul Émile-Weil attributed the delayed clotting in hemophilia to the presence of a clot-inhibiting substance in the blood (antithrombin). As American physiologist William Henry Howell astutely noted, the explanations offered by each investigator varied according to "the theory of coagulation adopted."[24] In 1910 Howell began actively researching the known anticoagulant peptone (i.e., a substance known to inhibit clot formation when exposed to blood); he did this on the assumption that this work might help advance his own general theory of blood coagulation. Within a year, Howell concurred with those investigators who maintained that normal blood plasma contained a native clot-inhibitor called antithrombin.[25] Most importantly, Howell's research on anticoagulants led to his idiosyncratic interpretation of clotting events in the bloodstream, which in turn greatly influenced how he and other American physicians interpreted the defect in hemophilia in the years between World War I and World War II.

Between 1912 and 1914, Howell made his first sustained studies of the blood defect in hemophilia and did so with the aim of clarifying a general theory of blood coagulation. Howell could not determine the "ultimate cause of the condition," but he rejected the explanations of Morawitz and Weil and even endorsed the possibility that Addis's notion that a qualitative deficiency in the prothrombin might be correct. Because platelets supplied the prothrombin in the blood plasma, Howell said a defect in either the platelets or plasma was likely; though he clearly favored the latter between 1914 and 1916.[26]

Howell's influence on American interpretations of hemophilia derived from his position as chair of Physiology at Johns Hopkins Medical School, the preeminent site in the United States for clinicians to learn about the potential for laboratory research for their practice. Howell also established himself as the leading American authority on hematology by writing the most influential physiology textbook in the United States. Between 1904 and 1946, Howell was sole author of *A Textbook of Physiology for Medical Students and Physicians*, which was widely used as the basis for all hematological as well as physiological subjects taught in American medical schools. Howell regularly revised his textbook, often to make major updates to the sections on hematology (his specialty). His thoughts on matters related to blood clotting became highly influential in the United States in the late 1910s and 1920s. In fact, not only did American physicians and medical students treat Howell's general theory of blood coagulation as gospel, but most hematologists in the United States felt compelled to do so as well.[27]

Inspired partly by Howell, Harvard physician and hematology enthusiast Roger Irving Lee and his junior colleague George Richards Minot began investigating the cause of hemophilia (ca. 1916). In their bench studies, Minot and Lee decided that they would separate the red blood cells from the yellow-greenish liquid portion of the blood known as plasma. The process involved putting the blood in a test tube and using centrifugal force to separate the opaque, heavier portion containing the red blood cells from the translucent, lighter plasma. Then, in one of their trials to determine the source of the defect, these investigators added the platelets of hemophilic blood to normal blood plasma and found that it produced a delayed clotting time. Conversely, when they combined normal platelets with hemophilic blood plasma, they found that the clotting time approached normal. By this measure, the platelets rather than the blood plasma seemed to be the key to the delayed clotting time found in hemophilia patients. Minot and Lee then concluded from their laboratory observations that hemophilic bleeding resulted from "an hereditary defect in the blood platelets." They reasoned that the hemophiliac bled longer because of the "slow availability of the platelets for the purposes of coagulation."[28]

Minot and Lee—like Wright, Addis, and others before them—committed themselves to finding the best technique for measuring the clotting time of hemophilic blood. In 1913, before Minot and Lee embarked on their study of "Blood Platelets in Hemophilia," Lee and his intern Paul White had devised a simple and reliable technique that could determine the whole blood clotting time at room temperatures. They tested their technique on 125 patients with a wide variety of diseases (including hemophilia) and found it to be a simple and reliable measure of prolonged clotting. In fact, Minot and Lee's 1916 hemophilia study further confirmed the usefulness of the Lee-White clotting time and helped establish it as a standard tool in experimental and clinical laboratories throughout the United States.[29] But while Minot and Lee's findings fit within Howell's existing conceptual frameworks for understanding blood clotting, their laboratory practice was based on a different set of assumptions about the purpose of blood clotting research. Harvard was then at the vanguard of clinical science in North America, and its investigators had been trained to integrate laboratory discipline into their clinical research and practice. The emphasis of Minot and Lee's experimental work was clinical, with a focus on diagnosing and correcting the pathology. Howell's focus, on the other hand, was reversed. He primarily concentrated on understanding "normal" physiological functions as they were revealed by pathological investigations. His goal was to advance a general theory of blood clotting even as he taught clinicians their physiology.

The clinical focus of Minot and Lee's blood clotting experiments was most evident in their interest in using blood transfusion to treat hemophilia patients. The 1910s saw a surge of interest in making blood transfusions a safe and effective therapy, and 1916 proved to be a pivotal year in advancing the prospects of transfusions for hemophilia patients.[30] Included in Minot and Lee's 1916 report of their bench studies on the defect in hemophilia clotting was a clinical case that these investigators called "of especial interest." After gaining "the enthusiastic approval of the patient," surgeon Beth Vincent transfused the hemophiliac with 600 cubic centimeters of whole blood drawn from a compatible donor. Before the transfusion, the donor's blood had a normal clotting time of 7 minutes. The patient's clotting time was 150 minutes. Afterward, the patient's blood clotted in only 8 minutes. As Minot and Lee put it, "in view of the fact that normal platelets in small amounts in vitro could shorten the hemophilic coagulation time, it was thought that the transfusion of normal blood might shorten the coagulation time of the hemophilic blood, and that the lasting effect of such a procedure would be evident as long as the life of the normal transfused platelets." The experiment confirmed their reasoning by this account. The prolonged clotting time had been normalized by whole blood transfusion. And, as they expected, the patient's clotting time began to lengthen in the coming days; it first reached 100 minutes on the fifth day. Then, on the seventh day, the patient suffered a spontaneous hemorrhage into his right knee joint. The full-blown pathology had returned.[31] Interestingly Minot and Lee's 1916 paper, "The Blood Platelets in Hemophilia," devoted little more than a paragraph to the transfusion experiment. Yet 1916 witnessed the first widely circulated reports of transfusion for hemophilia since Lane's precocious but risky transfusion experiment of 1840.

Unlike Howell, Minot and Lee did not have a stake in the fight over the best general theory for explaining blood clotting. As clinicians, they saw their own laboratory work on hemophilic blood as adding nothing substantially new to the debates about the pathophysiology of blood. Rather, their focus was explicitly on better diagnosis and treatment of the hemophilia patient. Given that so many clotting experts pointed to the platelets as a source of the prolonged clotting of hemophilic blood, Minot and Lee quite reasonably chose to study the role of the platelets in hemophilia. Yet, when referencing Howell's own inconclusive study of the pathological defect in hemophilia (ca. 1914–16), they felt compelled to say that their promotion of the platelet hypothesis did not contradict Howell's general theory of clotting, noting that Howell "does not deny to the blood platelets a share in this deficiency."[32]

Minot and Lee displayed great tact by not challenging Howell's general theory of clotting in 1916 because Howell's influence in American medicine only grew in the interwar years (1919–39). By 1917 Howell's general theory of blood coagulation was changing radically in favor of the idea that inhibitory substances, native to the blood at low levels, were key mechanisms in normal and pathological blood clotting. With respect to hemophilia, this meant that he was less committed to endorsing either the platelet hypothesis or the prothrombin hypothesis. This remarkable shift came after his student Jay McLean recovered a clotting inhibitor from dog livers and hearts that Howell famously dubbed "heparin."[33] By the 1920s Howell frequently said that a native anticoagulant (akin to heparin) circulated in normal blood. He called it antiprothrombin because he now believed that this inhibitory substance kept prothrombin from changing into thrombin in the presence of calcium. It was an idiosyncratic theory that not only lacked definitive proof but contradicted Morawitz's classic theory. In an effort to confirm his general theory, Howell returned to active hemophilia research in the mid 1920s; if his general theory was correct, he could no longer maintain the possibility (as he did in his last hemophilia publication of 1914) that Addis was correct. In 1926 he therefore concluded that "prothrombin in hemophilic blood does not differ from that of normal blood either in its concentration or its properties."[34] Much to his chagrin, however, his hemophilia research produced no evidence to confirm his hope that heparin was involved in the defect in hemophilia. Howell thus had little choice but to endorse the platelet defect hypothesis advanced in different ways by Morawitz, Minot, and Lee. As Howell now explained it, the platelets in hemophilia patients were excessively stable, and their slow disintegration in shed blood accounted for the delayed clotting time. Howell's final judgment on hemophilia helped stabilize the platelet hypothesis as the dominant theory among American hematologists for the delayed clotting time in hemophilic blood.[35]

In a relatively short time span, hematology had become essential to the practice of modern medicine. The discipline went from having relatively little clinical relevance in 1900 to being a routine, seemingly ubiquitous feature of hospital care two decades later.[36] Blood testing was introduced into clinical diagnosis between 1900 and 1925. Blood transfusions were increasingly practicable after World War I. And the hematologist's "conquest of pernicious anemia" in 1926 was, by many accounts, one of the greatest medical breakthroughs of the twentieth century. In fact, Minot and William Murphy earned a share of the 1934 Nobel Prize in Medicine for demonstrating that a regulated diet of liver cured the vast majority of their pernicious anemia patients.[37] In short, increasing numbers of physicians were placing tremendous faith in laboratory-based hematology for the discipline it afforded their clinical practice. And with the growing popularity and acceptability of blood transfusions between the two World Wars, clinicians increasingly saw the possibility for treatment as well as diagnosis.

Intractable Bleeding and Innovations in Blood Transfusion

As previously hinted, blood transfusion—for all its risks and troubled history—became especially enticing as a potential treatment for hemophilic bleeding in the second decade of the twentieth century.[38] It was a key element in establishing Minot and Lee's findings about the role of blood platelets in hemophilia in 1916. Thomas Addis had also secretly (and innovatively) experimented with it in 1910 with his hemophilia patient William Webb.[39] Generally, these investigators hoped that their mix of laboratory and clinical experimentation on hemophilia could explain why hemophilic blood clotted slowly while simultaneously showing how a hitherto dangerous clinical intervention like blood transfusion could be safely and effectively employed to correct the specific mechanism responsible for the delayed clotting in cases of hemophilia.[40]

Yet, at the turn of the century, it was clear that the practice of blood transfusion continued to face serious obstacles before it could make any appreciable impact on clinical medicine. Fortunately, one of the longstanding problems no longer seemed so formidable. Transfusionists had had long grappled with the local and systemic infections that patients often developed following a transfusion. The rise of germ theory made it all too apparent how dangerous the transfusionist's equipment could be, but the growing acceptance of aseptic as well as antiseptic practices in the 1880s and 1890s gave physicians and surgeons the confidence they needed to begin experimenting with blood transfusion in ever greater numbers. By the early 1900s, sterile methods were routine, and surgeons took the lead in promoting transfusion by perfecting instruments and techniques for moving blood directly from donor to patient while reducing the risk of infection and addressing another, intractable problem: the premature clotting of the blood.

Transfusionists had always been stymied by the fact that the donor's blood would immediately clot as it came into contact with the air, the patient's body, and the physician's tools. Addis himself had hoped to solve this problem in 1910 when he added a low concentration of sodium phosphate, an anticoagulant, to his donor's blood before successfully transfusing it into his trusting hemophilic patient, William Webb.[41] Although Addis did not immediately publish his ground-breaking transfusion experiment, his innovation was building on the work of scientists who had begun in the 1890s to test the degree to which various anticoagulant substances might be capable of keeping donor blood fluid in transit to the patient. All the best candidates had proved toxic to recipients, including the sodium citrate solutions that laboratory scientists commonly employed as an anticoagulant in their bench work with blood. The lack of easy insights from the laboratory seemed to stymie blood transfusion research at the turn of the century. In 1906, however, the American surgeon George Washington Crile created a vogue in direct transfusions by connecting a donor's vein to a patient's artery using a method pioneered by Alexis Carrell.[42] Crile was interested in using transfusions to treat surgical shock, but his technical innovation circumvented the problem of clotting. Yet, even as the direct method spurred enthusiasm for blood transfusion among American physicians during the 1910s, immediate progress was hampered by the remarkable surgical skill necessary to carry it out. No one appears to have used it to treat a hemophilia patient, presumably because surgical cutting on a bleeder—even for the purposes of getting blood into him—would have been wildly irresponsible.

The surgical vogue for direct transfusions encouraged Richard Lewisohn (1875–1961), a surgeon at New York City's Mount Sinai Hospital, to investigate whether the old anticoagulant, sodium citrate, might be safely added to transfused blood if administered in very low concentrations. His idea proved sound in studies with dogs and thereafter in human patients. In fact, Lewisohn's solution—0.2 percent sodium citrate, 99.8 percent blood—emerged as the standard mixture for transfusable blood after his 1915 study of the problem became widely appreciated in the interwar years.[43]

Lewisohn's colleague, pathologist Reuben Ottenberg (1882–1959), did not wait on medical consensus to apply the innovation of anticoagulated blood to hemophilia. In early 1916, Ottenberg seized on Lewisohn's discovery and successfully transfused a hemophilic patient at Mount Sinai Hospital using citrated blood.[44] Addis, sensing an opportunity, immediately published his secret transfusion of William Webb from 1910 in the same medical journal as Ottenberg's article.[45] Addis thereby called attention to the fact that he had been the first experimental physician to successfully transfuse a hemophiliac using anticoagulated blood (sodium phosphate in his case).[46]

Roughly concurrent with these developments, the final and most mysterious obstacle to safe and practicable blood transfusions was the question of blood compatibility between donors and recipients. Until the early 1900s, no one had been able to explain why some patients benefited from transfusion while others suffered violent, sometimes fatal reactions to transfused blood. Then, in 1900–1901, German pathologist Karl Landsteiner noticed the tendency of one patient's blood to cause another patient's blood to clump together when brought into contact at the laboratory bench. He subsequently discovered that the individual differences in human blood (rather than bacterial contamination) accounted for the so-called agglutination phenomenon, and he then determined that patients could be grouped into three blood types, A, B, and C. Two of Landsteiner's students discovered a fourth blood type, AB, a year later. (Type C was later renamed Type O.)[47] Landsteiner's serology work demonstrated that transfusions between patients with the same blood group did not destroy blood cells (hemolysis), but that such destruction occurs along predictable lines when a person is transfused with donor blood of an incompatible blood group. Landsteiner learned that transfusion recipients experienced an allergic response when their blood cross-reacted. While briefly noting the implications of his serological work for transfusion problems, Landsteiner and others did not actively promote this work to transfusionists. Unfortunately, most transfusionists ignored this research or failed to appreciate its relevance to their work. The practical implications of Landsteiner's blood group and cross-reaction discoveries were not fully worked out until the 1920s and 1930s.[48]

Paradoxically, it was the advent of "total warfare" in the 1910s that gave medical professionals and the public the strongest opportunities and incentives to render transfusions practicable. World War I witnessed trauma on a hitherto unprecedented scale and helped transfusionists innovate their practice in an environment where extreme risk taking was a truly acceptable norm. Beginning in 1917, military surgeons and physicians in the

Allied forces began using blood transfusion for the treatment of shock and blood loss among injured soldiers. There were many difficulties: the unsanitary conditions, the crude tools, the difficulties of unwanted clotting, and the problem of "agglutination and hemolysis from admixture of incompatible bloods."[49] There was great ingenuity in handling some of these problems, including the introduction of citrated blood, syringe-cannula administration, and the application of Roger Lee's quick procedure for screening blood compatibility.[50] On the whole, the greatest difficulty derived from the highly perishable nature of whole blood and the great difficulties of supplying preserved blood to the battlefront. Even under the most sterile and refrigerated conditions then available, red blood cells could last no longer than three weeks. Military physicians initiated efforts to use stored blood on the battlefield, but they could not overcome the difficulties of supplying the perishable substance on the necessary scale. In the later stages of the war, soldiers were pulled aside at mobile depots to donate blood to wounded comrades. In other words, transfusable blood was typically carried to the front "on the hoof"—literally *in* the men.[51] The wartime practice of blood transfusion was often makeshift, prone to inefficiency, and relatively limited given the scale of killing; but there was much to be praised as well. For a few hundred souls, the results proved dramatic and lifesaving. And for medical observers, it was clear that blood transfusion would thereafter be indispensable to the well-being of both warring and peaceful nations. The total warfare occasioned by the Great War made risk taking necessary while providing a rationale for relevant sectors of European and American society to take the laboratory and clinical contributions of hematologists to heart.

The interwar years (1919–39) also witnessed a variety of successful efforts to render transfusion medicine practicable for civilian as well as military populations. Toward this end, a few influential physicians who served in World War I communicated their transfusion experiences afterward. Geoffrey Keynes, a British surgeon and brother of economist John Maynard Keynes, became a forceful advocate of the practice after American physicians introduced him to the use of citrated blood for the treatment of shock as well as blood loss. In 1922 he published *Blood Transfusion*, which helped medical professionals throughout Great Britain initiate voluntary blood donation during the 1920s.[52] The interwar years witnessed other significant developments in transfusion medicine that helped demonstrate its practicability across broad sectors of medicine and society. During the Spanish Civil War (1936–39), for instance, the Republican Army Medical Corps operated the first large-scale transfusion service and effectively supplied wounded soldiers in frontline positions with stored blood drawn from a civilian population.[53] More famously, beginning in 1937, the first blood banks began appearing in civilian hospitals throughout Europe and North America. Effective blood banking was the last serious obstacle to making blood transfusion a readily available treatment for patients. Spurred by the exigencies of World War II, the early 1940s witnessed the standardization of blood transfusion services. The public experienced blood transfusion as a safe, routine, and life-saving practice.

The advances in transfusion medicine that occurred in the first four decades of the twentieth century were undoubtedly hard fought. There were plentiful opportunities for failure, and many of the successes gave rise to vexing questions about balancing the risks of patient safety against the need to innovate. Ultimately, however, it was a commitment to hematological discipline in the laboratory that helped the "practical" transfusionists sustain progress through the turbulent years of the twentieth century. In short, blood transfusion would not have become a routine treatment for bleeding and shock between 1910 and 1940 were it not for laboratory-based research on immunology and blood groups, procoagulants and anticoagulants, blood storage, and many other blood matters that could be assayed using biochemical know-how.

Hemophilia played little to no role in the rise of transfusion medicine, but the future of hemophilia management—as heralded by the publicized hemophilia transfusions of 1916—would soon hinge on this innovation. That is not to say that transfusion pioneers ignored hemophilia. Occasional hemophilia researchers such as Roger Lee were quite integral to making blood transfusion practicable in the early twentieth century and voiced cautious optimism throughout this era about the potential of blood transfusion to make a difference for people with bleeding disorders. In fact, Lee and White had developed their whole blood clotting-time technique at Massachusetts General Hospital (ca. 1913) in order to help surgeon Beth Vincent evaluate the blood clotting science in advance of his own researches into the practicability of blood transfusion. Lee later recalled that it was still "considered dangerous to insert a needle into a vein" when they were experimenting in the 1910s. This era stood in marked contrast, he said, to the subsequent period of the 1920s and 1930s when blood chemistry not only rendered transfusions practicable but "proudly promised to tell us the secrets of human life."[54] Such optimism proved justified only where experimentalists integrated laboratory and clinical perspectives into their handling of both blood and hemophilia.

The Quantitative Turn in Blood Clotting Research

The interwar years were a particularly vital period for blood coagulation science because the promise of biochemistry and its technologies sustained hopes among blood researchers that their work could lead to future cures. In the 1930s in particular, these investigators began demonstrating how the power of the laboratory might be harnessed to transform the way clinicians treated hemophilia, jaundice, and a variety of other diseases that were characterized by abnormal bleeding. The desire to create blood tests that could measure quantitative (rather than qualitative) defects in abnormal blood was especially motivating. Like the earlier studies of Wright, Addis, and Howell, clotting studies of the 1930s drew on the promise of novel laboratory assays for testing the blood and a ready supply of hemophilic blood drawn from subjects in clinical cases of hemophilia and other bleeding disorders. The practices of the so-called Iowa Group were indicative of the importance of the quantitative turn in studies of normal and abnormal clotting.

In 1930 the pathologist Harry Pratt Smith (1895–1972) had just been recruited to the University of Iowa and appointed its chair in pathology.[55] Previously, Smith had trained and collaborated with pathologist George Whipple at the Hooper Foundation in San Francisco and later at the University of Rochester. Whipple's demonstration that liver extract could alleviate pernicious anemia in the dog earned him his share of the 1934 Nobel Prize with Harvard's Minot and Murphy. Smith arrived in Iowa City with plans to form a research group based on the model of Whipple's work.[56] He devoted his research program to understanding the mechanisms responsible for hemostasis (including blood clotting), and he recruited Emory Warner and a few other promising young men, including Kenneth Brinkhous, Charles Owen, and Walter Seegers, to work with him.

Together, Smith's team of researchers became known in the field of hematology as the Iowa Group.[57]

Over the course of the 1930s, the Iowa Group researchers conducted many laboratory studies aimed at characterizing the functions of the known proteins in blood plasma. They isolated these complex proteins, purified them as best they could, and tested them in a variety of ways to see if these plasma factors could correct samples of blood suspected of having clotting or other hemostatic deficiencies. The Iowa Group's emphasis on quantification and purification techniques was central to its success.[58] Specifically, the group's techniques for measuring the clotting action of various substances presented hematologists with a meaningful way to evaluate clinical efforts to correct hemophilic bleeding. On the model of breakthroughs in diabetes and pernicious anemia research, the Iowa Group interpreted bleeding disorders as metabolic deficiencies that could be corrected by the administration of whatever functional substance was absent in the patient's body.[59] Using this approach, for example, members of the Iowa Group discovered that the bleeding often found in newborns was a correctable deficiency of vitamin K.[60] But the approach was practicable only for bleeding disorders where investigators had reliable laboratory techniques for measuring the functional properties of blood.

The first laboratory assays that simply and reliably measured the functional activity of prothrombin in the blood plasma appeared in the mid-1930s. Such tests not only were suitable for clinical laboratories but also made it much easier for hematologists to investigate the hypotheses of Addis and a few others that the clotting defect in hemophilic blood lay in the conversion of prothrombin into thrombin. In 1935 Armand Quick (1894–1978) of Marquette University in Milwaukee unveiled the first and simplest of these assays (the prothrombin time or PT), which has long been used in clinical laboratories throughout the world.[61] Shortly thereafter, Iowa pathologists Emory Warner, Kenneth Brinkhous, and Harry Smith announced that they had developed their own assay for measuring prothrombin.[62] These assays soon became widely known among hematologists as the one-stage and two-stage prothrombin consumption tests, because the Quick test merged the two stages of prothrombin conversion described by Morawitz, while the Iowa test kept them separate.[63]

For the two decades after the appearance of their prothrombin consumption tests, Quick and the Iowa Group fought vigorously for the preeminence of their respective techniques. Quick's approach had the advantage because his one-stage assay was simpler to employ in clinical settings, and, in most cases, the tests produced identical results. There were, however, discrepancies between the tests under certain conditions (e.g., when used with blood drawn in early infancy or when used to test refrigerated blood).[64] The debates between the two groups, while heated, were mostly collegial, and their disagreements actually proved productive in the years after World War II. Specifically, the discrepancies in the assays made it possible for hematologists to see that the conversion of prothrombin to thrombin (by tissue thromboplastin) was dependent upon the presence of other plasma factors. This helped establish the fact that there were many coagulation factors in the plasma beyond those elaborated in Morawitz's classic theory of blood clotting. Taken together, the prothrombin tests of Quick and the Iowans would help clinical investigators in the 1940s and 1950s to identify with greater perspicuity what was typical or atypical about the blood of their bleeder patients.[65]

Laboratory assays were not the only critical instrument that clotting researchers at Iowa used to further their research program. In the course of their studies of various bleeding conditions, the Iowa Group frequently used blood samples drawn from bleeder patients. On occasion, the Iowa Group also employed dogs in blood clotting studies, both as sources of organ tissue and blood plasma and as subjects for testing dietary supplements and plasma components. Brinkhous, in particular, found numerous experimental uses for the laboratory's dogs. In one series of experiments, he prepared bile-fistula dogs identical to those used by George Whipple in his Rochester studies of bile formation and function. A bile-fistula dog is "fabricated" by tying the common bile duct of these dogs so as to retain all the bile in the gallbladder. The procedure allows the researcher to collect the bile via an opening (or fistula) in the abdominal wall of the dog and thereby subject the substance to laboratory testing.[66] As a side effect, many bile-fistula dogs acquired a tendency to bleed. Brinkhous was interested in the latter phenomenon and determined that the acquired bleeding tendency in these dogs was due to a prothrombin deficiency. Following Whipple's model of a metabolic deficiency, the Iowa Group subsequently fed the dogs bile and vitamin K (extracted from alfalfa) to normalize their metabolisms. These dog studies were part and parcel to the Iowa Group's successful treatment by vitamin K of adult patients with obstructive jaundice and of newborns with hemorrhagic disease. Within the group, it was Kenneth Brinkhous who singled out hemophilia for his personal attention.

Brinkhous's initial attempts to study hemophilia were makeshift. Between 1935 and 1938, he teamed up with a medical student to obtain fresh samples of hemophilic blood. The medical student would check hospital admissions to find out whether a hemophilic patient was admitted the previous day. When a patient was available, Brinkhous would go to his bedside to determine whether the hemophiliac would be willing to donate blood. Brinkhous soon found this "hodge podge" approach to be an unsatisfactory way of doing research, relying as it did on an unpredictable passage of materials between clinic and laboratory. Fresh hemophilic plasma was necessary for his studies, but its supply was always dependent, in his words, upon whether "a patient with hemophilia was unfortunate enough to have to come to the hospital."[67]

In 1938 two critical events occurred at the University Hospital in Iowa City to help Brinkhous stabilize his laboratory studies of hemophilia. First, the hospital established a blood bank for its transfusion service, allowing Brinkhous to conduct his bench studies on a schedule that was no longer dictated by the highly perishable nature of his blood samples. Second, Brinkhous obtained a reliable donor of hemophilic blood when Jimmy Laughlin became a patient at the University Hospital. Laughlin, a twenty-four-year-old taxi driver with severe hemophilia, was admitted for a life-threatening bleed following a fistfight with a passenger who refused to pay his fare. Brinkhous approached Laughlin at the bedside and conveyed to this patient his concern about the dangers of taxi driving for someone with hemophilia. He then offered Laughlin a position as a dishwasher and helper in the Iowa Group's laboratory. Laughlin agreed to the career change and soon began working full time in the laboratory with Brinkhous, Smith, and the others (fig. 2.2). Thus, through a strategy of opportunism, Brinkhous was able to remedy the shortage of hemophilic blood for study by taking advantage of blood banking and by bringing a "hemophiliac" into his laboratory.

This practical organization of the laboratory soon grew complicated. As Brinkhous accumulated experience with Laughlin's condition, he became increasingly confident that he could manage Laughlin's bleeds and might even prevent them. Like many patients with severe hemophilia, Laughlin suffered from toothaches because he could not properly maintain his teeth

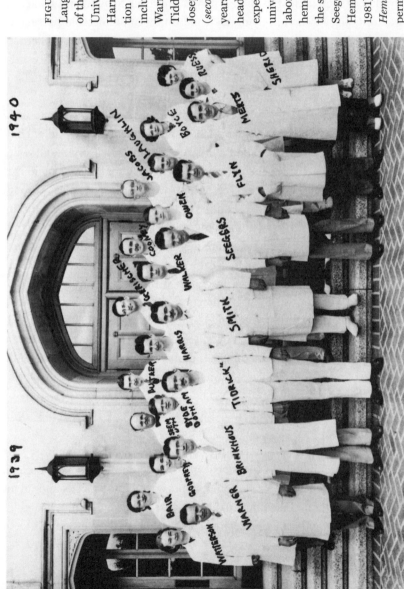

FIGURE 2.2. Iowa Group with Jimmy Laughlin. This faculty and staff photo of the Department of Pathology at the University of Iowa, 1939–40, depicts Harry P. Smith's Iowa Blood Coagulation Research Group. The core team included (*first row, left to right*) Emory Warner, Kenneth Brinkhous, Robert Tiddrick, Smith, Walter Seegers, Joseph Flynn, Edwin Mertz, and (*second row*) Charles Owen. In later years, most of these pathologists headed their own laboratories for experimental hematology at other universities. Jimmy Laughlin, the laboratory technician with severe hemophilia, appears next to Owen in the second row. *Source:* Walter H. Seegers, "A Personal Perspective on Hemostasis and Thrombosis (1937–1981)," *Seminars in Thrombosis and Hemostasis* 7 (1981): 178 (reprinted by permission of Thieme Publishers).

without risk of bleeding. Brinkhous proposed extracting the offending teeth and controlling Laughlin's bleeding by using measured transfusions of whole blood given before the surgery and at predetermined intervals of time after it. This proposal led to the first blood transfusion to a hemophiliac in Iowa City, and Brinkhous remembered the traumatic experience that followed as testament to his bravado and overconfidence. "Lo and behold," he recalled, "[Laughlin] continued to bleed the first four days . . . in spite of transfusions" planned in advance.[68] After Laughlin nearly bled to death in the first forty-eight hours, Brinkhous decided to divert from his experimental protocol and shift to transfusions given more frequently and at smaller volumes.[69] Laughlin's condition stabilized, and over the next few days, the bleeding finally stopped. In light of this traumatic experience, Brinkhous tempered his desire to manage hemophilic bleeding clinically. Instead, he returned to his laboratory studies with greater appreciation of the difficulties involved in translating blood work using test tubes and centrifuges into reliable clinical practice. Jimmy Laughlin continued to work as a lab assistant for the Iowa researchers, but Brinkhous now limited Laughlin's participation in his hemophilia work to the occasional sample of hemophilic blood drawn from Laughlin's vein.

Given his experimental goals, Brinkhous was largely ambivalent about keeping his clinical and laboratory life distinct. The point was to bridge the gap, to make laboratory science applicable to the clinical management of hemophilia. Yet his tooth extraction experiment indicated the dangers of such ambivalence. The near loss of Laughlin forced Brinkhous to consider the uncertainties and risks of his experimental pathologist's perspective, while also reinforcing the need to study hemophilic bodies as well as blood. Brinkhous knew that the use of laboratory animals presented the safest solution to the problem of correcting hemophilic bleeding experimentally. The examples of Whipple's anemic dogs and the Iowa Group's own bile-fistula dogs (used in their vitamin deficiency work) all suggested that a therapeutic breakthrough in the laboratory was possible for hemophilia given the right circumstances and experimental organism. However, researchers knew too little about the clotting defect in hemophilia in the late 1930s to create the condition in a laboratory animal, and no nonhuman hemophiliacs were yet known to exist in nature. In short, without animal organisms to study, Brinkhous returned to his samples of hemophilic blood and hoped that the solution lay there.[70]

"Experiments of Nature"

Since the mid-1910s, when Minot and Lee first envisioned the clotting defect in hemophilia as a consequence of a deficiency in the blood platelets, there had been little compelling evidence to confirm either the controversial findings of Thomas Addis or the more systemic accounts of William Henry Howell. As World War II was breaking out in Europe, most American hemophilia researchers still conceived of the condition as a platelet deficiency with some involvement of the circulating plasma. But even within this paradigm, there was substantial progress being made that capitalized on the availability of hemophilic blood and patients for study as well as increased quantitative focus on the chemistry of blood clotting. In an important 1939 article, for instance, Brinkhous utilized readily available blood of Jimmy Laughlin (with confirmation in four other hemophilia patients) to explain that hematologists could measure "the speed with which prothrombin converted to thrombin in hemophilic blood" using techniques devised by the Iowa Group. Indeed, Brinkhous had found not only that the "prothrombin conversion rate" in hemophilic blood was delayed but that the delay was correctable with addition of minute amounts of tissue thromboplastin. This result confirmed the existence of a measurable physiologic mechanism that (presumably) no other investigator had sufficiently interrogated, and it promised normalization of the hemophilic defect at a biochemical level with renewed focus on the roles of tissue thromboplastin and other possible plasma factors in converting prothrombin to thrombin. Unfortunately, it still did not tell hematologists the exact nature of the defect. Because Brinkhous had been transfusing Laughlin regularly at this point, he concluded his article by stressing the promise of blood transfusion in its relation to the evolving science of measuring blood clotting activity: in his opinion, "the cells and platelets of the donor's blood supply the missing element . . . [and a] simple explanation is that the element so supplied is thromboplastin . . . [but this] possibility needs further study, both because of its theoretical importance, and because of its therapeutic implications."[71]

After World War II, Brinkhous and other blood clotting researchers would finally get their opportunity for further exploration. The postwar era would witness a veritable eruption of new insights into the mechanisms of blood coagulation that were, in part, due to the Depression-era efforts by the Iowa Group, Armand Quick, and others to visualize, quantify, and correct the coagulation defects found in a variety of other bleeder patients. Those advances came with increased quantitative focus on the qualitative abnormality in prothrombin (that Addis had foretold). But the shift away from the platelet hypothesis of hemophilia was also substantially aided after 1936 by research that looked at blood clotting in its relation to the actual biochemical composition of blood plasma.

In light of the fact that contemporary medicine defines hemophilia as a deficiency of one or another plasma factor, it is usually said that the platelet hypothesis prevailed for some years despite earlier evidence to the contrary. Between 1927 and 1937, at least three separate laboratories in Germany, Belgium, and the United States performed experiments strongly suggesting that the clotting defect in hemophilia was localized to the plasma.[72] In the United States, two laboratory studies conducted by hematologist and internist Arthur J. Patek at Harvard's Thorndike Memorial Laboratory helped turn the tide definitively against the platelet hypothesis of Minot and Lee. The insight came from seemingly unlikely quarters because Minot, who directed the Thorndike Laboratory, gave Patek permission to challenge his assumptions about hemophilia. In 1936 Patek and his colleague Richard Stetson demonstrated that the addition of normal plasma to hemophilic plasma could actually correct the prolonged clotting time typically found in hemophilic blood. Patek initiated his studies of hemophilia on the assumption that blood transfusion had shown that it could correct hemophilic bleeding and that previous laboratory studies of hemophilia not only had been conducted under artificial conditions (i.e., in vitro systems of calcified blood) but also had been understood in terms of blood clotting theories whose "varied nomenclature" had possibly "served to confound rather than clarify understanding of this disease."[73] Minot was soon converted and even developed an appreciation of Addis's work that he had long viewed with suspicion.

Later that same year, Patek turned to biochemist F. H. Laskey Taylor to help him localize the corrective property to a crude fraction of normal plasma and test it in a living patient (i.e., in vivo). It was later said that "the something" that Patek and Taylor found in 1936 was a previously unknown globulin substance, although they did not say this in print.[74] It took a decade before investigators widely appreciated this breakthrough. What Patek and Taylor did write in 1937 was that "one may conclude at this juncture only that the clotting substance is precipitated with globulin, but there is no proof that it is the globulin itself." In any case, Patek believed that he and Taylor had definitively shown that the hemophilic defect was not in the platelets and that his in vivo study had come closest to realizing the desire for a specific treatment for hemophilia. He concluded: "The fact that normal globulin substance [i.e., their crude plasma fraction] reduces the clotting time *in vivo*, we believe changes the complexion of the disease from an abnormality that was immutably fixed to one that is amenable to change."[75]

For many experimental hematologists, Patek and Taylor's work encouraged efforts to examine the plasma more closely and determine what role, if any, hitherto unrecognized plasma proteins might play in normal and abnormal clotting. Hemophilic blood made itself opaque to human understanding by inexplicably freeing platelets into surrounding plasma, thereby making it difficult for the hematologist to discern whether it was the platelets or the plasma factors that were the culprit.[76] Following the work of Patek, Stetson, and Taylor, the powerful Minot withdrew his support of the platelet hypothesis, encouraging American investigators to actively investigate the plasma as the site of the defect in hemophilia. During World War II, the attention and resources of most blood researchers were diverted to problems of immediate consequence to the war effort. As soon as they returned to active peacetime research in the late 1940s, however, experimental hematologists immediately addressed the promise of the plasma factor hypothesis, laying the platelet hypothesis to rest.

Brinkhous returned from his wartime service in 1946, accepted the chair of the pathology department at the University of North Carolina Medical School, and immediately took up his interrupted bench studies of the clotting defect in hemophilic blood. He published this work in 1947, confirming his provisional conclusion of 1939 that "in hemophilia there is a deficiency in a plasma factor required for platelet utilization" that delays the conversion of prothrombin into thrombin. By 1950 Brinkhous and colleagues were calling the missing plasma factor "antihemophilic factor" (AHF) because its absence accounted for the delayed clotting times found in most hemophilia patients. Later, in 1958, hematologists widely agreed to call it factor VIII.[77] In effect, the immediate postwar period initiated the search for deficient plasma factors in hemophilic blood. Hemophilia and other bleeding disorders were then conceptualized as pathologies of delayed blood clotting that could each be effectively normalized by plasma fractions tailored to address the bleeder patient's specific plasma factor deficiency.

None of these advances would have been possible without the cooperation of a few trusting hemophilia patients. Time and again, experimental hematologists of the 1930s and 1940s relied on the assistance and cooperation of hemophilia patients to provide the bodies, blood, and tissue they needed to advance their studies and scientific careers. Most famously, Harvard's George Minot brought a twenty-three-year-old hemophilia patient named Russell White into his laboratory in 1932. As described by physician Francis Rackemann in 1956, White was "much interested" in the Thorndike laboratory's work and "more than cooperative" over the years. Rackemann, who was also Minot's cousin and biographer, characterized White's participation with Harvard blood research as vital to all of Harvard's hematological endeavors in the mid-twentieth century:

> White's blood, studied so extensively, is used again and again to test the plasma of patients who bleed from unknown causes. If a small amount of plasma (say 0.10 cc.) from the specimen will clot 2.00 cc. of White's blood, the patient has "antihemophilic activity" and is normal. If, however, no clot forms, then the patient may have hemophilia. During World War II, both the army and the navy sent samples of blood to be tested at the Thorndike, and White's blood was almost an essential tool.[78]

In the context of the Thorndike laboratory, White became a necessary instrument to the advance of hematological science. His blood even functioned as a norm for determining whether blood samples that came through the laboratory were "hemophilic" or "normal." It is hardly surprising, then, that Arthur Patek and Richard Stetson acknowledged their indebtedness to White and three other "hemophilic patients" for "their ready cooperation" with the Thorndike's important hemophilia study of 1936.[79] White probably deserves some share of the credit that Patek, Stetson, and Taylor garnered for their demonstration that the prolonged clotting of hemophilic blood was due to a hitherto unknown plasma factor deficiency.

Russell White was likely the first professional hemophiliac in the United States. Like Iowa's Jimmy Laughlin a few years later, White made himself an integral part of the research enterprises conducted by his physicians. In fact, White publicly acknowledged that he had benefited greatly from the attention and care he received among researchers at Harvard's Thorndike Laboratory. In 1954 White (then forty-five) recalled the Depression-era research at Harvard to *Boston Globe* reporter Frances Burns:

> When I came here, I was at a low ebb. Today I am perfectly well. Tomorrow I may feel a muscle sore and tight and a joint aching, and I know I'm bleeding in the joints again. . . . Dr. Minot wanted to have someone always in the ward that could be used for his blood experiments. That's why I've stayed here . . . I remember Dr. Minot warmly. He was a kind man. He'd sit beside a patient and listen to him, let him tell him how he was feeling. He was soft-spoken. Like all the research workers, he'd usually end up by referring back to knowledge he'd got from reading, right back to the Bible.[80]

Minot, Patek, and other researchers at Harvard's Thorndike laboratory would have undoubtedly been pleased with White's assessment of their work. These prominent investigators saw their work as a cooperative enterprise that served the public good as well as the private interests of their patients. Moreover, as White astutely observed, these researchers even shared their Judeo-Christian religious sensibilities with their patient-subjects as a justification for their actions.

Modern hemophilia management, including the use of blood and plasma transfusions, became possible only after the disorder had been recast from a constitutional malady to a blood disease (generally) and a bleeding disorder (specifically). This transformation was laborious and complicated. Yet, in its reliance on bleeder patients, novel instrumentation, and sustained hematological discipline, hemophilia's transformation into a manageable blood disease undoubtedly reflected the technological ethos of experimental medicine in the first half of the twentieth century. This fact was obvious to prominent researchers in the field of blood coagulation studies. As hematologist Oscar Ratnoff once put it, progress in regard to the basic pathologies of hemophilia and other bleeding disorders reflected a commitment to seeing every aspect of these diseases as a problem that could be elucidated by "a continual cross-fertilization of ideas and techniques between clinic and laboratory" and by "studies of individuals with defective coagulation."[81]

For practical purposes, advancement in blood research required twentieth-century hematologists to treat the bodies and blood of hemophilia patients in the most instrumental of terms while negotiating the fact of their humanity. The experiences of Russell White and Jimmy Laughlin suggest that the relationship between research subject and experimenter was also symbiotic and that investigators did their best to observe the Hippocratic ethic to "do no harm" even as they tried to advance their science. Yet there was also a moral economy operating by the mid-twentieth century that reflected a complex blend of the need to innovate as well as respect the interests of different participants (doctor-researcher, patient-subject). This moral economy, along with the technological ethos that supported it, would play a critical role in how hemophilia diagnosis and treatment developed after World War II.

Paradoxically, the war years (1939–45) proved to be a pivotal era of advancement for hemophilia management even though most explicit hemophilia research was interrupted. Blood and plasma transfusions emerged as a routine, relatively safe procedure at this time. Mass blood donation also became an enduring reality of modernizing societies as the United States, Great Britain, and their allies embraced transfusion medicine as a priority in the war effort.[82] Many hemophilia researchers in these countries took a necessary hiatus from concentrated investigations of hemophilia as they devoted themselves to caring for soldiers, gaining experience with transfusion medicine, and helping integrate transfusions, blood banking, and mass donation into clinical practice. Of course, wartime innovations in clinical hematology directly benefited hemophilia patients and their physicians as these innovations made their way into routine medical care. In fact, as more hemophilia patients came to rely on transfusion services in the 1940s, they came into more sustained relationships with hematologists. This, in turn, served to facilitate further cooperation between hemophilia researchers and their subjects as each sought even greater control of bleeding after the war.

Reflecting back on the immediate postwar era, Pittsburgh hematologist Jessica Lewis penned a short article for the *Journal of the American Medical Association* in 1962 about the path-breaking contributions in the field of blood coagulation research in the previous three decades. She noted the importance of the two kinds of laboratory tests—the "prothrombin type" that proliferated in the 1930s and 1940s and the "thromboplastic type" that emerged in the 1950s—but she also titled the essay "Experiments of Nature" to emphasize the critical role that the clinical identification of bleeder patients had played in advancing the field.[83] In characterizing bleeders as "experiments of nature," Lewis effectively captured the fact that clotting researchers had resolutely committed themselves in the twentieth century to treating the blood and bodies of their bleeder patients as a natural resource.

Vital Factors in the Making
of a Masculine World

In November 1953, the *Saturday Evening Post* published a six-page il-lustrated essay bearing the provocative title: "I've Got the Lonesomest Disease!" (fig. 3.1). In most respects, this essay resembled many other jour-nalistic treatments of hemophilia in the two decades after World War II. It highlighted the importance of blood donation and transfusions for hemo-philia patients, recent efforts by hematologists to understand and treat the bleeding disorder, the social isolation that patients often experienced, the hereditary and sex-linked nature of the condition, and even the familial challenges of raising afflicted boys into well-adjusted men. Yet this maga-zine feature was also unique, in that its author, Helen Furnas, was a self-described "bleeder." Written at a time when hematologists reserved hemo-philia diagnoses for boys and men, Furnas's essay provided a firsthand female perspective on a condition that physicians and scientists had tradi-tionally framed as a male problem.[1]

This chapter explores how hemophilia's development into a treatable bleeding disorder was intimately related to its status as a male disease. Helen Furnas's bleeding disorder was what hematologists today call a clotting fac-tor XI deficiency. It is sometimes categorized as a rare type of hemophilia—hemophilia C—although hematologists in the 1950s debated if this new pathology should really count as a true form of hemophilia. A key point of contention was the fact that the disorder, unlike the two more common forms of hemophilia, occurred equally in both male and female patients.

I've Got the Lonesomest Disease!

By HELEN FURNAS

The author has to carry a physician's certificate in her handbag, to prove to strange doctors that she's really a "bleeder" and not a neurotic female. Here's what is now being done for her and thousands of others who suffer from an ailment that can turn a minor cut into a major tragedy.

THE rarest version of one of the world's rarest ailments—I've got it. It seldom harms me and it just bores or annoys doctors, except a few earnest researchers exploring the mysteries of hemophilia and allied conditions. They can be counted on to take me big. While working on this article, I mentioned to one of them that I am a "PTA-type hemophiloid." He reacted like Julius Caesar when Cleopatra unrolled from that rug. His eyes gleamed, his hands clutched.

"You don't get out of here alive," he said, "without leaving us a nice sample of your blood to work on." I was the second specimen of the breed he had ever seen.

He got the blood. The more science learns about these troubles the better for us "bleeders"—our unscientific if graphic traditional name. Besides, exploration of our peculiarities promises new help for many others facing more common heart and blood ailments.

In the dictionary, hemophilia is a "morbid condition, usually congenital, characterized by a tendency to bleed immoderately . . . caused by improper coagulation of the blood." That does for a starter. It sounds inconvenient, and my difficulty is all of that. I have to carry in my already overstuffed handbag a specialist's elaborate analysis of my condition, with instructions about what to do if accident strikes or surgery is needed. Without that paper, any strange doctor whom I warn that I'm a bleeder just tickets me as neurotic. Chances are he never

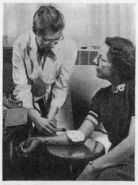

Mrs. Ruth Holland, a medical technologist, tests the clotting factors of the author's blood.

saw a bleeder in his whole professional career. All he knows about hemophilia is that the book says only males have it.

So he says soothingly, "You can't be a bleeder. You're female," and disregards the analysis. Or he raises an eyebrow, checks the clotting time of my blood, which is often deceptively normal, and then does his disregarding on a scientific basis.

How can I, who am not a doctor, tell him that I'm no book-type "classic" hemophiliac, but a PTA, and that my trouble affects both sexes? Unless he spends too much time on highly specialized articles by hematologists—blood specialist—he never heard of PTA standing for anything but Parent-Teachers Association. It's no reproach. Surgeons and general practitioners can't be experts on everything, and are often well advised to let patients' wild tales go in one ear and out the other.

Only this tale isn't wild, as several doctors have found to their sorrow and mine. Long ago, before modern ways of coping with the condition were known, I almost died of inexplicable hemorrhages following the simplest kind of gynecological operation. My surgeon, a famous doctor and an utter lamb, was frantic with bewilderment and frustration. I have equally ruined the peace of mind of dental surgeons after tooth-pullings, and once kept our family doctor up all night because of uncontrollable bleeding from a small internal nose operation.

Yet—here is the treacherous part—in between and since, I have had teeth out and serious surgery

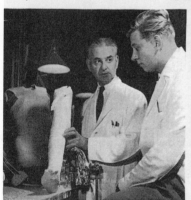

Dr. Henry Jordan and orthopedist Paul Schumacher discuss the cast of a hemophiliac's leg prior to making a brace.

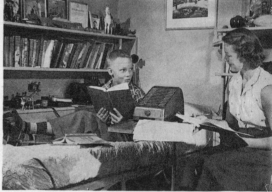

A traveling teacher, Mrs. Bette Manarel, instructs Lee Henry, a hemophiliac, in his Syosset, Long Island, home. Lee also has a microphone and receiver hookup with a schoolroom.

FIGURE 3.1. "I've Got the Lonesomest Disease!" *Saturday Evening Post*, 1953. *Source*: Helen Furnas, "I've Got the Lonesomest Disease!" *Saturday Evening Post*, 226 (November 21, 1953): 24. Reprinted with permission of The Saturday Evening Post Society, Inc. (© SEPS licensed by Curtis Licensing, Indianapolis, IN. All rights reserved).

First described in early 1953 as "plasma thromboplastin antecedent (PTA) deficiency," factor XI deficiency manifested as a mild-to-moderate case of classical hemophilia. Nosebleeds and bruising were common among the handful of known patients, and some female victims experienced prolonged bleeding during menstruation or following childbirth.[2] These patients lacked the debilitating joint bleeds that were so common in severe hemophilia, but their condition was far from innocuous because trauma or surgery could lead to a life-threatening bleed.

Before the discovery of PTA deficiency, hematologists were content to identify patients such as Furnas quite simply as "bleeders." The meaning of the hematologist's technological ethos for *female* and *male* bleeders in postwar America stands out today because the 1950s were a pivotal decade in the making of the world of modern hemophilia management. The spirit of progress associated with this era is readily apparent in Furnas's account and indicates how laboratory and clinical research on blood clotting was beginning to make a discernible difference in the way bleeder patients experienced both modern medicine and society. In fact, the title of Furnas's essay pointed astutely to the tension between the loneliness experienced by bleeder patients in the mid-twentieth century and the way hematologists—bolstered by transfusion medicine and the recent discoveries by blood coagulation researchers—could help combat the estrangement occasioned by any serious bleeding disorder. Postwar hematologists envisioned the promise of their specialty in their capacity to help patients and families achieve some normalcy in their lives. They believed that their expertise and technologies could help bleeder patients cope with a risky world and better integrate themselves as productive members of society.

In short, Furnas's perspective on this emerging world was unique as well as representative. Her identity as a female "hemophiliac" was marginal in the sense that her gender, sex, and age put her at the periphery of an emergent treatment community that focused largely on a male pediatric population. Yet, as Furnas herself acknowledged the sickly boys and young men with classical hemophilia had greater need than she and other female bleeders did. The title "I've Got the Lonesomest Disease!" thus had a double meaning. On the one hand, it emphasized the loneliness experienced by the young boys who suffered from the severest of all bleeding disorders (classical hemophilia); on the other hand, it highlighted Furnas's marginal status within an emerging hemophilia community that often did not provide equal recognition or treatment for bona-fide female bleeders like her. Both meanings reflect attitudes that were instrumental to the social and medical governance of the hemophiliac's world in the second half of the twentieth century.

The Rule of Linking Hemophilia to Sex

Throughout most of the past century, hematologists and geneticists endorsed the idea that hemophilia was predominantly a male bleeding disorder. Though "endorse" may seem too overtly conscious, I use it advisedly—hereditary experts such as William Bulloch and Paul Fildes put considerable work into making the statement that "only males get hemophilia" ring true. As detailed in chapter 1, these eugenicists reviewed more than nine hundred sources and compiled more than six hundred pedigrees for Karl Pearson's *Treasury of Human Inheritance* in 1911.[3] On one level, they were scientists devoted to objective interpretation of the data. The extant medical literature on hemophilia contained a significant number of female cases, but none fit neatly with the dominant portrait of the malady. On another level, however, these heredity experts were actively promoting the idea that physicians should be suspicious of any attempt to identify congenital or hereditary bleeding in a female patient as true hemophilia. Bulloch and Fildes were neither the first nor the last authorities to recommend that sex be used as a cardinal criteria for distinguishing hemophilia from other forms of bleeding.[4] This investment in maintaining a link between hemophilia and sex had profound implications for how both experts and the public would treat people with bleeding disorders in the twentieth century.

Together with the rise of Mendelianism and the discovery of sex-linked inheritance in the early twentieth century, this influential study by Bulloch and Fildes established a hereditarian orthodoxy with respect to hemophilia, one that called on physicians to limit application of the diagnosis almost exclusively to males (fig. 3.2).[5] There is little in the medical literature of the 1920s or 1930s to suggest that hematologists were actively questioning the axiom that only males had hemophilia or that they worried much about how to define hemophilia when they discovered cases of unusual bleeding in their female patients. Geneticists—few of whom had medical training—agreed in characterizing hemophilia as a sex-linked disorder. Hematologists assumed that sex linkage was a general rule to be enforced until there

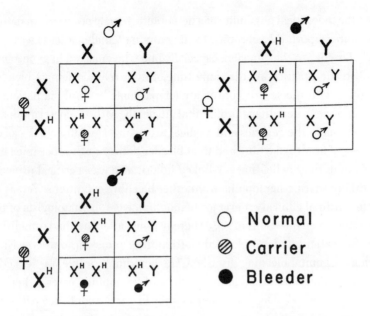

FIGURE 3.2. Mendelian Sex-Linked Inheritance of Hemophilia, 1955 Illustration. Geneticists began using hemophilia's characteristic transmission from unaffected women to their sons to illustrate the principles sex-linked Mendelian inheritance by the 1920s. By the 1950s, hematologists such as Theodore Spaet continued to educate physicians about genetics even as they sought to promote state-of-the-art hemophilia care. As shown in the mating at the bottom-left of the figure, there was a 25 percent chance that the crossing of a male "bleeder" (X^HY) and a female "carrier" (X^HX) would produce a "female bleeder" (X^HX^H). The "H" represents the hemophilia gene. *Source*: Theodore Spaet, "Recent Progress in the Study of Hemophilia," *Stanford Medical Bulletin* 13 (February 1955): 26.

was clear evidence against it. Most other learned physicians followed the lead of the geneticists and hematologists by reserving the hemophilia diagnosis for male patients with congenital bleeding. Paul Clough of the Johns Hopkins Medical School said in 1929 that the disease "is (practically) limited to males."[6]

Clinical hematologists in the 1920s and 1930s endorsed hemophilia's status as a sex-linked disease more out of convention than a conviction that females could not have the disorder. Hematologists had ample justification for this attitude. The classic model of Mendelian sex-linked inheritance left open the theoretical possibility of a hemophilic female occurring in nature. But more importantly, chronic bleeding among female patients was relatively familiar to the clinician, especially one who engaged in gynecologic or obstetric practice. At the same time, only rarely did female bleeders manifest with the severity of the archetypal male hemophilia patient or exhibit a clear hereditary profile that fit neatly with the descriptions of hemophilia in the genetics and medical textbooks. Hematologists—as the arbiters of how to diagnose and treat bleeder patients—thus became fairly uniform in their belief that sex-linked inheritance was a critical principle for differentiating hemophilia from other bleeding conditions. Yet, as far as the cardinal clinical criteria for hemophilia went, hematologists of this era entertained questions of sex or heredity only after they had established that the patient had a prolonged clotting time and symptoms consistent with a congenital bleeding disorder.[7] The hereditary profile was less critical, particularly because a large minority of hemophilia cases either was unprecedented (*de novo*) or lacked a family history to confirm a pattern of inheritance.

Yet, there were dissenters outside of hematology. In 1937, for example, University of Illinois hematologist Carroll Birch explained that a significant number of physicians were still employing the word "hemophilia" as a synonym for congenital bleeding. "Whether or not a female may have hemophilia depends largely upon one's concept of the disease. To some, all who bleed are 'bleeders' and all 'bleeders' are hemophiliacs. Especially in textbooks of gynecology, hemophilia is usually listed as one of the causes of uterine bleeding."[8] By linking hemophilia to sex, Birch was expressing something more than the hematologist's usual claim to authority over matters of bleeding.

Carroll LaFleur Birch (1895–1969) agreed with the hereditarian orthodoxy that characterized hemophilia as a "recessive, sex-linked character," but she was also a leading advocate in the United States for saying that hemophilia might best be characterized as a "sex-limited disease" (i.e., as occurring only in males due to nongenetic factors). Biological sex, she theorized in 1931, potentially held the key to controlling hemophilic bleeding, but not through the mechanisms of sex-linked heredity. Her theory built upon the idea that female transmitters of hemophilia were immune to the disease: "Hemophilia is limited to the male sex while it is transmitted through the unaffected female. Hence she must potentially have the disease. There are two possibilities. Is the disease manifest only in the presence of the male sex organs or are its symptoms held in abeyance in the presence of the female sex organs?"[9] More importantly, in arguing that hemophilia may be sex limited, Birch posited a relationship between sex hormones and the control of blood clotting. As one British hematologist later described Birch's thesis, "Women don't get hemophilia; therefore, if you feminize a male by means of a sex hormone, he will stop having hemophilia."[10]

Carroll Birch was among the first American physicians to specialize in the problem of hemophilia in the twentieth century, and she was unique for being the first female physician in the United States to gain an international reputation for this work. She earned her M.D. in 1925, graduating first in her class from the University of Illinois College of Medicine. Following her residency year, Birch accepted an instructor's position at the college to teach general medicine to undergraduates where she also began a career as an active clinical investigator in the university's Research and Education Hospital. In 1928 she established a division of hematology within the college's Department of Medicine and received an eight-bed ward at the hospital for hematological cases. Birch's goal, in part, was to establish herself as an academic specialist in hematology by conducting a formal study of hemophilia. In the spring of 1931, Birch reported some success alleviating bleeding in two brothers using material extracted from human ovaries. The college promoted Birch to assistant professor of medicine that year on the basis of her promising research. As reported by the Associated Press, "medical school authorities" regarded her recent hemophilia discoveries "as a distinct advance in physiological chemistry."[11]

The professional and media attention that Birch received focused initially on her early success in using ovarian extract to control the bleeding of two "high-grade hemophiliacs." Even before her first paper appeared, the Associated Press identified Birch's patients as brothers from a "family of hemophiliacs in Southern Illinois." She told the AP reporter that an "injection of the extract on one of them resulted in no symptoms of the disease for eleven months." The older brother, whose hemophilia was more severe, reportedly had no bleeding for five and half months after a transplant of the ovarian extract to his abdominal wall. Birch's use of ovarian extract to treat hemophilia was not entirely novel; she got the idea from reading a 1904 paper by a Dr. Grant in London.[12] Her colleague, surgeon Henry Bascom

Thomas, then proposed the transplant option and performed the actual operation. But it was Birch's sustained research program—based on the idea that sex hormones might hold the key to controlling hemophilia—that garnered most of the attention.

In July 1931 Birch published her preliminary data in the *Journal of the American Medical Association*. She had tested the urine of five of her (male) hemophilia patients, and all of them appeared to have lower than normal levels of the "female sex hormone." The result confirmed Birch's belief that "there must be something in the female organism which holds the disease in abeyance."[13] By the end of 1932, Birch reported the full results of her experimental hormone treatments to the *Journal of the American Medical Association*. Nineteen of the hemophilia patients she had treated with ovarian extract had a "good response," while nine others had shown "definite but less marked improvement." Birch maintained that the hormone treatments had lowered the number and severity of her patients' bleeding episodes and could even shorten clotting times. Nevertheless, she remained cautious. Even if the administration of female sex hormones could help control hemophilic bleeding, Birch insisted that ovarian extract treatments were no substitute for a blood transfusion.[14]

Although there was a good deal of enthusiasm for Birch's findings in the early 1930s, subsequent study of her sex hormone thesis failed to confirm her claims that ovarian extract reduced the frequency or severity of bleeding episodes in hemophilia patients.[15] As Birch concluded in 1937, some "hemophiliacs were improved by . . . ovarian extract while others showed no alteration in symptoms or laboratory findings." Moreover, Birch's hypothesis ran against the grain of existing knowledge of female biology. "If the presence of the female hormone inhibits or reduces the symptoms of hemophilia, then we might expect the [female] transmitters to show symptoms [of bleeding] after menopause;" yet, as Birch admitted, the incidence of postmenopausal bleeding in these women was no greater than any other group chosen at random.[16]

Even though Birch's work on sex hormones did not end as hoped, she maintained a strong interest in hemophilia's characterization as a "sex-limited disorder" through the 1930s. Between 1926 and 1935, Birch examined ninety-eight different male hemophilia patients, many of them regularly over that period (two patients for all nine years; thirty-seven for two years or more). None of her bleeder patients were female. However, in conducting extensive family histories of her male patients, Birch "inquired especially for a history of bleeding in female [family] members." She found twenty-five cases of female bleeders among the seventy-five families included in her pedigrees. In each and every case of female bleeding that Birch found, her retrospective diagnosis of the available health histories and clinical criteria fell short of true hemophilia.[17]

Birch published her decade's worth of clinical findings in *Hemophilia: Clinical and Genetic Aspects* (1937), one of the first American monographs devoted exclusively to hemophilia. Her book aimed to clarify the diverse features of hemophilia for any physician or dentist who might encounter a patient with intractable bleeding. In this sense, Birch's study had a prescriptive as well as descriptive dimension to it. Birch did not rule out the possibility of hemophilia in females or draw any conclusions about the question of hemophilia in the female sex. She was not trained in genetics, which made her presentation of the hereditary aspects of hemophilia idiosyncratic and a little dated to those who were. Still, Birch's assumptions and conclusions were entirely consistent with contemporary, Mendelian classifications of hemophilia as a sex-linked recessive trait as well as Bulloch and Fildes's hereditarian definition of hemophilia as "an *inherited* tendency in *males* to *bleed*."[18] Her hypothesis that sex hormones or other nonhereditary factors might play a critical role in the expression of hemophilic bleeding merely suggested that the disease might *also* be characterized as "sex limited." *Hemophilia: Clinical and Genetic Aspects* thus gave additional weight to the evolving sciences of human heredity that affirmed the rule of linking hemophilia to sex.[19]

During the 1940s, a history of sex-linked inheritance remained a critical rule by which the clinician could identify hemophilia in his patients and distinguish it from other forms of bleeding. The principles of Mendelian genetics now provided the rationale for linking observations about the relative incidence of hereditary bleeding among males and females to a truly causal explanation for the pathologies evident in the hemophilia pedigrees of scientists such as Bulloch and Fildes (1911) and Birch (1937). Consequently, if one was to speak of hemophilia scientifically—to be within the bounds of truthful discourse regarding this pathology—one had to give credence to the fact that biological sex was an essential aspect of hemophilia's identity. For all practical purposes, medical science defined hemophilia as a disease of the male sex in the first half of the twentieth century.[20]

Despite the consensus on a practical definition of hemophilia, there was still considerable speculation in the 1920s and 1930s as to whether "true" sex-linked hemophilia could occur in a female (fig. 3.2). As hematologist Paul Clough explained in *Diseases of the Blood* (1929), the theoretical possibility that the "union of a hemophilic male and a female conductor" could produce a female hemophiliac certainly exists, but "the chance of this happening accidentally is very small, and no authentic case of hemophilia in a female is on record."[21] There were occasional reports in the medical literature of a female experiencing severe bleeding. These cases were all questionable hemophilia, and none met the Mendelian requirement of being a female offspring of a male hemophiliac (X^HY) and a female carrier (X^HX). A few scientists theorized that the X^HX^H combination was lethal.[22] Others, such as Birch, suggested the X^HX^H genotype might exist but not manifest as a bleeding tendency because of nonhereditary factors. This debate about the X^HX^H genotype would not be settled until two key discoveries in the early 1950s. In the first, pathologists Kenneth Brinkhous and John Graham bred hemophilic dogs at the University of North Carolina to determine the practical consequences of a mating between a male hemophiliac and a female carrier. The beauty of the laboratory had always been its capacity for creating conditions that were improbable in the everyday world, and the new availability of hemophilic dogs allowed Graham and Brinkhous to breed female dogs with hemophilia in 1949 and thereby demonstrate the viability of this "theoretical genotype."[23] A little over a year later, British investigators resolved the debate for good when they confirmed the "nigh impossible" X^HX^H genotype in a clinical setting by discovering the cases of two female patients with classical hemophilia (factor VIII deficiency).[24]

Not until the discovery of PTA deficiency in 1953 did the rule of linking a hemophilia diagnosis to the male sex receive its first serious challenge. This disorder, an apparently mild form of hereditary bleeding, appeared in females as well as males. Recall that Helen Furnas was newly anointed as PTA deficient when she penned "I've Got the Lonesomest Disease!" for the *Saturday Evening Post*. Robert Rosenthal of Brooklyn's Beth Israel Hospital first discovered the "slight to moderate" bleeding tendency that he called PTA deficiency in "two sisters and their maternal uncle." In publishing his case reports, he enrolled the help of Herman Dreskin at Cincinnati's Jewish Hospital and his father, Nathan Rosenthal, a distinguished hematologist at New York City's Mount Sinai Hospital. Rosenthal's group demonstrated that the clotting factor deficiency responsible for this atypical form of hereditary hemophilic bleeding was previously unknown.[25] By 1956 Robert Rosenthal had completed extensive studies demonstrating that PTA deficiency was very similar to a mild case of classical hemophilia; only the clotting factor involved and the inheritance pattern differed. He characterized this new form of "hemophilia" as an autosomal dominant trait on the basis of its equal appearance among his female and male patients.[26]

Today's factor XI deficiency, or hemophilia C, was largely captured in Rosenthal's original findings, and while the condition is exceedingly rare (with an estimated incidence of 1 in 100,000 births in the United States), it is known to be more prevalent among Ashkenazi Jews than other groups. As much as 9 percent of the Ashkenazi Jewish population is a heterozygote carrier of the disorder, making it one of the most common genetic disorders in Israel.[27] It thus seems that geography, demographics, and other nonbiological factors can significantly impact how this "rarest" form of hemophilia is perceived and treated. After all, if the current epidemiological data are correct, cases of hemophilia C (factor XI deficiency)—whether female or male—are hardly marginal to medical practice where Jewish people of Ashkenazi descent are concentrated.

Thus, there was a time in the 1950s when blood coagulation researchers unwittingly found themselves questioning the rule of defining hereditary hemophilia as wholly sex linked. This unusual moment in the history of hemophilia reflected the new opportunities and resources available to hematologists after the Second World War. Many of the new cases of bleeding disorders closely resembled classical hemophilia in the male but differed in important and often confusing ways. Hematologists in the 1950s occasionally found themselves in the uncomfortable position of having to decide whether to endorse the rule of sex linkage that medical science had overwhelmingly embraced for more than a century. It became a problem that hematologists—for the sake of their specialty as well as their patients—could hardly ignore.

Engendering Beneficial Diagnoses in the Golden Era

The conditions that made it possible for 1950s-era hematologists to wonder whether they should confine their diagnoses of hemophilia to the male sex were undoubtedly related to the technological innovation that was so characteristic of the decade after World War II. Above all, the postwar hematologist's technological way of looking at blood plasma allowed clinicians to manage female as well as male bleeder patients in new, increasingly powerful ways. In the early 1950s, a combination of recent insights and new laboratory assays made it possible for hematologists to identify a growing number of clotting factor deficiencies among their bleeder patients—some of whom were women. PTA Deficiency was among the new finds. Yet, there was no one technology or class of technologies that entirely explains how this innovative era of blood coagulation research provided hemophilia management with its scientific rationale in the pivotal years between 1947 and 1964. Rather, it was the technological redescription of congenital bleeding in the era that prompted participants to later christen this innovative era the "golden age of blood coagulation research."[28] If innovation temporarily brought into question existing rules like "only males get hemophilia," it also gave experimental hematologists an unparalleled opportunity to transform how doctors managed bleeding patients of both sexes.

Serious questions about how to define hemophilia and other bleeding disorders initially arose in the early 1950s as hematologists in North America and Europe fully explored the insights of clotting science in the years immediately preceding and following World War II. This exploration often involved the introduction of new kinds of blood clotting assays that proved capable of measuring the activity of an array of different plasma factors involved in the blood samples of their bleeder patients. The most important of these clotting tests was the thromboplastin generation test introduced in 1953 by Oxford University hematologists Robert Gwyn Macfarlane, Rosemary Biggs, and Stuart Douglas and the partial thromboplastin time (or PTT) developed in the same era by University of North Carolina pathologists Robert Langdell, Robert Wagner, and Kenneth Brinkhous.[29] Each of these tests was a means for measuring the amount of time necessary to produce thrombin, a necessary precursor for forming clots. Unlike the prothrombin time assays of the 1930s, these new assays had the capacity to identify plasma coagulation factors in the absence of tissue thromboplastin (which allowed the hematologists using them to localize clotting factors that were hitherto obscure). Use of these laboratory assays in the 1950s greatly facilitated the biochemical isolation of clotting factors VIII and IX, which are now identified as the specific plasma factors that are deficient in patients with hemophilia A and B, respectively. The Oxford test achieved wide use in Britain and the Commonwealth for a time, whereas the PTT became a standard fixture of clinical and experimental laboratories in the United States. The PTT was the simpler procedure, a one-step technique, whereas Oxford's thromboplastin generation test involved a two-step procedure. Along with Quick's one-stage prothrombin consumption test (the PT), a modified form of the PTT would emerge by the 1970s as a standard screening tools for detecting bleeding disorders in clinics throughout the world.[30]

The new assays were only part of the reason that hematologists were seeing novel differences among their bleeder patients and witnessing a proliferation of bleeding disorders in the 1950s. For instance, Rosenthal discovered PTA deficiency without the aid of such novel blood assays. More critical to innovation than the more sensitive assays that leading experimentalists were introducing in the 1950s was the conceptualization of blood plasma (as opposed to whole blood) as an innovative site for treatment as well as clinical differentiation. As told in chapter 2, the latter movement effectively began in the preceding half century when hematologists and chemists rendered blood plasma into a substance whose components could be measured, manipulated, and even engineered. The new "thromboplastic" laboratory assays of the 1950s were therefore a potent refinement of an older desire to transform blood from a mysterious, obscure fluid into a malleable and increasingly perspicuous substance; they fulfilled the 1930s-era promise that blood clotting experts would one day have a quantitative measurement for visualizing all the qualitative (i.e., functional) differences in the blood plasma of their bleeder patients.

Thus, when Harvard researchers Arthur Patek and Richard Stetson reported in 1936 that a crude fraction of normal plasma could correct the abnormal clotting time in hemophilic plasma—both in test tubes and in patients—hemophilia research took on new importance in the rapidly advancing field of hematology. Although Patek and biochemist F. H. Laskey Taylor could not determine what specific "globulin substance" in the plasma fraction was responsible for the correction, their experiments reportedly demonstrated that a plasma factor found in normal plasma was functionally deficient in hemophilic plasma. Definitive understanding of the plasma defect in classical hemophilia took a decade to emerge, but these studies at Harvard were enough to suggest that plasma, rather than blood platelets, was the actual site of the defect in hemophilic blood. By localizing the defect to plasma, the Harvard studies also framed fresh plasma transfusions as a more precise treatment for hemophilia than whole blood transfusions.[31] Then, with the introduction of blood banking in 1938, support for the platelet hypothesis dwindled rapidly as blood and plasma transfusions became readily available treatments for hemophilia patients throughout the United States. By the early 1940s, clotting researchers were principally arguing about whether the prolonged clotting times were due to a deficiency in some plasma clotting factor or due to some inhibitory substance in the plasma (i.e., antithrombin). But it was clearly all about the plasma.

The development of plasma fractionation during the war years (1941–45) dramatically embodied the American effort to better understand blood plasma and capitalize on its therapeutic uses. Plasma fractionation is a biochemical processing technique designed to take blood plasma—that is, blood without its red cells—and separate it (with the aid of centrifugal force and ethyl alcohol) into its functional components. Harvard biochemist Edwin J. Cohn was the dominant personality behind the U.S. Navy-funded effort to fractionate plasma, a massive project during World War II that involved researchers at Harvard, Columbia, Wisconsin, and Stanford as well as several pharmaceutical firms.[32] Cohn's process divided blood plasma into five major groups or fractions. The first of these, Cohn fraction I, was rich in fibrinogen and other serum proteins (globulins) that facilitated clotting.[33] In fact, the technique yielded more than a dozen therapeutic products—including albumin for the treatment of shock and renal disease (fraction V) and gamma globulins for passive immunizations against measles and variety of other communicable diseases (fractions II and III).[34] Cohn began patenting his plasma fractionation projects during the war years. He and his associates also promoted the therapeutic properties of plasma fractions—aka "blood derivatives"—widely at the war's end.[35] Cohn's patent efforts were controversial in the 1940s because Harvard and many other universities barred their researchers from patenting their therapeutic discoveries. Yet as historian Angela Creager has revealed, Cohn and his allies argued persuasively that patents on plasma fractions by not-for-profit actors were necessary not only to ensure quality control but also to protect the public from mercenary interests. On these terms, Cohn continued to collaborate with companies like Armour Laboratories and Sharp and Dohme in the late 1940s as the pharmaceutical industry explored the profit potential of marketing therapeutic plasma fractions.[36]

While it would be more than two decades before plasma fractions for the treatment of hemophilia would be a profitable enterprise for pharmaceutical companies, the significance of plasma fractionation for hemophilia research was already apparent in the immediate postwar period. During the 1940s, the hemophilia research of George Minot, Laskey Taylor, and others at Harvard revolved around testing the procoagulant properties of Cohn fraction I on patients with classic hemophilia.[37] In the late 1940s, pharmaceutical firms such as Squibb and Armour were also producing Cohn fraction I for use by hemophilia researchers throughout the United States. Because fraction I was rich in procoagulant proteins (later called clotting factors), it became an important tool in the hemophilia researcher's attempts to determine why clotting in hemophilic blood was delayed. It also benefited the few lucky patients whose clinicians had access to this research tool. But more generally, the very existence of Cohn fraction I gave hope to researchers that they would soon understand the plasma factors involved in hemophilic bleeding and that an even more potent plasma fraction might be developed to normalize the specific clotting defect found in hemophiliacs and other bleeder patients.

There were nevertheless significant problems with Cohn fraction I. While it sometimes seemed miraculous in its ability to stop hemophilic bleeding, other times it proved no better than fresh plasma at controlling hemophilic bleeds, and occasionally it did not work at all. No one knew exactly why in the 1940s. But hemophilia researchers could nevertheless see the future in an innovation that demonstrated the potential for developing a potent plasma fraction that the pharmaceutical industry might one day produce for widespread use among hemophilia patients.

For blood clotting scientists, a more tantalizing finding for the treatment of both female and male bleeders came from the wartime research of Paul Owren, a hospital physician in Oslo during the German occupation of Norway. In 1943 he was called upon to treat Mary, a twenty-nine-year-old woman with a lifelong but obscure bleeding condition that had partially blinded her in her first bleeding episode at age three. Mary's prothrombin time did not behave as expected when Owren assayed it using Quick's prothrombin time test. The theory behind Quick's test held that prothrombin conversion rate was proportional to the amount of normal plasma. Owren reasoned that Quick's test was not actually specific for prothrombin. He then removed all the prothrombin from a sample of normal plasma (using an asbestos sterilization filter offered by a bacteriologist colleague). On adding this prothrombin-free plasma to Mary's blood he was pleased to see that it normalized Mary's prothrombin time. This result not only accelerated prothrombin conversion in Mary's blood but suggested that there was some procoagulant factor in normal plasma beyond the four factors described in Morawitz's classic theory of blood coagulation (i.e., fibrinogen, calcium ions, prothrombin, and tissue thromboplastin).

Mary's presentation did not meet the requirements of classical hemophilia: she was female, and there was no evidence initially that her condition was hereditary (though a family history of bleeding was later discovered). Owren therefore called the patient's bleeding disorder *parahaemophilia* and the plasma component she lacked *factor V*. Owren actually had to wait until the end of the war to determine the full significance of his findings. The isolation imposed by the German occupation meant that he was not wholly familiar with the existing science on these matters. In 1946 he therefore traveled to the Lister Institute in London and, reading the relevant literature for the first time, discovered that his case and research were unique. He published his results in English a year later and shocked the hematology establishment with the first conclusive evidence that more clotting factors existed in the plasma than were accounted for by Morawitz's well-studied theory.[38] Hemophilia experts, on the other hand, found little in Owren's discovery of parahaemophilia (factor V deficiency) to perturb their understanding of hemophilia, as Owren's findings hardly seemed to relate to the "hereditary tendency of males to bleed."

A more ambiguous but potentially ground-breaking wartime discovery in the science of hemophilia and clotting factors was that of Alfredo Pavlovsky, an Argentinean hematologist working with a large population of hemophilia patients in Buenos Aires. Pavlovsky and two colleagues were studying what proportions of normal plasma were capable of correcting the delayed clotting time in hemophilic blood when they unexpectedly discovered that plasma drawn from a hemophilia patient "with a greatly prolonged clotting time (1 hr. 20 mins.)" corrected the abnormal clotting time of the plasma from another patient "with a much shorter clotting time (40 mins.)." Pavlovsky also reported that plasma transfused from this hemophilia patient with the longest clotting time shortened the clotting time of eight other patients as if the recipients had been infused with normal plasma. For Pavlovsky, these were "paradoxical" findings that argued against the existence of a specific clotting factor (or globulin) for hemophilia—the theory then being most prominently advanced at Harvard by Patek, Taylor, Minot, and others.[39] Although the true significance of Pavlovsky's findings would not be fully appreciated until the early 1950s (in part because Pavlovsky insisted that hemophilia was due to an inhibitor rather than a clotting factor deficiency), investigators who sought to replicate his findings soon discovered that occasionally the blood of hemophilia patients was mutually corrective when mixed in vitro. In other words, this phenomenon suggested to some clotting experts that there could be more than one kind of hemophilia, even among males with the classic presentation.

These wartime studies provided postwar blood coagulation researchers in North America and Europe with incentives to engage in the study of hemophilia and other bleeding disorders, and even to interrogate female cases of bleeding more closely. Since the mid-1930s, researchers had largely assumed that there was only one plasma defect responsible for all cases of hemophilia, an assumption reinforced by the seeming effectiveness of Cohn fraction I. For adherents of the new theory that hemophilia was due to a deficiency of a clotting factor, the findings of Owren and Pavlovsky suggested that there were probably one or two plasma clotting factors still waiting positive identification, possibly many more, and that these unknown factors might appear in any case of a suspected bleeding disorder, including among patients who were previously categorized as classical hemophiliacs. An international race among experimental hematologists ensued.

Now that experimental hematologists more readily conceptualized their bleeder cases in terms of plasma factors, they were looking at these patients in a relatively novel, and certainly more focused, way. In fact, in the Anglophone world, investigators who worked with bleeder patients and their blood plasma gave implicit recognition to the technological ethos driving their activities by referring to themselves informally as "coagulationists" or "clotters." Clotters viewed the bleeder patient technologically in the sense that their expanding array of laboratory tests allowed the investigator to characterize the patient's pathology in terms of faulty mechanisms. The patient's initial presentation—male, female, severity of the bleed, a family history of bleeding—was less important to their work than the means to identify and quantify specific clotting factors. The more creative clotters engineered new assays to test and explore their theories about normal and abnormal blood coagulation while demonstrating that laboratory tests could be used to differentiate bleeder cases whose symptoms were indistinguishable by standard clinical criteria.

The critical breakthrough year for hemophilia and blood coagulation research came in 1952, when three different research groups demonstrated the existence of hemophiliacs whose symptoms were identical to "classical hemophilia" but evidently did not have the predominant form of the disease because they had a different clotting defect (later called factor IX deficiency).[40] In April 1952 Paul Aggeler's research team in San Francisco published the case of a "16-year old Caucasian male" with clinical symptoms of hemophilia and a record of more than 100 hospitalizations for "major hemorrhagic episodes." What was unusual about the boy was that the prolonged clotting time of his blood could not be normalized by in vitro methods known to correct hemophilic blood (including Cohn fraction I, which was by then known to contain the antihemophilic factor or "globulin" missing in hemophilic plasma). However, normal serum and plasma did correct the boy's clotting time. Using Pavlovsky's technique, the researchers also found that the child's blood and the blood of a typical hemophiliac were mutually corrective. This result helped clarify the importance of Pavlovsky's paradoxical wartime observation and pointed the San Francisco researchers to a definitive conclusion: there were at least two "hemophilias," each related to a discrete clotting factor deficiency in the blood plasma. Aggeler's accompanying laboratory investigation identified the factor missing in the boy's plasma as a "plasma thromboplastin component."[41]

After Aggeler's investigation, in August 1952 New York hematologist Irving Shulman reported a similar case in an eleven-month-old boy of Italian ethnicity. Shulman also differentiated the mechanisms of this boy's condition from classical hemophilia using Pavlovsky's technique, but he moreover noticed that the child's family had no history of bleeding. Shulman suggested the names *parahemophilia* or *pseudohemophilia* for nonhereditary bleeding that could be corrected by hemophilic plasma.[42]

Then, in December 1952 a group of British hematologists headed by Oxford's Rosemary Biggs and Robert Macfarlane identified seven additional cases of a hemophilia-like disorder that they recommended should not be classified as *true hemophilia*. The Oxford group identified these patients as different on seeing that their blood was mutually corrective of the majority of their hemophilia patients, but they also went farther than previous investigators by showing that "concentrated preparations of anti-haemophilic globulin are ineffective" in treating this new form of hemophilia.[43] Here, the Oxford Group was making a diagnosis on the basis of its patients' response to treatment—a now common way of defining a disease that was a relatively new phenomenon at the time.[44] Biggs and her colleagues decided to call this newly discovered disorder *Christmas disease*, and the plasma factor responsible for it, *Christmas factor*, after both the name of one of the patients (Stephen Christmas) and the timing of their publication (December 1952).[45]

Taken together, these three distinct groups of investigators effectively demonstrated that there were cases of bleeding among the hematologists' population of patients whose sex, symptoms, and family histories might indicate classical hemophilia but whose plasma could potentially tell a different story. Moreover, Owren's work had demonstrated that similar problems with clotting factors might be at work in the plasma of bleeders who did not meet the traditional requirements for *true hemophilia*. These cases thus initiated a controversy over the identity of hemophilia and other bleeder states. Christmas disease was only the beginning of a seemingly exponential increase in the number of bleeding disorders and clotting factors in the 1950s. Many clotters applied technical names to the disorders and biological factors they discovered; others chose to name the disorders and factors after the patients they had studied. At times, investigators lacked agreement on what entities they were actually studying or what to call them. In other words, as postwar hematologists subjected bleeder patients to their new disciplined perspectives and tools, their results raised numerous issues: questions about the traditional classifications, the best assays, appropriate treatment for different types of bleeding disorder, and so on. These uncertainties generated more studies and an increased need to scrutinize the blood of patients with bleeding disorders.[46]

Unfortunately, clotters were not always inclined to clarify their findings for nonspecialists. Indeed, as the atypical cases grew and the new findings proliferated, most hematologists and certainly most physicians grew troubled by what they saw in the medical literature on blood coagulation and bleeding disorders. The vast majority of medical practitioners could hardly begin to make sense of the growing incidence of atypical "hemophilia-like" conditions that clotting specialists had discovered by the mid-1950s. Hemophilic bleeding among female patients was only one among many sources of misunderstanding.

From a Hematological "Tower of Babel" to the Promised Land

Informally known as clotters, the blood clotting researchers who frequently uncovered atypical cases of bleeding in males and females during the 1950s oftentimes seemed more interested in complicating diagnostic practice than in simplifying things for clinicians; or, as one medical editorial put it, "those engaged in [blood clotting research] have been more interested in the problem for its own sake than in practical application."[47] The traditional axiom that said "only males get hemophilia" was among the clinical truisms that clotters seemed increasingly willing to jettison in their interest to clarify the mechanisms of normal and pathological clotting for themselves. By 1955 clotters were even going so far as to tell physicians that the classical clinical criteria for hemophilia were no longer sufficient for a diagnosis; only expert knowledge of blood coagulation was.[48] Here, clotters were not only asserting that diagnostic expertise was as much a function of laboratory insight as clinical training but behaving as if they alone had the skills required to achieve a definitive diagnosis. "Although it may sometimes require clinical skill and judgment to suspect hemophilia," argued Stanford University hematologist Theodore Spaet in 1955, "the diagnosis can be established with certainty only by modern laboratory methods."[49] In effect, the medical profession was being told that blood clotting science held the key to understanding hemophilia and related bleeding disorders. And for clinicians who were uncomfortable with the new clotting science and its technologies, there was little choice but to turn to a clotting expert to achieve the correct diagnosis for their bleeder patient.

This tension between clotters and clinicians fully surfaced in the medical literature in 1954. Early that year, the editorial office for the American hematology journal *Blood* received a manuscript from Paul Aggeler's coagulation research group in San Francisco. This paper described the "hemophilia-like disease," called plasma thromboplastin component (PTC) deficiency, which Aggeler's group had first described in 1952.[50] According to William Dameshek, the executive editor of *Blood*, this manuscript was "the trigger mechanism" that led him to enlist "aid from a number of authorities in the field of coagulation."[51] Aggeler's paper became an occasion, in other words, for coagulation specialists to clarify the fundamental nature of hemophilia in a published symposium. Such clarification seemed necessary to Dameshek because hematologists were being overwhelmed by the growing literature on blood coagulation. Between 1949 and 1954, at least four hundred articles were published each year on blood coagulation, and that literature was confusing to many clinical hematologists in its diversity, style, and substance.[52]

In introducing *Blood*'s March 1954 symposium on hemophilia, Dameshek noted that medical understandings of hemophilia had become increasingly ambiguous since World War II. "Until recently, hemophilia was easily defined and readily recognized," he said. "However, in the last few years, various active workers in the field [of blood coagulation] have unearthed new facts, developed new hypotheses, and have even had the temerity to claim that hemophilia may not actually be what it seems!" Of all hematologists, claimed Dameshek, "probably the most highly specialized is the coagulationist, one of the few subtypes [within hematology] whose members like to band together at certain meetings, if only to disagree." Dameshek then pointed beyond these "most highly specialized" blood experts to describe the majority of hematologists "who struggle as best they can through the intricacies of the coagulation factors, old, new, hypothetic, and synonymous," for they "have become confused and have begun to wonder 'What actually *is* Hemophilia?'"[53]

Hemophilia still had a relatively uniform appearance to clotters between 1937 and 1946. Although the nature of that defect was contested, most of these experimental hematologists reasoned that they were looking for a single functional anomaly in the blood plasma. By 1953, lab-based discoveries of atypical bleeding disorders that either were clinically indistinguishable from "classical hemophilia" or closely resembled a mild to moderate form of the disease made the terrain surrounding hemophilia look very different.[54] The proliferation of bleeding disorders was so rapid that Dameshek opined in 1954 that the "hematologic rialto" now included "not only hemophilia, but pseudohemophilia, hemophilia-like disease, parahemophilia, deuterohemophilia, hemophilia A, B, C, hemophiliod disease A, B, C, Christmas disease, and the 'literature' knows what else!"[55] As physicians of all kinds turned to hematologists for help in negotiating their bleeder cases, hematologists in turn struggled to make sense of what the blood coagulation specialists were saying. As such, there was increasing pressure on the clotting experts to clarify their science for hematologists and clinicians alike.

Ironically, it was hemophilia's reputation as a "time honored and apparently well-stabilized disease" that engendered so much confusion among hematologists and other physicians in the 1950s.[56] Throughout the first half of the twentieth century, hematologists taught their fellow physicians that a "typical case of hemophilia offers no diagnostic difficulties."[57] They said that a clinical diagnosis of the disorder could be readily determined from the bleeding, sex, and heredity characteristics of the patient.[58] Many hematologists even assumed that they could confirm or deny the ambiguous diagnosis by employing a simple laboratory test known as the whole blood clotting time. That changed after 1952, as clotters introduced their colleagues in hematology to new assays for identifying hemophilia and other bleeding disorders, such as the partial thromboplastin time. The new assays, along with the prothrombin time, emerged as powerful diagnostic tests for hemophilia and other bleeding disorders. They gave order to the otherwise disorderly experience of bleeding by relating it to the moral economy of the clotter's laboratory—that is, its working concepts, technologies, resources, and findings. The clotter's world thus emerged as an important, but esoteric specialty in the 1950s. Yet, as clotters innovated, hematologists were increasingly asked to put this esoteric subspecialty into context for clinicians. By 1955 the need to clarify the state of blood coagulation science was becoming acute because the diversity of concepts, techniques, and findings that clotters had created since 1947 had the paradoxical effect of putting hemophilia's long-standing status as a stable clinical entity into question.

By 1954, hemophilia had clearly become a source of considerable controversy among clotters and a source of confusion among rank-and-file hematologists and other medical professionals. Obviously, Dameshek hoped that his 1954 symposium of clotters would generate some consensus on the question, What is hemophilia? Unfortunately, he found "no great uniformity in either the type of response received, nor in the writers' interpretations of the problem at hand." Some of the papers even raised the disturbing possibility that hemophilia might best be considered a bleeding "syndrome" rather than a specific nosological entity.[59] Despite every indication that the confusions ran deep and the "lines of communication [were] thin," Dameshek refused to acknowledge the dangers this situation posed for the specialty of hematology or for the patients labeled with any number of diseases.[60] He chose instead to dwell on the positive. "Out of confusion," he rather glibly concluded, "often comes new clarity."[61] On its surface, the clarity that Dameshek and other hematologists sought from these clotters in the 1950s was confirmation that they could identify and treat hemophilia patients and other patients with bleeding disorders in a uniform way. However, the character of discussion between these clotters was so contentious that physicians who were not clotting specialists were harboring deep anxieties about their ability to recognize and differentiate bleeding disorders accurately.

The traditional concept of hemophilia had become, at once, too wide and too narrow for it to be an unambiguous diagnostic guide to the rank-and-file hematologist in the United States, and for many clotting specialists a standardized nomenclature seemed the most efficient way to address the problem. Thus, in July of that year, New York hematologist Irving S. Wright attended the International Conference on Thrombosis and Embolisms in Basel, Switzerland, and gave an introductory address to a distinguished audience of clotters entitled "Chaos or Communication."[62] Wright described the "strange and irregular" history of blood coagulation studies and proposed that the central difficulty facing their community was not a strictly scientific problem but a practical problem of language. He noted that many laboratory scientists had "described the action of what they have considered to be new factors which contribute to this process, and unfortunately have given them names without knowledge or consideration of the work of others who preceded them." He noted that some clotting factors were known by as many as ten to fourteen different names, which was even "confusing to the experienced investigator." Wright concluded, "A scientific Tower of Babel has thus been erected. The situation appears discouraging, if not chaotic, to the physician who is not a specialist in the field, and even more so to the medical student."[63] Afterward, Wright's proposal to create a nomenclature committee was positively received, and the International Committee on Blood Clotting Factors was born.[64]

The enthusiasm with which his fellow hematologists greeted Wright's suggestion is as noteworthy as the ultimate outcome.[65] Clotters were very aware that their work was troubling for clinical hematologists. They knew that without some standardized way of talking about coagulation research and bleeding disorders, it would become even more difficult for frontline hematologists to identify who, among their bleeder patients, were actually hemophilia patients. In fact, on the basis of what clotters had already reported in the literature, it was possible for hematologists to exclude some who were previously identified as hemophilia patients and to include others who were traditionally excluded from a diagnosis of hemophilia. Among those patients whom some clotters now included among the ranks of the hemophilia patients were female bleeders such as Helen Furnas, whom hematologists would have systematically excluded from a hemophilia diagnosis before the first half of the twentieth century.

As for resolution of the tensions between clotting science and clinical practice, it took three years of contentious meetings on the issue before the committee met in Rome in 1957 and finally agreed upon a uniform nomenclature for the known blood clotting factors.[66] In recognition of the meeting's setting, the committee decided to endorse Fritz Koller's Roman numeral system for identifying the blood coagulation factors.[67] The nosologic categories for classical hemophilia and the other known bleeding disorders thus became rooted in a classification system whereby each clinical bleeding syndrome could be identified by the coagulation factor that was functionally absent in the patient's blood plasma. Classical hemophilia or hemophilia A became factor VIII deficiency. Hemophilia B (previously known as Aggeler's PTC deficiency and Oxford's Christmas disease) became factor IX deficiency. The committee was also charged with establishing standards for identifying each clotting factor and thus clarifying the mechanisms underlying distinct bleeding disorders that had long been indistinguishable because they manifested in the clinic in remarkably similar ways.

The question, What is hemophilia? was not a question that the nomenclature committee formally posed for itself. Nor was the question of whether a hemophilia diagnosis should be reserved to females. However, these questions were implicitly addressed when the committee forged its standardized language for identifying the clotting factors involved in the diagnosis of hemophilia and other bleeding disorders. Factor VIII and factor IX deficiencies shared a sex-linked inheritance pattern and manifested in more severe forms than other clotting factor deficiencies. Disabling joint bleeds, for instance, were seldom found outside of male patients with one of these two conditions. As such, it seemed only natural to call these two clotting factor deficiencies hemophilia because their features were all readily captured by the traditional concept of hemophilia that had evolved since the early nineteenth century. But many of the milder bleeder types, each associated with a different clotting factor deficiency, also varied in at least one important way from the traditional hemophilia concept as it was defined for most of the twentieth century. For instance, the rare bleeding disorder known by the late 1950s as Stuart-Prower factor deficiency (factor X deficiency) occasionally presented with the kind of nosebleeds and the joint bleeding that one would see in classic hemophilia, but the patients' blood exhibited a prolonged prothrombin time (unlike classical hemophilia).[68] Most importantly, except for factor VIII and factor IX deficiencies, all other hereditary bleeding disorders were autosomal conditions that manifested equally in males and females. To say that any bleeding disorder other than factor VIII or factor IX deficiency was a form of hemophilia was to disregard what many then saw as a long tradition of saying that hemophilia was an entirely sex-linked phenomenon.

What, then, did this committee of distinguished hematologists decide to do with Rosenthal's PTA deficiency and, by extension, patients like Helen Furnas? There was nothing definitive—beyond inheritance patterns and clotting assays—to distinguish cases of PTA deficiency from milder forms of classical hemophilia. Moreover, clotting assays did not by themselves necessitate that the hemophilia concept be reserved for only bleeding disorders with a demonstrated sex-linked inheritance pattern. After four more years of study and debate, the nomenclature committee voted to recognize PTA factor as a distinct procoagulant substance in the plasma and assigned a Roman numeral designation to it. Thus, in 1961, PTA deficiency became factor XI deficiency. The committee did not rule on whether it should be classed as a form of hemophilia. It left the decision up to individual hematologists to decide what to tell clinicians, their patients, and the public. Since the 1961 vote, some hematologists have counted factor XI deficiency as a third, atypical form of hemophilia (hemophilia C) because of its clinical similarities to milder forms of classical hemophilia. More frequently, medical and popular discussions of hemophilia have followed tradition and reserved the hemophilia label for the sex-linked clotting deficiencies (factors VIII and IX).

By the early 1960s, hemophilia was once again a stable, well-defined nosological entity within biomedical thought and practice. Hematologists could now identify hemophilia and its allied bleeding disorders in highly specific, biochemical terms; and they had developed a system—however faulty—for facilitating constructive exchanges in the clinic between physicians and a growing variety of bleeder patients. The clotters had also delivered on their promise to understand the mechanisms responsible for normal and pathological bleeding. In doing so, these experts affirmed the promise of hematological discipline to render hemophilia and other bleeding disorders into conditions that could be normalized. After all, it made sense for hematology to ally itself with the normative discourse of genetics and therefore solidify hematology's claims to be a science of the first order. In the first half of the twentieth century, the science of heredity played a constitutive role in elevating hemophilia into a popular object of study (as suggested by the legacy of Bulloch and Fildes). For most clotters, the principle of sex linkage seemed both historically and biologically essential to their notion of what hemophilia was—this despite their laboratory and clinical experiences in the 1950s.

The Bleeder's Turn to the Specialist, for Better or Worse

"I've Got the Lonesomest Disease!" appeared in the Thanksgiving week issue of the *Saturday Evening Post* in 1953 and signaled for readers how medical authority and recognition mattered for bleeders in the postwar United States. In fact, the editor's lede—like the feature's title—pointed readers to the central tension in Furnas's encounters with her physicians: "The author has to carry a physician's certificate in her handbag, to prove to strange doctors that she's really a 'bleeder' and not a neurotic female. Here's what is now being done for her and thousands of others who suffer from an ailment that can turn a minor cut into a major tragedy." The message was clear. Furnas was battling not only a bleeding disorder but a medical system that was often dismissive of female bleeders even as it was beginning to give much needed attention to hemophilic boys. On this account, the "physician's certificate in her handbag" played a critical role in Furnas's ability to gain proper medical care. Why exactly was her certification as a bleeder necessary? Furnas's sex was clearly an issue. Yet, in many respects, her situation was not radically different from that of the classic, male hemophiliac. The *Post* story indicates that the relationship between hematologists and their bleeder patients could be mutually beneficial in the postwar era but also suggests that this symbiosis was filled with its own dramas and dilemmas.

What did Furnas's designation as a "PTA-type hemophiliod" actually mean to her? First of all, it prompted her to publicize the emerging world of hemophilia management so that the public could see the medical and scientific factors that were beginning to affect persons diagnosed with classical hemophilia and similar bleeding disorders. The opening of Furnas's essay captured the productive moral economy that existed between patients with bleeding disorders and the specialists who studied them. Just as Iowa City's Jimmy Laughlin or Boston's Russell White did, Furnas learned that her status as a "hemophiliac" made her blood a precious commodity in the eyes of the experimental hematologist.

> The rarest version of one of the worlds' rarest ailments—I've got it.
> It seldom harms me and it just bores or annoys doctors, except a few earnest researchers exploring the mysteries of hemophilia and allied conditions. They can be counted on to take me big. While working on this article, I mentioned to one of them that I am a "PTA-type hemophiliod." He reacted like Julius Caesar when Cleopatra unrolled from that rug. His eyes gleamed, his hands clutched.
>
> "You don't get out of here alive," he said, "without leaving us a nice sample of your blood to work on." I was the second specimen of the breed he had ever seen.

Furnas was largely optimistic and cooperative when it came to the esoteric world of the blood researcher. "He got the blood," she reported: "The more science learns about these troubles the better for us 'bleeders.'" Furnas then related one of the standard arguments that the era's blood researchers often used in their grant applications: "Besides, exploration of our peculiarities promises new help for many others facing more common heart and blood ailments." She readily understood that hematologists wanted to explore her unusual pathology for clues about the intimate workings of bleeding and clotting.

Furnas also appreciated what better scientific understanding of hemophilia entailed for bleeders of all sexes, and this fueled her enthusiasm for hematology. Before receiving her diagnosis of PTA deficiency in 1953, she tried on several occasions to tell her caregivers that she was a "bleeder." But physicians and dentists often dismissed her efforts to warn them. Typically, they would say "soothingly, 'You can't be a bleeder. You're female.'" Furnas fared no better with those skeptical (but thorough) doctors who put her claim to the test. When checked in the lab, the clotting time of her blood was often deceptively normal. In other words, she was fighting an uphill battle. Most medical and dental professionals in the mid-twentieth century were men who had little to no contact with hemophilia patients over the course of their professional lives. What they knew about hemophilia was usually limited to what they learned about it in school or from a recent medical text. Furnas observed that "all he [the doctor] knows about hemophilia is that the book says only males have it." For this reason, she explained that her episodic bleeds not only threatened her life whenever she underwent medical treatment but also bewildered, frustrated, and humbled her doctors. There was a lot of misunderstanding between Furnas and her caretakers over the years, "to their sorrow and mine," she said ruefully.

Furnas had good reason to welcome a certified diagnosis by a hematologist in the postwar climate. It could be authoritative as well as clarifying. It could facilitate proper medical treatment as well as diminish misunderstanding and mistakes. At its best, the blood specialist's diagnosis was an instrument of empowerment for both the patient and the treating physician. Hers is a portrait of hematology as a life-promoting discipline. It remains a vital trope for hematology today, and versions of it are found in every medical specialty. But her path to respectable care was not without its difficulties.

Furnas believed in the power of the hematologist's diagnosis, both in its essential correctness and in its authority, but she quickly learned that the value of that diagnosis could be redeemed only under the right conditions. Her identification as a "PTA-type hemophiliod" initially gave her no better standing in her caregivers' eyes than her earlier claims to be a "bleeder." As she explained, "How can I, who am not a doctor, tell him that I'm no book-type 'classic' hemophiliac, but a PTA, and that my trouble affects both sexes? Unless he spends too much time on highly specialized articles by hematologists . . . he never heard of PTA standing for anything but Parent-Teachers Association." Here Furnas was expressing another troubling dimension of her medical condition, this one cultural. She found it difficult to challenge the doctor's authority in those instances when he might be reluctant to believe her. Little wonder that Furnas resorted to carrying the blood specialist's elaborate analysis of her bleeding disorder in her "already overstuffed handbag" along with instructions about what to do in case she suffered an accident or needed surgery. Without it, she said, "any strange doctor whom I warn that I'm a bleeder just tickets me as neurotic." Furnas was clearly counting on the specialist's word to legitimate her claims to be a "bleeder." Potentially, her certified diagnosis as a "PTA-type hemophiliod" allowed less informed physicians to recognize the unusual nature of her pathology and treat her properly. It could help them get beyond their out-dated conceptions of hemophilia and might even play a significant role in combating the stigmatizing effects of sex discrimination in clinical settings.

"I've Got the Lonesomest Disease!" bears witness to the currency of Furnas's diagnosis in the early 1950s. The value of her diagnosis clearly depended on its credibility in the eyes of the physician who later employed it as a norm for treatment. What would have happened, however, had the specialized diagnosis lacked validity in the eyes of any physician Furnas might encounter? What if that diagnosis seemed incoherent or produced confusion? What if he judged it to be well intentioned but clinically mean-ingless? Unfortunately, this was not a hypothetical question in the 1950s. The guidelines for handling bleeder patients lagged behind the advancing science of blood coagulation research. Blood clotting researchers were just beginning to generate consensus among themselves about the meaning of bleeding disorders that manifested as atypical forms of hemophilia. Furnas's essay rightly highlighted that hematologists had an opportunity in the 1950s to reeducate medical practitioners, to publicize their latest findings for the benefit of all bleeder patients, including the fact that hemophilia was no longer an exclusively male disease even as it impacted a predomi-nately male, pediatric population. Yet, for the most part, they did not.[69]

Bleeder, "You Aren't Alone"

The twentieth-century physicians and scientists who promoted our re-strictive definition of hemophilia were not malicious in their sexism. They did not intend harm to females when they excluded them from a hemo-philia diagnosis. Indeed, quite the reverse. Hematologists were invested in all bleeder patients, but they advanced a masculine concept of hemophilia because it highlighted the severest type of hereditary bleeding that they were seeing in clinical settings.[70] Indeed, it is hard to imagine what hemophilia experts would have gained by insisting on the prominence of severe bleeding disorders in males at the expense of females. But there has been some harm done, and probably more than Furnas's testimony suggests.

Unlike today, hematologists in the 1950s did not make a concerted effort to inform physicians and the public that hereditary bleeding was a significant problem in females as well as males. Yet, as Furnas attested in 1953, they had that opportunity as advances in hematology revealed the diversity of hereditary bleeding in females as well as males. For example, after the discoveries of PTA and PTC deficiencies, a few hemophilia experts did try to use this knowledge to help expand the emerging hemophilia community beyond just the ranks of male patients and their families. In 1954 the U.S.-based Hemophilia Foundation received instruction from its recently formed Medical Advisory Council that "the Foundation and all its chapters" should henceforth include "hemophiliod types such as PTA and PTC, including females," in all of its programs.[71] Five eminent hematologists made this recommendation, all of them literate in the growing complexities of coagulation research. Despite such awareness that hemophilia and its kin were a danger to females as well as males, neither the experts nor hemophilia management advocates demonstrated much commitment to inclusiveness. Throughout the 1950s, publicity by the National Hemophilia Foundation and other hemophilia associations continued to cast hemophilia as a male problem. In fact, as detailed in the next chapter, popular presentations of the 1950s suggest that most experts and advocates were aggressively committed to framing hemophilia as a male affliction.

Consider again the testimony of Helen Furnas and what it tells us about the gender order in 1950s America. In maintaining that she had "the lonesomest disease," Furnas intimated the possibility that things might be otherwise. But what did her essay actually advocate? Furnas was a woman living and reflecting on the margins of a male-centered world in the early 1950s, but that did not make her unsympathetic to the boys and men who suffered from "true" hemophilia. Despite its mildly feminist tone, "I've Got the Lonesomest Disease!" primarily emphasized the plight of the classic "hemophiliac" rather than the troubles of women like Furnas. "We PTA-types are lucky," Furnas asserted. "Classic hemophilia, of which our trouble is only a minor cousin, can be really heartbreaking." Furnas effectively translated her rarified experiences as a "PTA-type hemophiliod," and troubles with dismissive doctors, into an explicit concern for the largely male, pediatric population of hemophiliacs who were the focus of concern in many hospitals around the country. Furnas wholeheartedly endorsed efforts by hematologists and afflicted families to advance themselves. And during the 1950s, that meant framing hemophilia as a truly pressing problem for boys.

For many reasons, the focus on hemophilic boys was the right message for the postwar era. The American public was only beginning to learn fully about hemophilia's nature and effects in 1953. The postwar years witnessed a significant cultural shift in how the disease was presented to the American public. As hospitals more readily provided transfusions, advocates of hemophilia management spoke more openly of the disease. Calls for blood donors helped democratize the content of those discussions as well because hemophilia's widespread characterization as a royal disease did not suit the afflicted boys and men who were commonly in need of fresh blood or plasma. Thus, in turning from her own plight to that of America's thousands of hemophilic boys, Furnas explained: "So it's often called 'the royal disease.' It's nothing of the sort. It hits taxi drivers, machinists, waiters and professors, as well as princes and millionaire bankers."

In its title and emphasis, Furnas's narrative also reminded Americans that the boys and young men with the disorder were experiencing unnecessary isolation. Her article then related important aspects of post–World War II research on hemophilia to recent advocacy efforts by a "500-member Hemophilia Foundation," whose aim was to organize hemophilia patients, their families, and physicians into a recognizable and influential community. Furnas added, "The experience of the pioneer New York chapter [of the Hemophilia Foundation] shows that the prime contribution of such organizations is *personal*, getting the word to hemophilia patients and their families: 'You aren't alone.'" Indeed, drawing on her own experience as a rare type of hemophilic bleeder, Furnas claimed that without an organized community of patients, families, and medical professionals "this hemophilia, both statistically and personally, is the lonesomest disease in the world."[72]

Read today, this portrait of hemophilia is ironic. The isolation invoked by Furnas's title was not just her own but predominantly that of the male hemophilia patient and his family. In other words, "I've Got the Lonesomest Disease!" effectively publicized the loneliness experienced by the young

boys who suffered from classical hemophilia at the same time that it highlighted Furnas's marginal status within an emergent hemophilia treatment
community that often did not provide equal recognition or treatment for
bona fide female bleeders like herself. Both of these senses reflect attitudes
in modern medicine and society that structured the governance of the
hemophiliac's world in the second half of the twentieth century.

Furnas and her contemporaries were also committed to seeing the future as bright. In 1955, for instance, Stanford University hematologist
Theodore Spaet claimed not only that hemophilia had become the "subject
of numerous reviews in the medical literature and lay press" but that it had
even "been elevated to the stature of poliomyelitis, heart disease, cancer
and tuberculosis by the development of an organization to promote the
interests of sufferers."[73] Spaet was part of the younger generation of clotters and had recently joined forces with University of San Francisco's Paul
Aggeler to help isolate "PTC factor" (factor IX).[74] He was well positioned
to comment on the landscape surrounding hemophilia. Spaet even cited
Furnas's article from the *Saturday Evening Post* as an example of the publicity generated for hemophilia in the "lay press." He clearly thought of
Furnas's piece as representative of a future trend, even if he overestimated
the attention that hemophilia was receiving.

These publications—one by a bleeder patient (Furnas), another by a
hematologist (Spaet)—point to the novel relationships developing between
patients with bleeding disorders and medical specialists in postwar America. Hemophilia patients, their families, and advocates were reaching out
to specialists in the late 1940s and 1950s. That is why, at the height of the
controversies surrounding postwar coagulation research, the Hemophilia
Foundation established a medical advisory council that was largely composed of top clotting specialists in the United States.[75] Advocates for hemophilia management sought ways to facilitate communication between
experts such as Spaet and the patients and families represented by Furnas.
Spaet and Furnas were excited that professionals and laypeople were join-
ing forces and fashioning themselves into a community whose ultimate
focus was to understand and cure hemophilia and related bleeding disorders. In their writings, however, each voiced cautious optimism with
respect to ongoing hemophilia research. Thus, after describing postwar
attempts to create an insulin-like injection that might enable the hemophilia patient "to lead a close-to-normal life," Furnas admitted that "this is

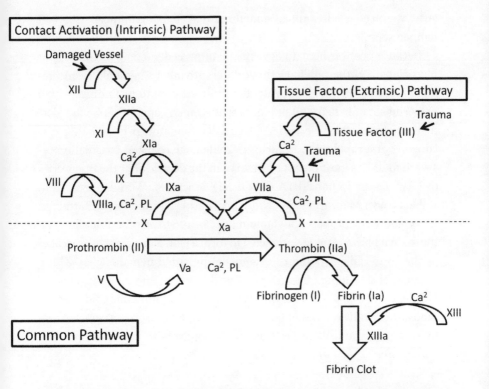

FIGURE 3.3. The Blood Coagulation Cascade, 1964 to the Present. The cascade hypothesis of blood coagulation portrays the chemical action of blood clotting factors involved in the formation of a fibrin clot. Blood coagulation normally begins after traumatic injury to the lining of the blood vessel (which initiates the tissue factor pathway), but the process can also be activated by contact with damaged cellular matter (the contact activation pathway). Hemophilia A results from a deficiency of factor VIII circulating in the blood; hemophilia B from a deficiency of factor IX. The absence of VIIIa or IXa in the coagulation cascade leads to delayed clotting (hence the prolonged clotting times characteristic of hemophilic blood).

Key: Roman numerals represent standardized names of clotting factors, a lowercase *a* indicates the clotting factor in its activated form; Ca^2 = calcium, PL = platelet phospholipid. Factors V, VIII, XI, and XIII are each activated by the release of thrombin (IIa), which amplifies the process. Ca^2 is sometimes called factor IV. Factor VI is unassigned for historical reasons. For simplicity, this illustration omits several factors involved in the initial contact activation and also omits the anticoagulants or inhibitors that regulate the activation of various clotting factors (including factor VIII).

strictly a bleeder's dreaming," something that "barring miracles . . . won't happen soon."[76]

Because postwar hematology created unprecedented opportunities for physicians and the public to think differently about hemophilia and related bleeding disorders, it presented those attuned to its findings with a powerful set of beliefs and practices that seemed capable of one day normalizing the clotting factor deficiencies that hematologists were then discovering at a rapid pace. In fact, the golden age of blood coagulation research found its most potent expression in the decade after the discoveries of PTC (factor IX) and PTA (factor XI) deficiency. Working separately, Robert Gwyn MacFarlane in Oxford and Earl Davie and Oscar Ratnoff in Cleveland each proposed a viable model in 1964 for describing how all the known plasma factors interacted to form a clot. Known as the "cascade" or the "waterfall" hypothesis, this model provided hematologists with a schema for developing treatments as well as perfecting their diagnosis of bleeder cases (fig. 3.3).[77] One thing was clear throughout this golden age of innovation: individuals and families with bleeding disorders were looking to hematology and the experts as they grappled with their past, present, and future.

CHAPTER FOUR

Normality within Limits

In 1955 the producers of the early television medical drama *Medic* devoted an entire half-hour episode to the story of Davey Stinson, an eleven-year-old hemophiliac who had cut himself badly after landing on a glass of milk that he inadvertently knocked from his bedside table. At the hospital, the doctors eventually stop Davey's bleeding with the help of a hematologist and three transfusions. As Dr. Styner informs Davey's parents that their son has pulled through, the father asks about his son's future.

DR. STYNER: Your boy's alive, Mr. Stinson. Twenty years ago, he would have been dead.

MR. STINSON: Alive? Alive for what, so he can spend his life in hospital beds with braces and wheelchairs?

Sensing that Davey is waking and conscious of their conversation, Styner asks the parents to step outside, so that he can tell them "the truth."

DR. STYNER: There's a man in Michigan, and another one back in Massachusetts. They've isolated the normal protein in the blood that your son lacks. There are a lot of problems with it. It may be months or even years before it can be used clinically. But there it is. Somebody's doing something about David's trouble. . . . You've got a sick boy, but you are not alone with him. . . . Tomorrow, maybe a year from tomorrow, the man in Michigan or maybe the man back in Massachusetts, maybe they'll finally hit on the right answer. . . . Kids like Davey can jump on their bikes and not worry about bumps, bruises.

But unlike Mr. Stinson and Dr. Styner, the scientific men in Michigan and Massachusetts were real. As *Medic* portrayed in surprising detail, the hemophilia patient's future lay in the hard work and continued progress of experimental hematology. When Mr. Stinson pressed Dr. Styner on whether Davey would live another five years, melodramatic music cued, and Styner responded: "maybe five, maybe fifty."

Like most popular accounts of hemophilia in the 1950s, this episode of *Medic*, revealingly titled "A Time to Be Alive," highlighted the new hope and inspiration that the present and future held for hemophilia patients and their families even as it reminded viewers that the natural course of hemophilia remained grim. Most boys and men with hemophilia still faced dismal prospects. Yet the story suggested that changes in postwar medicine and society were transforming the expectations of and for people with hemophilia.[1] The message was clear. Something like a normal life would one day soon be possible for the hemophiliac in postwar America. But was this true?

Beginning in the 1950s, the improving fitness of the "hemophiliac" in the United States was often judged in terms of idealized visions of American boyhood and manhood, mirroring the therapeutic focus on a predominantly male, pediatric population. Simply put, the goal of postwar hemophilia management was oriented toward transforming sickly boys into men who were capable of leading productive and fulfilling lives. Talk of normality served this goal. Professional writings about hemophilia in the first half of the twentieth century mentioned the word *normal* only in terms of what physicians judged typical of the malady. Journalists and other popular writers seem not to have used the concept of normality at all when speaking of hemophilia before this point. Beginning in the 1950s, however, Americans in the emergent hemophilia community began invoking the word *normal* when imagining the prospects of the hemophiliac. *Normal* became an expression of the ideal as well as the typical. The word—along with its linguistic kin *normality* and *normalcy*—provided advocates of hemophilia management with convenient shorthand for expressing a diverse range of goals, most of which were unprecedented in their optimism. Yet the goal of a normal life was a largely unexamined ideal in the 1950s and 1960s. Patients, parents, and their physicians did not usually say what they meant when they invoked the idea of normal. Nevertheless, whatever it was that patients, their parents, and their physicians sought by invoking the idea, it was undoubtedly critical to how advocates of hemophilia management believed the life of the hemophiliac should be governed.

The life experience of Americans with hemophilia changed significantly in the 1950s. A recognizable hemophilia community emerged within the United States and other developed nations as medical efforts to manage the disease progressed. This community developed its own culture and norms as it embraced the promises of post–World War II medicine. But above all, it was dedicated to seeing the hemophiliac as a boy or young man who was capable—*often through extraordinary means*—of living normally.

The impetus for forming hemophilia communities in North America, Europe, and the world transcended the patient's need to gain access to new medical services. It was also embedded in the complex personal challenges that boys and men with hemophilia confronted in their rapidly modernizing world. As Frank Schnabel, the founder of the World Federation for Hemophilia, put it in the 1960s:

> I wanted to be like everyone else. I didn't want to be different. So I
> never told anyone what was wrong with me. Then it occurred to me
> that if all hemophiliacs hid their problem, how could we ever expect to
> make any progress? I felt we had to educate people about hemophilia,
> and then push, and push hard, for better treatment and more career
> opportunities. So I went to the other extreme and just refused to stop
> talking about hemophilia.[2]

The utterly rational desire to fit in—to be judged as fit for life "like everyone else"—was what Schnabel and many other persons with hemophilia sought as the twentieth century progressed. Yet, if we are to understand the social origins of modern hemophilia management, it is vital to recognize how hemophilia care advocates of the era articulated this desire for a normal life and tried to realize it.

The hemophilia communities that first emerged in the 1950s represented a visibly paradoxical advocacy movement, one that was devoted to the production of the ordinary—normal lives, normal people—through investments in extraordinary means. However, the hemophilia patients' postwar prospects in the United States are also part of the larger story of American medicine and society in the twentieth century. In the closing decades of the twentieth century, these postwar expectations about the possibility of a normal life for persons with hemophilia would be partially fulfilled, altered, and eventually undermined by the scale and scope of the blood-borne AIDS epidemic. Schnabel was not only a founding member of a global hemophilia community but one of thousands of hemophiliacs who died from AIDS in the 1980s and 1990s.[3] For better and worse, these events were made possible by the heady meliorism of the 1950s that allowed interested parties to look at hemophilia's dismal past and imagine a different fate for present and future patients. Indeed, hemophilia's transformation into a manageable disease in the years after World War II would not have been possible without the availability of blood and plasma transfusions for hemophilia; nor would ensuing developments take the form that they did without the accompanying realization that each hemophilia patient represented a significant if not overwhelming demand on scarce blood resources. In short, these and other postwar developments dramatically changed how Americans with hemophilia and their advocates thought about blood, disease, and health.

Thus, beginning in the 1950s, hemophilia patients and their families sought to influence, resist, and change how medical professionals and laypeople in the United States envisioned the hemophilia patient's prospects for a healthier, if not normal, life. They did this initially by constituting themselves as an identifiable community.

Creating a Community

The hemophilia patient's stake in effective medical treatment had always been a life or death matter. But increasingly, as transfusion medicine increased the likelihood that hemophilic boys would reach adulthood, attention shifted to the problem of life, and how best to live with illness. In postwar America, patients and their families were confronting hemophilia in a new way—as a chronic, manageable disease—and they responded in innovative ways that mirrored American understandings of medical and social progress in the era. An identifiable hemophilia community materialized in the 1950s on the basis of these shared concerns.

Notably, no one thought of persons living with hemophilia as a "community" until the postwar era. Before 1940, hemophilia patients were told that their condition was rare and difficult to treat, and most of these patients were the only "hemophiliac" their physician had ever treated. Where physicians had some experience treating hemophilia patients, it was uncommon for them to be treating more than one or two at a time. The growing availability of state-of-the-art hematological services brought patients and families to certain hospitals in ever greater numbers, helping remove the cloak of invisibility and isolation that had previously surrounded patients.

Although the reliance of hemophilia patients on hospitals predated World War II, the availability of safe and reliable transfusion services improved how these patients experienced these institutions.[4] Traditionally, hospital care meant little more than compression or cautery for bleeding, ice for swelling, narcotics for pain, and a bed for rest. As surgeons and internists advanced transfusion medicine in the 1920s and 1930s, people with hemophilia were increasingly persuaded to go to the hospital, and patients and families often found reasons for encouragement in the services they found there. As hospitals began offering more reliable transfusion services in the late 1930s and 1940s, the demand for clinical hematologists also grew. Blood banks became integrated into hospital routines at this time, benefiting bleeders of all kinds. Hemophilia patients witnessed these changes most acutely because they relied heavily on these services.

Once blood banking and wartime advances made blood and plasma transfusions routinely available in the 1940s, hemophilia patients and their families began viewing their life prospects differently. An untimely death was more easily avoided by the 1950s, and dismal outcomes—like severe crippling from repeated joint bleeds—could increasingly be alleviated by the modern transfusion and orthopedic services that were available at many hospitals. This change in perspective, in turn, made it abundantly clear to people with hemophilia why communal forms of action were necessary. The growing availability of effective medical services provided meaningful incentive for hemophilia patients to turn to specialists in hospitals, to meet other patients there, and to experience their rare condition as something shared. Thus, when patients and their families cast hemophilia as a lonesome disease in the postwar years, they were emphasizing the isolation occasioned by their rare condition at a moment of profound change.[5]

Nevertheless, there was growing concern that medical advances did not benefit hemophilia patients as they should. High costs and blood shortages, among other burdensome problems, made it practically impossible for patients to take full advantage of the medical understanding and treatments that hematologists trumpeted in the postwar years and that increasing numbers of physicians could now offer. Although such burdens were undoubtedly a better option than the prospect of little to no treatment, blood's emergence as a precious commodity in the late 1940s and 1950s served to heighten the patient's sense that his fate hinged not merely on what transfusion medicine could do for him but also on society's willingness to promote blood donation as well as access to these services.[6] The promise and the challenge of hemophilia management called for an advocacy movement that could address the problems associated with the medical management of their disease. In the 1950s, voluntary hemophilia associations became the public face of the emergent hemophilia community and established themselves as the backbone of a small but meaningful social movement that sought to improve the circumstances of hemophilia patients and their families.

By 1950 patients and their families were beginning to view the hospital's hematologists and local blood bankers as potent allies. Meanwhile, the need for alliances was growing more apparent because the promised benefits of transfusion services were proving hard to deliver to those who needed them repeatedly. Patients with hemophilia typically required multiple pints of blood or plasma to control a single bleeding episode. A severe hemophiliac could use dozens of units in any given hospital stay, hundreds of units in the span of a few years. The most troubling problem to emerge for heavy users of blood services in the late 1940s was the dramatic drop-off in voluntary blood donation after World War II. As Americans sought a return to "normalcy" in peacetime, they had to be encouraged to donate their blood. The American Red Cross sought to encourage wartime levels of voluntary blood donation by casting blood donation as a show of civic duty and patriotism as well as a relatively painless form of self-sacrifice.[7] The linkage of voluntary blood donation to symbolic forms of citizenship occasionally proved potent. When the need for blood seemed acute—say, in the event of a tornado or an explosion at a chemical plant—the American public often responded promptly and admirably. More typically, however, peacetime calls for blood donation received a tepid response from Americans unless there was an identifiable recipient with whom potential donors could link their sacrifice. These circumstances gave hemophilia patients and blood bankers shared cause to promote the other's interests.

Hemophilia patients and their families were increasingly called upon to publicize their illness as they tried to recruit blood donors for their multiple transfusions. This demand to identify themselves publicly was a new and significant burden for people with hemophilia. They had to overcome their legitimate fears of being stigmatized to benefit from the transfusion services that were increasingly available. Ideally, hemophilia patients and families wanted not only blood donors but donors who viewed them with understanding and compassion, as ordinary people with unusual needs. At its best, the challenges of the hematological revolution became an opportunity for people with hemophilia to translate their illness experiences into forms of sharing and action that were more transformative than self-pitying.

In an effort to round up civic-minded donors, newspapers in postwar America also ran stories about hemophilic children. The Red Cross and blood bankers encouraged such coverage beginning in the 1940s, and so did hemophilia associations as they began to emerge in the 1950s. In January 1949, for instance, the *New York Times* reported the case of fourteen-year-old Vincent Viviano, who was being discharged from a Brooklyn hospital after his teacher, classmates, and local magistrate had solicited 109 pints from local donors, enough to send the boy home with the surplus blood "banked in case Vincent should need future transfusions."[8] Fifteen months later, the *Times* introduced readers to sixteen-year-old Angelo Giamona, a New Jersey boy who was lying in Columbia Presbyterian Medical Center awaiting blood donors as he reached the "eighty-pint mark" following a basketball injury. The boy had a "desperate fear of blood," according to his doctors, yet his "life or death depends entirely on blood." The *Times* personalized the effect of donor blood. Angelo "notes how much better he feels after every transfusion," the paper reported. "'Angi,' as the nurses call him, is losing this fear which, doctors believe, is the natural reaction of a young hemophilia sufferer."[9]

Such stories were more than moralizing reminders of the necessity of giving blood regularly. The rhetoric of voluntarism that was so characteristic of the postwar era represented a significant trade-off for patients. On the one hand, the frequent calls for blood donation stigmatized "the hemophiliac" as fundamentally unwell and vulnerable, casting him as a person whose continued survival depended on the generosity of others. Postwar stories of blood donation therefore put strict limits on what was possible for people with hemophilia even as they made the patient's chronic demands for blood sustainable. On the other hand, it was only through frequent reminders of the hemophiliac's unique need for blood plasma that such patients stood a chance of anything approaching normalcy. Thus, boys and men with hemophilia found good motivation to tolerate the constant reminders of their dependency in the era's steady calls for voluntary blood donation. At their best, public calls to donate blood to hemophiliacs affirmed ideas of kinship, community, and even patriotism for afflicted boys and men; stories like Angi's often allowed patients to embrace what they shared with their fellow man rather than requiring them to dwell on what marked them as different. But given the trade-offs involved in publicizing their plight, patients could be forgiven any ambivalence they had about their need for blood. In this era of mass blood donation, people with hemophilia had little choice but to publicize their vulnerability and dependence when they needed transfusions for their health and their quest for normalcy.

As patients and their families became increasingly dependent on transfusion medicine from the war years forward, their sense of community crystallized around voluntary blood donation as a fundamental expression of civic virtue as well as social acceptance and belonging. Charles Carmen recalled that "there are gracious people, good people, who really want to help a hemophiliac." As an adolescent in the 1950s, Carmen relied on businessmen and community leaders in rural Arizona to volunteer their blood for his regularly prescribed whole blood transfusions. In fact, he became friends with some of these regular volunteers and even considered them to be an extension of his tight-knit family.[10] Thus, even as illness isolated him from many of his adolescent peers, Carmen appreciated that his "bleeder" status provided him with a meaningful place in his community. He felt at home in his local community by virtue of people who voluntarily donated blood to improve his lot. While this notion of community has been a vital part of the life experience of hemophilia patients and their families since the advent of blood banking and donor networks, it did not constitute—in and of itself—a need for persons with hemophilia to think of themselves as a distinctive group. Rather, the idea of a hemophilia community initially arose from the persistent *failure* of traditional communities to commit to voluntary blood donation in a way that was adequate to the special needs of hemophilia patients.

The idea of a hemophilia community therefore found its formal expression with the creation of voluntary health associations dedicated to helping hemophilia patients and their families overcome their vulnerability to whole blood and plasma shortages.[11] In 1954, for example, journalist Pearl Puckett penned "Calling All Bleeders," a story for *American Mercury* that reported how Nebraskans were witnessing the growing visibility of hemophilia in their state. The catalyst of change was the establishment in Omaha of a hemophilia advocacy organization called the Foundation for Bleeders, but Puckett described hemophilia's new visibility in Nebraska as nothing short of a demographic revolution. "Recent statistics show that hemophilia has outgrown its old classification as a rare disease. Your town, community or city might not be full of bleeders but the disease is certainly on the increase. Since the new Foundation for Bleeders was established in Omaha, Nebraska, more than one hundred persons [with hemophilia] have popped up in and around the immediate vicinity." Don Gaughenbaugh, a retired jeweler and self-described "bleeder," helped found this local advocacy organization with the goal of building community and achieving greater recognition for persons with hemophilia. "You find bleeders everywhere you go . . . and most of the cases are pitiful," said Gaughenbaugh. "The ignorance about hemophilia is amazing, and this ignorance must be overcome." As Puckett's story emphasized, Omaha's hemophilia foundation was "calling all bleeders . . . to learn the identity of those suffering from the disease in order to bring benefits of the Foundation to them." The benefits that associations such as Omaha's Foundation for Bleeders promoted in the 1950s included direct financial aid. As Puckett stressed, "Hemophilia is a costly illness because transfusions are costly, and in order to live at all one must have hundreds of transfusions."[12]

The problems faced by hemophilia patients in the 1950s paralleled those faced by many other Americans with chronic illness (including those with polio or diabetes), but the hemophilia associations served patients and families best where they voiced the unique needs of this population. Don Gaughenbaugh, by the time he reached age fifty in 1954, had become "one of the best-informed persons on hemophilia in the United States." As Puckett noted, "Don has had more than three hundred transfusions, and estimated ten thousand hemorrhages, and knows the ins and outs of living with this affliction." Gaughenbaugh's treatments represented a hard truth about contemporary treatments for hemophilia: the patient's reliance on transfusion medicine was extraordinary. For emphasis, Puckett related the tale of another patient, twelve-year-old Kenny Holmstrom, whose tooth extraction "turned into a major catastrophe . . . [requiring] months to actually stop the bleeding." Among her points, Puckett noted that such patients not only needed lots of blood but also frequently needed fresh-frozen plasma and specialized attention that only people familiar with hemophilia could deliver. Thus, the primary benefit that Omaha's Foundation for Bleeders sought for its members in 1954 was the establishment of "a frozen blood plasma bank in Nebraska" that would be devoted to hemophilic patients. "Ordinary blood plasma, such as that collected by the Red Cross or in the average blood bank, is of no benefit at all—in fact, it is worse than nothing, due to the fact the coagulating agent is quickly lost unless it is immediately frozen." The emergence of the hemophilia community was thus effectively tied to the experience of improving hematological services that promised unique benefits to people with bleeding disorders.[13]

Most notably, the longest-standing U.S. organization devoted to advocacy of hemophilia awareness and management, the National Hemophilia Foundation (NHF), traces its origins to 1948 when Robert Lee Henry and Betty Jane Henry, the parents of a seven-year-old boy with hemophilia, first filed for incorporation of The Hemophilia Foundation, Inc., with the state of New York.[14] From its inception, the foundation had three fundamental missions. Its first publicized aim was "to render direct aid to indigent sufferers" (including negotiating access to blood services), and the second was "to sponsor and encourage research in hemophilia." Both of these aims reflected the needs that Robert Lee Henry identified as most important for hemophilic boys after the war, and each necessitated a third priority, that the Hemophilia Foundation promote awareness of the disease and its treatability. The hidden character of the hemophilia experience prevented the public (i.e., potential blood donors) from understanding the unique circumstances of affected patients and families. Greater visibility for hemophilia was the key not only to promoting research or securing blood for transfusions and other medical services but also to combating the unseen, multifaceted problems facing patients. Betty Jane Henry's own sense of the foundation's priorities was to address "the pain" that was so much apart of chronic bleeding.[15] Others stressed the need for hemophilia societies to combat stigma and loneliness. All of these priorities called upon the Henrys' foundation to publicize the "disease," its "victims," and their creditable character.

Robert Lee Henry was a tax attorney and certified public accountant from the North Shore of Long Island. His son, Lee, suffered from severe hemophilia at a time—during and immediately after the war—when the only relatively effective treatment for the control of hemophilic bleeding was a fresh blood or plasma transfusion. Blood was hard to come by for Lee because his B-negative blood type was rare. But once his father returned home from his wartime service, Lee finally had a reliable source of matched blood available. In the late 1940s, Lee was transfused with his father's B-negative blood dozens and dozens of times.[16] Despite the Henry family's personal hardships, both Robert Lee and Betty Jane understood how fortunate they were in comparison to most families burdened by hemophilia. The Henrys had a workable arrangement for getting blood to Lee that usually proved sufficient to his needs, but they were also acutely aware that most families with hemophilia received less of what they needed, particularly when they relied predominantly on the generosity of strangers for donor blood.

The Henry family was also relatively privileged. They could afford the best available care for their son, and New York City's medical institutions provided state-of-the-art services. In Helen Furnas's 1953 *Saturday Evening Post* feature on hemophilia, Lee Henry is pictured studying at home, safe in bed with a "traveling teacher" nearby to tutor him. Sitting beside Lee is also a microphone and receiver hook-up with a schoolroom, which allowed him to keep pace with his fellow students whenever he was bedridden (see fig. 3.1).[17] Close examination of the photograph also reveals that Lee's right leg is immobilized with a special orthopedic brace meant to alleviate the crippling effects of his hemophilic bleeds. By comparison, most parents of hemophilic boys lacked the kind of material resources, education, and connections of the Henrys. Few had adequate insurance, and many still had difficulties getting to clinics were appropriate treatment was available.[18] Even for the Henrys, the costs could be daunting. As Robert Lee Henry told one reporter, medical bills could place demands on even the "comfortable income" of his successful law practice and "cut it to pieces."[19]

Robert Lee Henry was initially inspired to organize a foundation for persons with hemophilia by a 1946 story in the *New York Daily News* about the plight and suffering of another hemophilic boy, from nearby Glen Cove, whose family could not afford proper care for their son. Indeed, the senior Henry's efforts to mobilize a foundation for people with hemophilia gained early momentum by virtue of the family's circle of friends and acquaintances, which included many well-to-do society people from the New York City metropolitan area. Susan Resnick's social history of the U.S. hemophilia community notes that the contributions of the "Henrys and their friends epitomized the spirit of voluntarism and *noblesse oblige* among upper-class Americans" after the war.[20] Publicity of the foundation and the Henrys' modestly successful fund-raising events encouraged groups across the country to begin forming their own local advocacy groups, particularly after *McCall's* magazine publicized the Henrys' efforts in 1951 in a feature entitled "His Parents Refused to Let This Boy Die." The *McCall's* article inspired what Resnick describes as a deluge of letters from around the country and world.[21]

Because the quality of services for hemophilia care varied widely in the 1950s, patients and their families were increasingly drawn to the larger towns and cities where higher standards of care were available. Because of the high quality of hematological services being offered at the University of Rochester Medical Center, the city of Rochester in upstate New York attracted many patients and families in the late 1940s and 1950s and had one of the earliest chapters of the NHF. In fact, local hemophilia associations tended to arise in places where hospitals possessed specialists with noticeable expertise in bleeding disorders and transfusion medicine. In the 1950s, the most innovative and experienced hemophilia specialists resided in the larger hospitals and well-established medical schools in cities such as Boston, Baltimore, Chicago, Philadelphia, Los Angeles, and San Francisco. Some specialists were also found in places such as Salt Lake City, Utah; Ann Arbor, Michigan; and Chapel Hill, North Carolina, where state universities were scaling-up their medical schools and teaching hospitals with the help of federal and state support. Whether patients and families chose to live in these places or just travel there for their care, these locations promised them physicians who could provide comfort in the form of visible diagnostic, prognostic, and therapeutic expertise. Such specialists also offered hope to hemophilia patients for a better future insofar as they utilized the patient's visits to the hospital as occasions for conducting basic research, employing new technologies, and evaluating treatments.[22]

The NHF's greatest successes in the 1950s were found in its efforts to combat the loneliness, isolation, and stigma that traditionally accompanied affliction by hemophilia. As Susan Resnick relates, NHF chapter meetings became a "forum where parents traded 'horror stories' over coffee, held tense discussions of how to recruit blood donors, and found a safe place to release pent-up anxiety." The NHF's promotion of local chapters undoubtedly prompted many hemophilia patients and their families to come together, identify themselves as part of a distinctive community, share their suffering, and devise strategies for transforming their experiences into something positive. It was constituted as a "community of fate," says Resnick.[23] Yet the Henrys' Hemophilia Foundation was not an entirely unique organization. Postwar patients and families organized around other diseases too—including muscular dystrophy (1950), familial dysautonomia (1951), and cystic fibrosis (1957). In every case, afflicted families certainly constituted their own distinctive "communities of fate" around shared hereditary illness and suffering.[24] Their needs and demands had many similarities because each group was responding to the promises of modern medicine and society. But in each case, patients and families saw their fate in terms of the lived experience of their particular disease.

In the emergent hemophilia community, patients and their families recognized that their collective fate depended on how effectively postwar American medicine and society could capitalize on the ongoing hematological revolution and deliver some normalcy into their lives. Building on growing media attention for recent advances in medicine, advocates cast transfusions and clotting science as therapeutic interventions that transformed the prospects of hemophilia patients and their families. The implicit goal was to render the hemophiliac into a socially creditable individual. As such, the emergent hemophilia community combated stigma, isolation, and loneliness not only where patients and families shared their horror stories but, even more effectively, where their advocacy successfully delivered hematological and other medical services that put patients on the path to greater physical and emotional independence.

The NHF and other hemophilia advocacy associations thus represented a concerted effort by patients and their families in the 1950s to bridge the gap between the promise and the reality of hematology in American society. After all, the unfortunate circumstance that typically motivated patients and families to organize into formal hemophilia associations was the inability of local communities—especially those with state-of-the-art health care—to live up to promises of transfusion medicine and the lofty rhetoric of voluntarism that the Red Cross blood collection services couched in terms of the American citizen's civic and patriotic duty. The hemophiliac's prospects for normalcy in the 1950s thus entailed a commitment to the melioristic, civic-oriented ethic that sustained mass blood donation in postwar America as well as trust in the continued progress of the century's hematological revolution.

Indeed, by forming visible hemophilia communities, patients and families were not only seeking out others with a shared fate but were also staking a claim in the hematologist's technological ethos. The hemophilia societies were simultaneously a manifestation of the patient's need to translate the physician's know-how into something that they would truly experience as life promoting and a normalizing vehicle for patients and families to overcome the stigma and loneliness of hemophilia. Although patients and families were largely responsible for forming hemophilia associations, their collective interests in improving blood and treatment services dictated their heavy reliance on medical experts to provide guidance as well as hope and services. Community building thus facilitated the hemophilia patient's need to be a socially creditable person, even if it simultaneously drew attention to his status as an invalid and dependent.

How Integral Were Experts to the Hemophilia Community?

People with hemophilia and their families relied more than most Americans on the guidance of specialists after World War II, but they were not unusual in their turn to the experts. To borrow a phrase from historian Elaine Tyler May, Americans were looking increasingly to the experts during the late 1940s and early 1950s "to make the unmanageable manageable."[25] Indeed, where Americans valorized the experts in the postwar era, they typically cast scientific endeavors in a romantic light, often speaking of science as if it were the embodiment of objectivity, certainty, or control. As one study of the postwar American psyche explained, experts "assumed a much broader and more important role in directing the behavior, goals, and ideals of normal people" in the two decades after the war. Experts became "norm-setters who would tell people how to approach and live life," and their authority to speak the truth on such matters was judged to be a function of their scientific objectivity and their capacity to approach the social and natural worlds without the popular passions that supposedly biased how laypeople managed their lives.[26] In this climate, the hemophilia patient's reliance on specialists was a common response to the particular challenges he faced. Yet, even if Americans with hemophilia had every incentive to rely on the experts as they constituted their sense of themselves and their community, they did not incorporate the experts into their growing advocacy movement uncritically.

The hemophilia community's turn to the expert in the 1950s was not without some difficulty for patients and families. As the Henry family's Hemophilia Foundation became a national advocacy organization in the early 1950s, it brought hemophilia patients and families into greater contact with the views and interests of experts, especially hematologists. Within the advocacy movement itself, the reliance on experts implicitly raised questions of who actually belonged to the hemophilia community. How inclusive of experts would the community become as advocates sought to secure some recognition, services, and progress for hemophilia patients and their families? Indeed, it remains an open question today—as it did in the 1950s—to what degree the views of hemophilia specialists should be privileged within the hemophilia community. To what extent should the experts be allowed to determine the interests of people with hemophilia, or to set priorities and agendas for the advocacy movement? In short, what stake did postwar patients and their families have in including the experts within their nascent community? In the first two decades of hemophilia care advocacy in the United States, the answer hinged on whether patients and families believed that leading advocates and their experts were fulfilling medicine's promise of delivering some immediate relief while also demonstrating progress toward achieving increasingly "normal lives."

The blood specialists were excited to have the understanding and support of families in the 1950s. People with hemophilia and experts alike were interested in their collective fate. And while it was fairly clear to everyone what the needs of people with hemophilia were, the experts often differed from the patients and families in how to prioritize the distribution of scarce resources to meet those needs. In short, a double bind emerged in the American hemophilia community during the 1950s: as the advocacy movement grew, investments in research were often pitted against calls for immediate, direct aid to individual patients.

Robert Lee Henry envisioned a special role for hemophilia specialists when establishing the Hemophilia Foundation. In the late 1940s, Henry reached out for guidance to local experts in the New York City area, principally to hematologists Peter Vogel, Frank Bassen, and Martin Rosenthal at the Mount Sinai Hospital and to orthopedic surgeon Henry Jordan of the Lenox Hill Hospital. These physicians had considerable hands-on experience with treating hemophilia patients, and they formed an informal expert advisory board for the foundation in the early years. As New York City's leading hemophilia specialists in the late 1940s and 1950s, these doctors divided their labor, coordinated their activities among themselves and with other clinicians, and even tried to manage the blood supply problems that came with providing hemophilia patients with transfusions in the era.[27]

The Hemophilia Foundation's ties to specialized medicine were most evident in the organization's earliest efforts to support hemophilia research. According to its original charter, the first stated mission of the foundation was "to make grants and donations for research and the clinical study of hemophilia, abnormal blood conditions, and similar ailments."[28] As suggested, this mission proved less of a priority in the early years of the organization than cooperative attempts by expert physicians and organized hemophilia families to coordinate care in their local communities. In a meager way, the foundation did support Benjamin Alexander's ongoing blood clotting research at Harvard University and the Children's Hospital in Boston in the late 1940s and early 1950s. Not until 1954, however, did the Hemophilia Foundation actually began to realize its mission of promoting hemophilia research and fostering ties to the larger national and international community of hemophilia specialists. It did so by establishing a formal Medical Advisory Council (MAC). Henry first constituted the MAC in late 1953. He designated Dr. Peter Vogel of Mt. Sinai Hospital as its temporary chairman. The original members were Drs. Benjamin Alexander, Kenneth Brinkhous, John H. Lawrence, Armand Quick, Leandro Tocantins, and Maxwell Wintrobe, all of them distinguished experimental hematologists. The MAC's first meeting took place at the Hotel Claridge in Atlantic City, New Jersey, at which time Brinkhous was elected its permanent chair.[29]

The foundation's concerted efforts to support hemophilia research after 1954 opened the way for specialists across the United States to play an increased role in the priorities of the organization. In 1954 Henry and the board appointed New York hematologist Martin Rosenthal as the permanent medical director to the foundation to be on call to dispense expert advice to its members. Rosenthal would be the voice of medical expertise for many years to come. But often after 1954, Rosenthal would consult with Brinkhous or other members of the Medical Advisory Council before making recommendations that related to the fruits of experimental hematology.

Meanwhile, the hemophilia advocacy movement continued to grow in a grass-roots fashion. In 1956 the Hemophilia Foundation officially changed its name to the National Hemophilia Foundation (NHF) to reflect its maturation into a "loose federation" of local hemophilia societies devoted to supporting hemophilia patients and families. There were seventeen active chapters in the United States and one in Montreal, Canada, that year.[30] Robert Lee Henry transformed his New York City–based Hemophilia Foundation into the head of a national advocacy network when hemophilia societies appeared in various cities, including Rochester, Chicago, and Los Angeles, in the early 1950s. As Henry envisioned it, the "members" of the Hemophilia Foundation were the "chapters," whose primary responsibility was to represent the local interests of patients and families.[31] Henry also believed a decentralized organization would "result in more understanding of hemophilia by members of the medical profession" and in more "medical minds" devoted to the development of "a cure."[32] In effect, with the establishment of a medical director and the MAC in 1954, Henry and the board of trustees assigned the national office with the task of communicating to the chapters what research and treatment initiatives its medical advisers thought the foundation should support. Though lay leaders always had a say in what initiatives to support, the strong ties between the experts and the national office frequently guided those decisions.

As the foundation grew, its leaders sought a steady flow of information from the New York office to the chapters, and from the chapters to patients, families, and their physicians. Particularly important between 1951 and 1956 were the foundation's efforts to educate the clinicians and family doctors who offered hands-on care to hemophilia patients. Most medical professions were unfamiliar not only with the rapidly evolving science surrounding bleeding disorders but also with a rudimentary understanding of the disease. As hematologist Peter Vogel put it in 1951, "the Henrys know more about hemophilia than most doctors."[33] Through its newsletters and bulletins, the national office sought to educate physicians about the patient and family's experience of illness, the special needs of these patients, and the hemophilia specialist's recommendations about clinical management. Chapter leaders tailored the information to their members (especially in their own local newsletters); at their local meetings, they encouraged patients and families to educate themselves and their physicians about the important developments taking place in hemophilia research and treatment.

By 1955, however, many chapter leaders had discovered that the foundation's organization arrangement was somewhat lacking in its responsiveness to the immediate needs of patients and their families. It was at the level of local chapters that most hemophilia patients received identifiable services such as physician referrals, blood credits, financial loans, orthopedic braces, and other enabling devices and services. Chapter leaders fully recognized that member families judged their effectiveness in terms of the tangible aid and services they could generate; many were themselves parents of hemophilic sons. So quite naturally, the chapters wanted the national office to provide more in the way of financial assistance and expert guidance for them and their constituents—the self-designated "sufferers." The direct loan program of the national office was a particular point of tension. Less than half of the moneys that the national office distributed to the chapters for distribution to patients were ever repaid in the early years. Henry's strong preference for investing the foundation's moneys in research after 1953 was strengthened by his observation that the direct loan program was a losing proposition. As significant differences of opinion about outreach, research, and fund raising emerged, some trustees became openly critical of Henry's plans and priorities.

The foundation's executive secretary, Margaret Hexter, was the mother of a hemophilic child who, like the chapter leaders, was personally committed to seeing that suffering families got as much tangible aid as the national office could provide. In her voluntary position, Hexter devoted a considerable amount of her time to the aid of isolated hemophilia patients who did not have the resources of a local chapter. As Hexter became personally involved in charity cases across the country, she saw a growing need for a national office that included a professional staff, some of whose members might possibly act as field officers. In one case from the summer of 1955, the mother of a twenty-four-year-old hemophilic patient from Kings Mountain, North Carolina, wrote the foundation after the state's Department of Public Welfare denied aid for vocational training for her son. Unfamiliar with North Carolina's policies in 1955, Hexter openly questioned the treatment of this family because she knew that hemophilia patients in the states of New York and New Jersey received public assistance through existing "crippled children's" programs. Moreover, as a parent herself, Hexter found it hard to imagine how any family burdened by hemophilia could manage without some form of public assistance. Advocacy, she thought, could entail securing services from the states that were adequate to the needs of hemophilia families.[34] Thus, over the course of 1955, Hexter and other leading parents envisioned the need for a larger and stronger national organization that could bring visibility to the desperate circumstances of hemophilia patients in places where existing state services did not recognize the needs of such patients and their families. The growth of the foundation, they reasoned, was the best way to get adequate care for hemophilia patients throughout the nation.[35]

As more chapters joined the Hemophilia Foundation between 1952 and 1955, the board meetings were filling with more patients or parents of hemophilic children who prioritized direct aid above the distant benefits of a "cure." While being generally supportive of the foundation's investments in research, many advocates began arguing that the national office's preoccupation with funding research should not be allowed to squeeze out efforts at direct aid for lack of resources. Leaders of the larger chapters— for example, Chicago and Los Angeles—concluded by 1956 that more than a name change was necessary to make the Hemophilia Foundation into an effective national advocacy association. As such, a consensus quickly emerged on the foundation's board of trustees that the NHF should transform itself from an entirely voluntary organization into a professionally staffed enterprise capable of conducting national fund-raising drives. Local chapters had asserted their desire for a national office that was primarily devoted to raising funds for hemophilia programs and services families could immediately use.

The year 1956 thus became pivotal in the history of the National Hemophilia Foundation, as the direction of the advocacy movement experienced some inevitable growing pains related as much to its rapid growth and prior successes as to differences in opinion about the best way to move forward. In January, the board of trustees not only approved the association's formal name change of the Hemophilia Foundation, Inc., to the National Hemophilia Foundation but also moved to hire a full-time executive director to lead the day-to-day operations of the NHF. The latter motion passed despite misgivings by Henry and others that their eighteen-chapter, two-thousand-member organization was capable of supporting a professional staff, even with the prospect of a national fund-raising campaign. Not wishing to scale back in any area, the trustees also agreed to finance the Medical Advisory Council's proposal to hold the first scientific symposium on hemophilia that August. On the surface, all of these actions were momentous steps forward, but they also exacerbated tensions among leading advocates regarding whether direct aid or research should be the organization's principal focus because the NHF proved unable by year's end to cover the expense of all these initiatives.

Henry was personally troubled by the ambitious direction the trustees were headed in 1956 and resigned from the NHF in September, leaving others to take up the challenge of resolving how to meet the financial and other demands to pursue both direct aid and research.[36] It was an unfortunate turns of events for everyone to see Henry completely relinquish his involvement with the foundation that his family founded, especially in light of the successful scientific symposium on hemophilia that the NHF sponsored with the guidance of its Medical Advisory Council in New York City that August. This conference, which included more than sixty distinguished researchers from nine different countries, was the first of its kind and was held concurrent to the biennial meeting of the International Hematology Society to ensure the attendance of a large audience of medical professionals.[37]

The growing pains experienced by NHF leaders reflected the enormous gap between promise and reality that confronted all disease-focused advocacy groups and voluntary health organizations in the mid- to late 1950s. The consensus among NHF trustees in 1956 was that a professional staff at the national office could orchestrate a national fund-raising campaign modeled on the widely known and celebrated model of the March of Dimes that the National Foundation for Infantile Paralysis (NFIP) had successfully employed to provide resources for both direct aid and research for polio. The successful approval of Salk's polio vaccine in 1955 had followed the NFIP's momentous field trials in 1954.[38] Unfortunately, every voluntary health organization in the United States was looking to the successful model of the NFIP; the American public had grown somewhat resistant to the frequent calls for donations from so many deserving charities—

including hemophilia associations. It was certainly true, as Henry argued, that the NHF, a society with only a couple thousand members, could not realistically compete with much larger health advocacy groups. And though the NHF would struggle continuously with these issues for years to come, most leading advocates of improved hemophilia care in the mid-1950s saw encouragement in the lofty promises of the era; they wanted to take the foundation to ever greater levels of success.

More important than the change in NHF leadership was the board of trustee's decision in 1956 to govern and organize the foundation in a manner that reflected the growing involvement of patients and families from across the country. The growth of the organization had been steady since 1952, but it had also been haphazard. Henry had never actively focused the foundation's efforts upon chapter building or recruitment. Now, with David Walsh as president, the NHF began to address the growth of the organization in a formal way. Walsh had been the president of the Midwest chapter in Chicago before moving to New York City in 1954 and becoming the NHF's executive treasurer in January 1956. As such, his sympathies were with the chapters and their need for professional and financial assistance. Notably, a group of four leading women from the Rochester and Metropolitan chapters in New York State proposed a series of successful motions that doubled the number of trustees to an upper limit of one hundred, expanded the committee of executive officers to nine members, and designated five hemophilia parents in the room as new trustees.[39] The group's successful motions reflected a clear desire among the mothers of hemophilic sons to democratize the organization further by making leadership positions at the national level more accessible to patients and affected families.

These organizational changes created a temporary rift between the NHF and hemophilia researchers. The tension grew out of specific financial commitments that Henry made to researchers at Mount Sinai Hospital and the Protein Foundation for 1956 but were not immediately honored by the new NHF leadership in late 1956.[40] The rift carried great weight for both lay and expert leaders within the U.S. hemophilia community during the late 1950s as they each worked to advance the cause of hemophilia management according to their own vision. The experts were not immediately comfortable with the idea that the NHF's resources should focus on direct aid to patients and families at the expense of their efforts to develop treatments, especially AHF-rich plasma fractions, that experimental hematologists widely believed might effectively control hemophilic bleeding in the near future.

In the late 1950s, Brinkhous and NHF medical director Martin Rosenthal thus found themselves emphasizing to the NHF's parent-leaders the need for patience and caution. For these top two medical advisers, the failure of the NHF's new leadership to support extant research commitments in 1956–57 highlighted the instability of grass-roots advocacy and the need for parents and patients to focus on the long-term solutions that only medical experts and broad public support could provide. As such, Brinkhous and Rosenthal decided that the MAC should scale up its efforts to develop a concentrated plasma fraction, rich in AHF (factor VIII) or other clotting factors. As they saw it, hemophilia families across the nation were growing needlessly impatient with the experts who could actually help them.

At the same time, hemophilia patients, their families, and their lay advocates were hoping for more than what postwar hematology had been able to provide. By 1960, hemophilia patients and their physicians had nearly two decades of experience with the forward-looking promises of modern hematology. Yet, by any measure, the life of a hemophilia patient was still "abnormal." One expert later described the patient's experience in the postwar period as follows:

> His life . . . is dominated by multiple hospital, clinic and emergency-room visits, unscheduled traveling at awkward times, interminable, depressing delays in hospital corridors, repetition of his long and complicated tale to medical personnel changing every few weeks, treatment lacking continuity or consistency, a succession of x-ray studies, blood tests, and other diagnostic procedures usually unnecessary, multiple venipunctures from young doctors still learning this skill, a bewildering deluge of hospital bills never current and seldom accurate, and endless harassment to recruit blood donors.[41]

Brinkhous and Rosenthal knew this illness experience all too well. They believed, however, that it would be best if the NHF were to broaden its organizational base to include more "non-hemophilia patients" (e.g., civic leaders, professionals, and even other types of "bleeders") and to focus the scope of the organization's research program on the need for "the development of a suitable preparation for use in hemophilia with a nationwide availability." Rosenthal not only favored recruitment of advocates from outside the ranks of hemophilia families but linked such recruitment back to traditional notions of community, civility, and voluntarism that facilitated mass blood donation as well as the NFIP's successful advocacy of a polio vaccine. This, too, was a question of how the hemophilia community should be constituted. He observed that "in areas where civic consciousness is high and where there are few demands from various competing organizations, individuals . . . have successfully contributed non-hemophilic leaders to Chapters working in those regions."[42] From the perspective of these postwar hematologists, lay leadership at the NHF had become too insular—not inclusive enough of civic-minded non-hemophiliacs—to advance the cause of hemophilia management as effectively as they, the experts, wished.

Who constituted the hemophilia community in the era of the expert? The hemophilia community in postwar America undoubtedly comprised not only patients and affected families but also experts who provided encouragement and aid. Indeed, the advocacy movement's efforts to advance some normalcy for hemophilia patients and their families in 1950s would not have been possible without the involvement of experts. But the early years of America's hemophilia community also suggest that the origins and character of the advocacy movement did not rely uncritically on the experts. Leading patients and families frequently resisted the expert's calls for "patience" and "caution," as they rightfully looked at the lofty promises of progress that American medicine and society held out to its citizenry. They readily expressed their interest in seeing the experts deliver some normalcy, both in the here and now and in the near future. And while the affected community was small in size and the resources for such disease advocacy groups were inadequate, the accomplishments of the American hemophilia community in the 1950s made a notable difference in the lives of many patients and families (particularly in delivering improving blood services and in overcoming the traditional isolation that accompanied severe bleeding disorders). The pursuit of normality, like other features of the hemophilia advocacy movement, predominantly reflected the patient's experiences and interests even as patients and families turned to the experts to help them negotiate what normality meant for them.

Give Him as Much Life as He Can Take

Even as advocates of improved hemophilia care embraced the pursuit of a "normal life," they linked a diverse array of goals, beliefs, and behaviors to their invocations of normality. From the standpoint of physicians, normal for the hemophilic patient was always a relative measure of physical and mental fitness. For the hematologist, it meant levels of clotting factor in the bloodstream that were capable of eliciting prompt blood coagulation. To orthopedists and physical therapists, it meant joints and muscles that allowed full and flexible movement without pain. For psychiatrists and social workers, it meant patients who were well adjusted to their circumstances and able to lead happy and productive lives whatever their physical limitations. All of these registers of the word "normal" mattered to patients and families, but they had their own diverse measure of what normality meant and how to pursue it in a modernizing society. Those meanings frequently extended beyond the matter of treatment to include all aspects of life. Thus, as *Reader's Digest* reported of Frank Schnabel's life and advocacy activities in the United States and Canada in the 1950s, advocates stressed that some semblance of a "normal life" was achievable for the hemophilic boy if he learned how "to accept as much life as he could take." Indeed, as compellingly told by journalist Robert Littell in 1959, Schnabel's personal story not only provided "new hope and inspiration" for patients seeking normal lives but also explained that the social promotion of normality entailed breaking "all the rules that are supposed to govern hemophiliacs" and doing everything possible to redefine expectations of what people with hemophilia could do.[43]

Greater visibility for hemophilia in its relation to blood donation in the postwar decades was critical to getting out the word that some normalcy was possible for people with hemophilia. It also meant, in the terminology of the day, that hemophiliacs were no longer just invalids. As Americans grew increasingly familiar with the clinical uses of blood and plasma, there were growing opportunities for advocates to impress upon the public that the "hemophiliac" was a creditable individual who—with the aid of transfusions—was capable of overcoming his disability and contributing to society.[44] Transfusion services adequate to the needs of chronic bleeders, advocates argued, not only were deliverable but benefitted everyone by giving hemophilic boys and men a solid chance of leading socially productive as well as personally fulfilling lives. In other words, the NHF's positive portraits of hemophilia encouraged civic-minded Americans that giving blood for the hemophiliac's transfusions was a worthwhile social and economic investment in which they could take pride.

One way advocates in the mid-1950s promoted a more vital, positive image of hemophiliacs was by circulating narratives and images that recognized the pain and hardships of hemophilia while stressing how degrees of normalcy were already possible. In 1956, for example, the NHF widely circulated *Mingled Blood*, an essay written by Ralph Zimmerman, a recently deceased hemophiliac "who joined the Foundation in its earliest stages." Zimmerman wrote the essay as a twenty-two-year-old college student, shortly before graduating from Wisconsin State College in Eau Claire and moving on to the law school at the University of Wisconsin at Madison. While Zimmerman's personal situation ended tragically, the foundation saw in his essay a message of hope as well.

The hope in Ralph Zimmerman's essay stemmed not only from medical science and faith that society would do right by hemophiliacs but also from the fact that treatments had already improved the lives of patients like himself. Thus, Zimmerman told of his own adult experience and his college years, which were relatively healthy and filled with "joy and a sense of achievement." He explained that he had excelled in "debate and forensics" and "been lucky in politics," even being elected as his college's student body president. "Like so many other American youths, I've worked my way through college as a clerk in a hardware store," he said. But most critically, Zimmerman stressed that, "except for periodic transfusions, my life is as normal as anyone else's, and my aims and ambitions are the same as anyone else's." He played golf on weekends—though he was no Ben Hogan. "And back home, a girl wears my wedding band," he proudly confided. As did much fifties-era publicity for hemophilia, Ralph Zimmerman's oratory came with an explicit moral for all Americans. It stressed that "a different type of social relationship needs to be found."

> Because a hemophiliac is so totally dependent on society during his early years and because his very existence is sometimes then precarious, society now tends to lag in recognizing the change. It sometimes fails to realize that this hemophiliac's life is no longer in serious question and that now his right to aspire to any new height should not be

frowned on by a society still vividly remembering the past. Now, he seeks neither pity nor privilege. He wishes only to be regarded not as a hemophiliac but rather a human being to be evaluated like any human being.

Thus, Zimmerman expressed his vision for the future: that American society would evolve to consider hemophilia patients as persons with normal lives and ambitions while helping young men like him to realize their dreams.[45] This vision was not unique to Zimmerman. Other advocates widely embraced and promoted such messages in the 1950s.

As advocates began to think of the hemophilic child as a boy who would likely grow into a man, it was not uncommon for them to take the next step and follow Ralph Zimmerman in imagining that child's potential to become a productive member of society. Unfortunately, as suggested by portrayals of hemophilia in fifties-era television and print media, the old stereotypes about the disease were pervasive precisely because bleeding episodes, pain, and the threat of an untimely death all remained harsh realities of the illness experience in the 1950s. In fact, on those rare occasions when people actually considered the hemophiliac's predicament, they usually imagined an individual who was prone to invalidism and an untimely death. Americans were not entirely wrong in their thinking, but what advocates were stressing to the public was that a growing number of hemophilia patients and families in the United States were dedicating themselves to the pursuit of a "normal life" and experiencing some success in that endeavor.

Thus, even as advocates in the mid- to late 1950s publicized the image of the hemophilic child as that of a sickly, lonely, and often crippled boy in order to drum up support for blood donation and financial aid, they also countered that reality with the fact that increasingly these boys had grown into productive young men whose lives were filled with surprisingly mundane pursuits: college educations, careers, and even happy marriages. No one delivered hard evidence in the 1950s that patients were living longer, but patients and experienced physicians knew that things had improved dramatically since 1940. In fact, we know today that in cities like Cleveland, where hospitals provided state-of-the-art care for hemophilia patients, that median life expectancy for severe hemophiliacs born in the 1940s and 1950s had risen to nearly forty years of age.[46] Though it might initially seem that advocates were promoting two contradictory images of the "hemophiliac," they were actually claiming on the basis of their lived experience that society had a say in how this patient—usually a boy—was going to turn out. Was he to be allowed to become an invalid for lack of treatment, or was he to be given the opportunity for some normalcy?

The tension between portraits of hemophiliac as both normal and invalid played out on television and radio as well as print media. Consider again the episode of *Medic* mentioned at the beginning of this chapter, this time as an illustration of how expertise was capable of altering the fate of young patients like the fictional Davey Stinson. The program gave an elaborate description of the child's treatment that was consistent with the show's theme of medical realism. Dr. Styner's voiceover explained the medical team's actions as they worked on Davey:

> On arrival at the hospital, he [Davey] was given two units of antihemophilic plasma. He's approaching shock. . . . Blood pressure seventy over forty. Pulse, one hundred and sixty. The cut on his arm is sutured, and a pressure bandage with fibrin foam applied. His face presents another problem. His lacerations are not as deep and can be easily sutured. But the application of the pressure bandage is extremely difficult in this area. Because the patient is a known hemophiliac, a cross-match is run immediately and six units of fresh blood are ordered. The blood must be fresh for the vital protein, anti-hemophilic factor, which is lacking in the patient's blood, the same protein which causes normal blood to coagulate, loses its effectiveness twenty-four hours after it is taken from the donor. In order to insure a sufficient supply of fresh blood on hand, a call is sent out to all available sources in the area requesting blood of the patient's type.[47]

The script's technical detail surpasses what the era's popular media usually volunteered about hemophilia care. Even by the standards of accuracy that *Medic*'s producers set for the series, the medical particulars occasionally seem overdone. Yet the scene well illustrates how this prime-time drama valorized the scientific and technological skill of the physician even to the point of alienating its viewers. The point was not just to showcase medical progress but to stress, as indicated in the episode's title "A Time to Be Alive," that the prospects for young hemophilia patients were at turning point. It was possible that lay and medical attention to the problem of hemophilia could give the Davey Stimpsons of America a real chance at normalcy. In effect, Americans were being told that they could invest credibly in the future of such sick children. Boys like Davey were far from hopeless.

Although *Medic*'s hemophilia episode is still a more highly idealized portrait of hemophilia care than most patients received in 1955, it can nevertheless be interpreted as a faithful rendering of how organized medicine and hemophilia care advocates were selling the transformative potential of hematology to the American public. Dow Chemical, *Medic*'s corporate sponsor, advertised the television show to the American public as making "no compromise with truth," and "A Time to Be Alive" dutifully reflected how the show's producers understood that slogan. Medical realism was the purported hallmark of the series. *Medic*'s creator, James Moser, saw drama in the day-to-day routines of professional work and despised the soapiness of existing medical dramas on radio, film, and TV where doctors seemed to practice medicine only in passing. So in creating *Medic*, Moser not only spent time with medical professionals at Los Angeles County Hospital to create authentic material but turned to the Los Angeles County Medical Association to help sell and produce the show.[48]

Davey's postoperative care in "A Time to Be Alive," is therefore emblematic of the promise and peril faced by hemophilia patients and their physicians in the 1950s. While Davey lies unconscious and still bleeding following his operation, Carl the intern enters the room to prepare another transfusion for the boy, Davey's third. The intern remarks, "Seems there's enough AHF in the blood to induce clotting." But Dr. Styner warns him: "Well, it's not quite that simple, Carl. Hemophiliacs not only lack the AHF in the blood, but they tend to resist it. Sometimes one of them will build up antibodies that fight the one thing that can save their lives. I read about a patient who took thirty transfusions and was still bleeding when he died." Here, the script delved ever so slightly into clinical difficulties seldom mentioned in the era's popular media. Hematologists understood by 1954 that fresh blood and plasma lacked enough AHF (factor VIII) to bring hemophilia bleeding under control and that—even with a plasma fraction rich in AHF—a significant minority of hemophilia patients would likely develop immune resistance to the clotting factors in the foreign blood plasma. Styner's polite reprimand did not dissuade Carl from posing a potential solution to these interconnected problems: "What about isolating the AHF, I mean so it could be administered in massive doses?" Styner responded, referencing the development of Cohn plasma fraction I for hemophilia: "Well, it's been tried experimentally. It's not too reliable yet. So far the best we've got is fresh blood and plasma. All we can do is what we are doing. I talked to George Fletcher, the hematologist. He agrees with the procedure we are following." There was no dramatic cure here, no obvious triumph of medical science. But it was clear from such exchanges that the continued progress of hematology held the key not only to controlling bleeding in hemophilia but to normalizing the lives of patients as well.

Not surprisingly, hemophilia families and their advocates openly embraced *Medic*'s treatment of hemophilia.[49] In February 1955 the Chicago-based Midwest chapter of the Hemophilia Foundation circulated a newsletter proclaiming *Medic* a "splendid" program and asked members to send letters of appreciation to their local TV stations for airing programs like this one. "Evidence that interest in Hemophilia is constantly growing," said the newsletter, "is shown by the number of television and radio presentations on this problem."[50] Robert Lee Henry also obtained a film copy for the NHF's head office that he screened and loaned for interested parties. Kenneth Brinkhous, the chairman of the foundation's MAC, judged it an "excellent film."[51] *Medic*'s portrait of hemophilia and its management were entirely consistent with the images and information that hemophilia associations were circulating in their publicity and fund-raising campaigns of the 1950s.

This overwhelmingly positive response to *Medic*'s hemophilia episode was predicated on the less than ideal television portraits of hemophilia that came before it. In 1954 television producers twice garnered the unwanted attention of the Hemophilia Foundation, first in a February broadcast of ABC's regular mystery series, *The Mask*, and later in an April broadcast of NBC's *Dragnet*. *The Mask* teledrama, entitled "A Royal Revenge," featured the murder of a man—a prince—with hemophilia. A reviewer writing for the Hemophilia Foundation newsletter commended the program for providing a "true description of the disease and its effect" and recognizing "blood transfusion" as a treatment, but she also bemoaned some of "the facts" as presented, including several misconceptions: "Hemophiliacs never have haircuts," "never handle glass," and "live in mortal fear of pin pricks." In fact, the program overstressed "the dangers of external cuts" while presenting the royal victim as untouched by the "major troubles . . . [of] internal bleeding and crippling" and beset on all sides by greedy and jealous family members who wished him ill. The reviewer seemed bemused by a plot that "gave the victim no chance at all" of survival, but she ultimately found "major fault" with the fact that the show's "errors fit in with a lot of emoting which created the feeling that a hemophiliac's chances are hopeless." She warned, "Such an impression could be demoralizing to young hemophiliacs, to the parents of young hemophiliacs, and to others who don't realize the disease is far from being a death warrant."[52] More damning was the criticism that *Dragnet*'s producers received from the Hemophilia Foundation and its Southern California chapter after they portrayed the villain of their telecast on April 8 as a hemophiliac. Although people with hemophilia were undoubtedly ordinary people ranging from heroes to criminals, the foundation did not wish its constituents cast in a negative light at a time when it was stressing that "hemophiliacs" were ordinary people whose aspirations for normality were creditable.

In their feedback to media producers, the NHF and other advocacy groups actively combated stigma by attempting to set public standards and attitudes about what life with hemophilia was like, and how it did not differ dramatically from the "normal lives" that most Americans strived for. Thus, in response to *Dragnet*'s inclusion of a hemophilic villain, the national office encouraged chapters and individual members to write television producers and remind them that "hemophilia is an unhappy fact and not a dramatic fiction." Indeed, there is circumstantial evidence to suggest that *Medic*'s fact-laden presentation of hemophilia in January 1955 was in part due to the foundation's response to the *Dragnet* episode. The foundation's complaints to *Dragnet*'s producers received a "gracious reply" assuring members of the hemophilia community that "any misleading references were unintentional" and that the letters and literature sent by the foundation to NBC had been "circulated among the writers and production staff." They even promised to handle hemophilia "in a proper manner" should it ever "again be a factor in a 'Dragnet' script."[53] Conceivably, James Moser, who wrote for *Dragnet* and wrote and produced for *Medic*, saw the complaint and literature from the Hemophilia Foundation in the spring of 1954. Moser and NBC produced *Medic*'s hemophilia episode later in 1954, and the degree of "accuracy" that is so evident in "A Time to Be Alive" suggests a producer who had incentive to stick to the facts.

The need for positive images of people with hemophilia—particularly ones that cast the patient as creditable (i.e., worthy of social and economic investment) was necessary in the 1950s for both the medical professional and the lay public to hear. Even though hemophilic boys and men were capable of "being normal" in some settings in the 1950s, most of their physicians and fellow citizens still discouraged them from expressing too much boyish vigor. For instance, it was common for physicians treating hemophiliacs to interpret a patient's demands to be treated like other boys as a self-defeating act. As Charles Carmen recalled of his teenage years in the era, an experienced surgeon once warned him that having hemophilia was like living in a glass house. "You should not venture out of that house," said the surgeon. Carmen replied that he was "sadly mistaken. That's not the kind of life I choose to live. I choose to live a very full impacting kind of life."[54] In fact, when it came to the clinical care of hemophilia in the 1950s, perceptive patients like Carmen oftentimes found that physicians were no better at treating them *normally* than were laypeople. This fact was wholly unacceptable from the perspective not only of many hemophilia patients but also of their advocates in the United States; their faith in the hemophiliac's capacity for a "normal life" was already becoming entrenched by the mid 1950s. Yet, as Carmen testified, even more troubling was the fact that many physicians still knew less about hemophilia than patients and their families.

Generally speaking, postwar medical advice characterized the hemophiliac as an extremely fragile being. As hematologist Salvatore Lucia pointed out in 1950 to readers of the physician's handbook *Conn's Current Therapy*, the therapeutic management of hemophilia should always include preventative measures "to temper the activities of [hemophilic] infants and children *as much as possible*."[55] Lucia was a pioneering hematologist who regularly transfused hemophiliacs. He had as much reason as any physician to feel confident about medicine's ability to control hemophilic bleeding, yet he recommended to physicians that it was always best if the hemophiliac enjoyed very limited physical activity. Doctors were instructed to restrict hemophiliacs from undertaking strenuous exercise or active participation in sports. For the majority of physicians who had little to no experience treating hemophilia, such recommendations were treated as common sense. As such, these doctors effectively encouraged the idea that the hemophiliac was a spectator on the sidelines of normal life.

As the 1950s came to a close, many hemophilia families did take such conservative recommendations to heart. They wanted their children to be spared the possibilities of crippling, invalidism or an early death. In "Two's Company," a 1960 photo essay from the *Saturday Evening Post*, hemophilic brothers Chris and David Daly were "forbidden such fun" as "roughhousing" with one another as most "natural" brothers do. Such examples were evidence that parents were generally expected to enforce the physician's proscriptions on the activities of afflicted sons. Hemophilia specialists in the 1950s viewed the hemophilic patient as "healthy" and "well-adjusted" if his bleeds were infrequent and crippling avoided. By this measure, "good" parents were those who often went to extreme lengths to ensure that their "fragile" child was guarded from every conceivable hazard. As Suzanne Massie said of her early years raising her hemophilic son, Bobby: "I began to develop a sixth sense, covertly watching, judging potentially dangerous situations before they became hazardous, staying alert without seeming to be, ready to let him move, but ready also to leap forward to catch him as he tripped. But it wasn't enough; even when his movements were still simple, there was always something I could not anticipate." Such anxiety was even expected of mothers (and to a lesser extent fathers). As the American Medical Association's *Today's Health* said of Edward Smith's mother in 1958: "Edward, with the help of his mother, tries to lead as normal a life as possible . . . but his mother must always accompany him when he goes out," keeping "a constant, close watch on him," knowing "what to do when her son suddenly begins hemorrhaging."[56]

Even as portraits of the fragile hemophilic boy persisted into the late 1950s and early 1960s, hemophilia specialists increasingly embraced a more liberal view of preventative care, one that figured the male hemophiliac differently from the stereotype—as having a tougher, more resilient constitution despite the tendencies toward bleeding and bruising. The physicians advancing this more durable image were typically those who had significant experience treating hemophilia patients because their clinical experiences gave them the confidence to say that patients could engage in most normal activities if they learned to moderate their behaviors. One of these specialists was Maurice Leonard of San Francisco. He believed that social isolation and stigma had as much potential to disable as did the patient's natural disposition for bleeding and crippling. In 1953 he warned parents and physicians, "Trauma must be avoided," though he stressed that "severe restrictions should not be imposed on hemophilic children. . . . Experience indicates that there is little correlation between episodes of bleeding and physical activity."[57] As Leonard saw it, hemophilic children were not nearly as fragile as people had been lead to believe. By 1956 he refined his preventive recommendations to say that "restrictions should not be of such a nature as to encourage invalidism."[58] Most importantly, Leonard was not alone in his more liberal treatment philosophy. Like Leonard, specialists who stressed moderate, "normalizing" behaviors among patients were prompting parents and physicians to encourage self-esteem and vitality among hemophilic boys and men.

Over the course of the 1950s, some experienced hemophilia specialists gravitated away from the tradition of highly restrictive preventative measures that seemed to encourage excessive forms of dependence in their patients. They gave consideration to the psychological and social effects of their actions and increasingly concerned themselves with the lasting effects of hemophilia and its treatment. As one orthopedist put it in 1957, the goal of hemophilia management was to raise hemophilic children into adults who had "learned to live with their affliction and protect their bodies." These mature patients had learned how to moderate their behaviors and, as a result, had "fewer hemorrhages."[59] In fact, medical advisers at the NHF and hemophilia management advocates began to embrace a more balanced approach to preventive care as the 1950s gave way to the more liberal 1960s.

Reflecting the patient's desire for some normalcy, advocates at the NHF actively involved themselves by the late 1950s in setting the standards for attitudes about "normal life," not just treatment regiments. Martin Rosenthal and Kenneth Brinkhous were not alone in hearing the pressing demands of patients and parent-leaders for some normalcy. The physicians and nurses treating hemophilia patients were also looking for ways to address the comprehensive needs of their patients because they too were hearing the same calls. One of these individuals was Dorothy White, a nurse who treated hemophilic boys on an outpatient basis in Rochester, New York's well-respected hemophilia clinic. She was also a leading advocate for families within the New York chapter of the NHF. In 1958 White authored an accessible treatment guide on hemophilia for parents and health professionals who were unfamiliar with the challenges faced at home by the hemophilic child and his family. With the support of Medical Director Martin Rosenthal, she published and distributed the NHF's first treatment guide for parents, a pamphlet entitled *Home Care of the Hemophilic*

Child. White's expressed goal was "to make known available comfort measures; simple treatments and aids for use when minor hemorrhage occurs; how best to handle the patient; to inform parents what measures can be taken to prevent deformity and to indicate the proper psychological approach to the problem."[60] On reviewing White's manual for the NHF, Brinkhous thought it "very valuable," telling Rosenthal that "Mrs. White appears to be well and soundly informed."[61] More importantly, the handbook clearly acknowledged not only that patients wanted some normalcy but that it was deliverable given contemporary resources and attitudes.

The therapeutic perspective outlined in *Home Care of the Hemophilic Child* recognized the critical role played by parents in the lives of hemophilic boys and called for a more active partnership between the hemophilia patient's family and physician. Recognizing the "widespread need . . . for knowledge of correct home care for the hemophilic child," White emphasized that hemophilia had "outgrown its previous classification of a rare disease" in recent years. Families did not need to suffer alone. Moreover, she stressed the advantages of "awakening . . . public interest" that allowed "young parents . . . to face the future" knowing that "hemophilia is more widely understood and more effectively treated than heretofore."[62] The home care guide emphasized the need for hemophilia parents to believe in the experts, to consult them, and to gain hope from the fact that they have been making progress toward more effective treatments.

Above all, *Home Care of the Hemophilic Child* recommended a "policy of 'normality within limits'" to parents raising a child with hemophilia. As White put it, "In every other respect he is a normal boy with a normal boy's desires. He should be encouraged to mix with other children and to make the most of his talents and aptitudes." Parents were thus warned of the dangers of protecting their son "like a hothouse plant," of the need to build up and maintain his general health, and of the necessity of remembering that the home is the child's "training ground." Moreover, in keeping with its policy of governance, the manual instructed parents to teach their hemophilic boy his limitations as soon as he is "old enough" and to cultivate behaviors that would allow him to adjust to his circumstances and "live as fully as possible with his handicap."[63] White and the NHF effectively told parents that their hemophilic son's psychology and social situation were of critical importance for his development into an adult male. "Normality within limits" became a must for the hemophilic child if he was ever going to make reasonable and independent choices about the risks of everyday life.

Despite their hemophilia, the patients and families described in the NHF's new *Home Care* manual were potentially normal in almost every respect. Indeed, what was expected of these boys was no less than what was expected of any other healthy boys in the United States. They were expected to become productive and fulfilled young men. It was a vision of the hemophilic child that resonated well with American hemophilia families in the late 1950s and early 1960s. One need only recall the unprecedented popularity of Dr. Benjamin Spock's *Common Sense Book of Baby and Child Care* (1946) in postwar America to understand what *Home Care of the Hemophilic Child* likely meant to the mothers and fathers of America's hemophilic sons.

Advocates of hemophilia management endorsed the "normality within limits" policy (ca. 1959–60) to promote confidence or self-worth among patients; and this typically meant that afflicted boys and men were encouraged to view themselves as normal, well-adjusted males. Thus, for instance, Dorothy White recommended that parents engage their sons in hobbies and sports fit for a "growing boy." Swimming, fishing, and boating were highly recommended. Basketball was not entirely forbidden if high top sneakers and knee-pads were worn. And there was value in allowing hemophilic boys to watch spectator sports like baseball or football that they could not play themselves. White encouraged most hobbies suitable for children, especially ones that might "occupy him happily when he must be alone." Model railroading and chess were recommended for their stimulating and absorbing natures. Chess could even be played "if the boy has no competition."[64] In fact, "normality within limits" would have been impossible for hemophilic boys and men of this era unless—as a rule—they felt comfortably masculine in their play as well as social interactions.

Of course, not every parent agreed with such putatively progressive recommendations for their child raising. In 1963, when Robert Massie advocated the importance of emotional as well as physical adjustment for the hemophilic child in the *Saturday Evening Post*, one mother from Massachusetts responded that she was willing to risk the emotional scarring of her son by keeping him out of school rather than expose him to "perilous classroom association" with other boys. She opined: "What earthly good is a child's emotional well-being . . . if that child, in adulthood is afflicted with stiff arms and legs?"[65]

The roles of fathers and mothers in the production of well-adjusted hemophiliacs faithfully mirrored many of the gender stereotypes in postwar American society. Advice literature often stressed the importance of the father's role as a stabilizing force within the hemophilic child's life. According to White, "The role of the father is most important. He can maintain a calmer and more practical attitude than the mother, who faces the problem twenty-four hours a day. At adolescence, particularly, the father's companionship becomes more than ever important. Overanxiety on the part of parents can not only prove destructive to the child, but may undermine the normal parent-child relationship."[66] This portrait also alludes to the pervasive image of the mother as someone whose presence threatened to overwhelm the hemophilic boy with feminine attention. Mothers, who were expected to spend their waking lives caring for their afflicted sons, were often cast—like the moms in Philip Wylie's infamous book *Generation of Vipers*—as overbearing, "feminizing" influences in their sons lives.[67] Hemophilia care advocates—Dorothy White included—tried to minimize the "momism" stereotype. But, their advice implicitly endorsed the common prejudice that hemophilic boys and men were frequently in danger of being emasculated.

White's call for "normality within limits," like much hemophilia advice of the era, called on parents and caretakers to achieve a balance in their hemophilic child's behaviors even as it reinforced the gender norms of the day. Another expert told the *New England Journal of Medicine* in 1965 that living with hemophilia "demands a delicate balance of sensible protection against injury while allowing the child enough independence to avoid his rebelling and incurring serious trauma in an attempt to 'prove' himself." Thus, as the 1950s gave way to the 1960s, a medical advice literature emerged instructing physicians on such topics as the "daredevil," risk-taking behavior in adolescent hemophiliacs as well as the necessity of well-considered male and female role modeling by parents.[68]

Given what went for normal male behavior in America during the 1950s and 1960s, there was a tendency among advocates to stress that the boys and men with the hemophilia were, as one treatment specialist observed a "tough group of people."[69] Pain was a serious problem for hemophilia patients. Even though bleeds or bruising could prove extremely painful or crippling, it was common for physicians to use narcotics sparingly with their bleeder patients because these painkillers carried the risk of addiction in the minds of many postwar Americans. That is why, in the 1940s, Frank Schnabel's pediatrician prepared his mother Mazie "to help her son endure long bouts of excruciating agony—without sedatives" because "once Frank began taking them, he would need them increasingly." By the 1950s, Frank was an adult raised in stoicism. As *Reader's Digest* put it, "Frank learned early that most unbearable pain can be borne." Hemophilia management in the postwar years was, in this sense, teaching afflicted boys that their "best chance of living" was to accept as much pain as they could bear.[70] Postwar advocates often expressed their ideas about normality in how they negotiated the gender issues raised by hemophilia and its management.

Where interested Americans thought along gendered lines about efforts to manage the lives of people with hemophilia, they were frequently expressing their ideas on the prospects of normality for such patients and families (fig. 4.1). In fact, the "normality within limits" concept captured this perspective from the standpoint of a patient's own experience and aspirations while invoking the progressive therapeutic idea that the hemophiliac required moderation in all things in order to thrive. Thus, even as progress-minded experts urged patients and their parents to set rational limits in their behaviors and expectations, they invoked a gendered rationale for such limits. They told parents, in effect, that their sickly boys could become relatively normal men, and the message resonated well with hemophilia patients and families.

An Extraordinary "Blood Brotherhood"

Invocations of normality—whether overt or coded in gendered norms—were the dominant way that advocates as well as medical professionals in the second half of the twentieth century framed the potential of hemophilia management for themselves and the American public. This framing, which often operated on an unconscious level, fit with the desires of many hemophilia patients and families to be at home in their own communities and to not feel as if their experiences were wholly different or apart from those of their neighbors. The paradox, of course, was that it usually took extraordinary measures for these patients and families to achieve what passed for ordinary within American society.

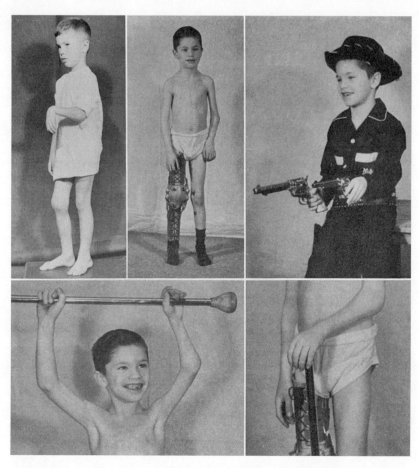

FIGURE 4.1. Orthopedic "Normalization" of the Hemophilic Child, Dr. Henry Jordan, 1958. *Source*: Henry H. Jordan, *Hemophilic Arthropathies* (Springfield, IL: Charles C Thomas Publisher, 1958), p. 103.

Newspapers, magazines, and radio were peppered during the 1950s and early 1960s with stories and appeals for voluntary blood donation that highlighted for advocates as well as the public what it really took for people with hemophilia (and other bleeding disorders) to thrive. In one widely reported case from January 1955, a thirty-one-year-old hemophilia patient named Willie Cook received 232 pints of whole blood and 168 pints of plasma while bleeding continuously for 422 hours at Duke Hospital in Durham, North Carolina. Included in this extraordinary effort to stem the tide of Cook's bleeding, Duke physicians flew in Cohn plasma fractions loaded with antihemophilic factor (clotting factor VIII) from Lansing, Michigan, and administered them to their patient intravenously. Yet even these well-regarded products proved insufficient to end Cook's hemorrhagic crisis. While setting a new record for the largest quantity of blood transfused to a single patient, this clinical intervention ended tragically with the patient's death.[71]

Cook's case points to a common problem faced by hemophilia patients in the two decades after World War II. Whether or not physicians were successful in stemming the tide of the hemophilia patient's bleeding, it was a given that the hemophilic patient would use disproportionate amounts of banked blood and blood products in the midst of being treated for hemorrhage.[72] Cook utilized more than usual, but the press frequently told of hemophilia cases that required a dozen units or more per visit. Added to the sheer amounts of blood involved were the details of the extraordinary efforts that certain communities made to insure that hemophiliacs in their midst had a fighting chance at life, including the mobilization of schoolchildren and teachers, fraternities and sororities, civic and business groups, unions and free trade associations, nuns and soldiers.[73] In spring 1956, for example, *Life* magazine profiled Jim Garner, a twenty-seven-year-old senior at San Francisco State University, who had a lifetime total of fourteen hundred transfusions and was then under the care of hemophilia expert Ted Spaet. Spaet was giving Garner a pint-a-day of plasma to help the young man get through college, and the photo-essay narrated how local student blood drives had raised more than 770 pints to shepherd Garner through his final year of college (fig. 4.2).[74] This *Life* portrait visually embodied the extraordinary means by which people with hemophilia achieved normality.

Of course, the extraordinary aspects of managing hemophilia in the two decades after World War II went well beyond what hematology and transfusion medicine could do. As told in this chapter, successful hemophilia management in the eyes of patients and families entailed the building of a hemophilia community across North America and the fashioning of new norms and expectations regarding people with hemophilia.

In breaking "the rules that were supposed to govern hemophiliacs," Frank Schnabel positioned himself as a role model within the emerging hemophilia community. His goal was to build recognition for hemophilia that

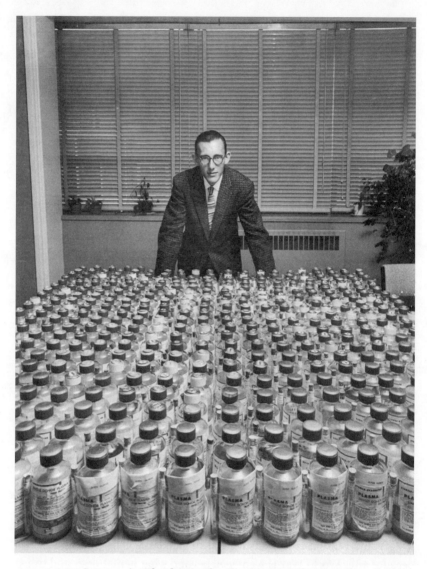

FIGURE 4.2. Community Blood Drive for Jim Garner, *Life*, 1956. The caption to this image read: "Jim Garner looking over 366 plasma bottles that are representing the number of daily transfusions he received during the past year." *Source*: "Daily Gift of Life: Student Blood Donors Keep Hemophiliac in School," *Life* 40 (April 30, 1956): 141. Reprinted with permission of Nat Farbman/Time & Life Pictures/Getty Images.

would improve services and opportunities for patients and their families. It was no mean feat. The need for collective action became apparent to him when he sought to fulfill his childhood dreams of travel (something hemophiliacs were usually barred from doing). After college at the University of Washington, this young American traveled to Los Angeles and England for graduate study and then to Costa Rica for work and adventure. When he finally settled in Montreal, Canada, in 1953, he soon realized that his braced legs might not go much further without good medical care. He had suffered a knee bleed that took the local hospital far too long to bring under control. By the time the physicians got around to transfusing him, his "knee was the size of a watermelon," he later recalled. Schnabel was disgusted that delayed care was the best that Canada's largest city could provide.[75]

Knowing that the United States had a Hemophilia Foundation, Schnabel created a Montreal chapter in 1953 and built relationships in the city between hematologists and patients. Schnabel soon transformed his Montreal hemophilia association into the Canadian Hemophilia Society, which by 1959 had chapters in Alberta, Ontario, and Quebec. Then in 1963, Schnabel founded the World Federation of Hemophilia (WFH), an organization that sought to coordinate hemophilia management advocacy and efforts around the world. Beginning with six founding members—hemophilia associations from Argentina, Australia, Belgium, Canada, France, and the United Kingdom—Schnabel built the WFH into the leading global association on all matters related to the management of bleeding disorders. The National Hemophilia Foundation joined the WFH as member association in 1965. Schnabel's advocacy efforts focused on bringing patients and families into sustained contact with the medical specialists who could help. Before Schnabel's achievement, a few experimental hematologists were the only people interested in hemophilia who traveled across national borders in the course of their work. Today, people with bleeding disorders travel the world with relative ease and can do so knowing the modern medical care is readily available in many countries and cities.

Families like the Henrys and the Schnabels had successfully devoted themselves to the production of ordinary lives through extraordinary efforts, and their efforts suggest just how hard fought the call of normality was. When Frank Schnabel died in 1987 at the age of sixty-one, he was remembered as having established a "great blood brotherhood" around the world "at great personal cost . . . for never having spared himself" when the need to travel on hemophilia business called.[76] The WFH's global "blood brotherhood" as well as hemophilia care advocacy in America were products of postwar society that embraced the idea of normality as a means for addressing the obvious gap between the promises of modern medicine and the difficult truth of living with hemophilia. Normality within limits proved achievable by the late 1950s. But as leading advocates demonstrated time and again in the two decades after World War II, it only came with extraordinary commitment.

CHAPTER FIVE

The Hemophiliac's Passport to Freedom

O n March 26, 1968, the front page of the *Wall Street Journal* featured the story of the seemingly miraculous recovery of Brooks Wright, a seven-year-old hemophilia patient from Greensboro, North Carolina. Wright had recently tumbled from a rocking chair onto his back. The fall produced continuous bleeding and swelling around Wright's spine that, in turn, incapacitated the nerves to his legs. Wright's doctors knew that his last serious bleed—two years earlier—had taken three days and more than nine transfusions of fresh plasma to stop. Believing that a comparable delay meant permanent paralysis for Wright, this time his doctors eschewed the conventional plasma transfusion in favor of an intravenous injection of a new high-potency, antihemophilic clotting factor concentrate.[1] Wright's bleeding stopped in a few hours. The swelling around his spinal cord diminished, and the feeling in his legs and his mobility soon returned. The headline read:

Hope for "Bleeders"

———

End to Hemophilia Peril
May Become Possible
With New Preparations

———

Bleeding Now Can Be Halted
With Injection of Clotting
Factor Missing in Victims

———

Baxter Lab Unveils a Drug

The story was of interest to the *Wall Street Journal* because Baxter Laboratories had announced plans to market its new antihemophilic (factor VIII) concentrate nationwide.[2] Dr. Kenneth Brinkhous, one of the concentrate's developers, explained to the *Journal* that "concentrates promise to revolutionize the management of serious bleeding in hemophilia patients."[3] More than a report about a promising new treatment, the story—and its claims—highlight a critical change in how entire generations of hemophilia patients and their families would conduct their lives and envision their future.

The 1960s witnessed the acceleration of a revolution in the experience of hemophilia—particularly in the hopes of hemophilia patients that they be regarded not as sickly and dependent but as normal persons, fully integrated into American society. As signaled by the promise of new treatments such as concentrated factor VIII, the revolution was partly technological. Yet, this transformation was driven not simply by medical and technical innovation. Properly understood, this revolution was social. Hemophilia patients were increasingly aware that they had a "manageable" disease. They had acquired a new and distinctive identity, in large part because of how Americans embraced medical and technical innovation in the two decades after World War II. Thus, as the 1950s gave way to the 1960s, a series of broad developments in American society helped patients and their families define for themselves what interests were critical to the "hemophiliac."

Beginning in the mid-1960s, clotting factor concentrates came to symbolize the patient's hopes for autonomy, fair treatment, and equal opportunity in an era when a growing number of Americans were embracing reform and activist government, a time when liberal legislation from the Civil Rights Act to Medicare/Medicaid highlighted nationwide inequalities between young and elderly, rich and poor, white and black. As one 1970 advertisement from Abbott Laboratories put it, concentrated factor VIII was the hemophilia patient's "passport to freedom."[4] On the one hand, this advertisement could be interpreted literally: with their new, portable treatments at their side, hemophilia patients could now travel, even to distant continents (fig. 5.1). Yet "freedom" presumably meant more than this to hemophilia patients in the United States. In many ways, the therapeutic developments of the 1960s were intended to deliver some much-needed

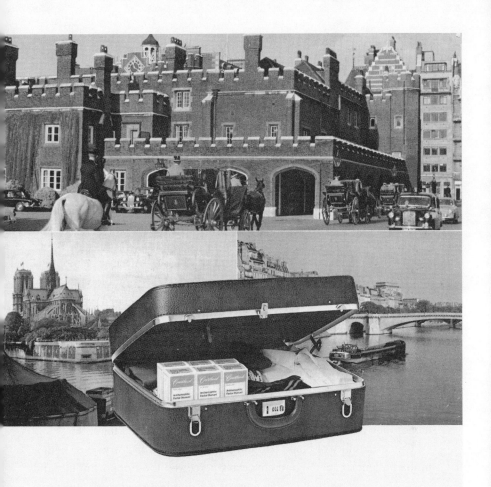

PASSPORT
TO FREEDOM
for the hemophiliac

FIGURE 5.1. "Passport to Freedom," 1970 Advertisement for Courtland's Factor VIII Concentrate (cover).

autonomy to hemophilia patients. They also promised to fulfill the postwar aspiration for normal lives, by removing some of the limits on such aspiration and easing the extraordinary burden that hemophilia management had always entailed for patients and families. Normalcy, in the progressive rhetoric of the era, was couched in terms of "freedom" for patients; but it remains an open question as to whether such talk really served the interests of greater autonomy for patients.

In 1970 hemophilia advocates were just beginning to portray clotting factor concentrates as a necessary rite of passage for boys and adolescent men with the bleeding disorder. Yet the growing availability of concentrates also highlighted a series of troubling issues—many of which were tied to access to treatment. The substantial biomedical and social developments of the 1960s raised vexing questions for the American hemophilia community in light of the nation's systems for delivering blood, plasma, and health care. How costly would the new treatments be? Would all hemophilia patients benefit? If not, who would? And, most critically, would the new concentrates help families escape the blood shortage problems that had been causing them so much distress since World War II? The answers to some of these questions would be worked out in the 1970s, but it was sixties-era developments in the science, industry, and delivery of blood products and medical services that prompted advocates of improved hemophilia management to view their prospects a little differently.

The availability of blood had long been a critical factor in how hemophilia patients, experts, and advocates perceived their opportunities and risks. However, with the emergence of clotting factor concentrates came important changes in the social and political economy surrounding blood. To many patients and families, it seemed by the late 1960s that their long-standing aspirations for some normalcy were finally coalescing with the hematologist's effort to bring the patient's bleeding disorder under control. The worry everyone shared by 1970 was how to deliver on this hematological achievement, given that it promised not only greater autonomy for patients but also considerable profit for the emerging biologics industry that was producing the new plasma concentrates. In essence, then, the American hemophilia community was beginning to realize that the patient's aspiration for more normalcy and autonomy was inextricably tied to blood plasma's emergence as a profitable commodity.

Living on Borrowed Blood

The "overriding concern" for parents of hemophiliacs during the 1950s and early 1960s was the difficulty of obtaining sufficient blood plasma for their sons.[5] The first-line treatment for hemophilic bleeding during this era was a transfusion of fresh or fresh-frozen plasma. The plasma usually came from voluntary blood donors. Thus, when journalist Robert Massie (himself the father of a hemophilic son) published a 1963 feature story on hemophilia for the *Saturday Evening Post*, the story's title —"They Live on Borrowed Blood"—gave top billing to this matter.[6] Often identified as "frequent" and "heavy" users of blood banks, hemophilia patients were more aware than most Americans that blood donation levels had dropped to dangerously low levels in many cities and towns.

Blood plasma shortages haunted parents of hemophilic children in the early 1960s because it seemed patently obvious that they were unnecessary. This was a generation of adults who could remember the society-wide blood drives of World War II and the Korean War and who widely embraced the concept that blood donation was the citizen's civic, if not patriotic duty. Yet throughout the 1950s, community blood drives, and the voluntary spirit that sustained them, had regularly failed to deliver supplies of blood that were adequate to the daily needs of either the nation as a whole or the American hemophilia population.

In the early 1960s, all indications suggested that the hemophiliac's blood supply problems were getting worse, not better. As one fund-raising pamphlet from the NHF put it in 1962, not only are there "an estimated 100,000 hemophilia patients in the United States today, putting up a determined fight to lead a normal constructive existence," but it now "takes 1,000,000 Americans, prepared to give blood each year, to meet the transfusion needs of the Nation's hemophilia patients."[7] As hemophilia seemed to be an increasingly manageable disease, the critical question for hemophiliacs and their families became whether Americans without connections to the hemophilia community were going to help them attain normal lives. Civic participation and a robust concept of citizenship lay at the heart of the struggle to increase levels of voluntary donation. Without it, advocates thought, the bleeding patient's need for affordable and timely blood services were unlikely to be met.

Not surprisingly, hemophilia was also playing a significant and increasingly visible role in debates about the blood supply. In March 1962, the *New York Times* ran a front-page story explaining the "worsening" nature of New York City's chronic blood shortage. City blood supplies were dwindling in the wake of increased demand for transfusions. The price of blood was rising. Voluntary blood donation was shrinking. To the dismay of some observers, for-profit blood banks and paid donors were flourishing as a result of the scarcity.[8] The 1962 blood shortage in New York City was judged so critical that one *Times* editorial chided New Yorkers for their apathy toward voluntary blood donation. "Blood," it said, "is too important a matter to permit the present disgraceful and dangerous situation to continue."[9] In covering New York City's 1962 blood shortage for the *Times*, David Binder explained that a significant portion of the new demand for blood in New York City stemmed from "advances in the treatment of hemophilia." He noted, for instance, that the Metropolitan chapter of the NHF supplied New York City's blood banks with the equivalent of "9,000 units" of blood plasma in 1962 to replace what the city's hemophilia population had used. This amount of blood plasma was three times greater than what patients had used in 1958. More importantly, the *Times* story explained that hemophilia patients and other transfusion patients in New York City were facing the possibility that their treatment needs might not be met in the current system. In fact, even though the city's blood banking establishment was insisting that "no one dies in New York for lack of blood," Binder pointed out that hemophilia patients and other heavy users felt the city's chronic blood shortage most acutely in the system, usually in the form of fees and replacement requirements.[10]

Binder's investigation uncovered a blood collection system plagued by apathy, waste, greed, confusion, and a general "lack of standards." He noted that volunteers gave less than half of the blood needed by the city's hospitals. To overcome shortages of volunteer blood in the years after World War II, for-profit blood banks began appearing in the United States in the 1950s. No one knew the true size of the nation's for-profit blood economy, but it was growing rapidly in New York City and other parts of the country. In 1956 volunteers in New York still delivered 60 percent of the city's blood. By 1962 less than half of the city's blood was donated voluntarily. Paid donation was becoming the norm, as paid blood donors were typically receiving payments of $5 to $200 per pint, depending on their blood type.[11]

There was legitimate cause for concern among proponents of the voluntary donor system. Indeed, the blood economy in the United States had evolved in the postwar era in ways that mirrored national debates about the delivery of health care to the entire nation: observers wondered if for-profit enterprises were the best means for delivering medical care to Americans or whether government programs were the better mechanism.

Concerns about profiteering in matters of blood arose rather predictably from the haphazard collection and distribution systems that had appeared in cities and towns throughout the United States in the 1950s. The majority of the nation's blood supplies had always come from voluntary sources. As told by historian Douglas Starr, "for-profit blood centers never constituted more than a fifth of the nation's collection capacity"; in the late 1950s, however, they became critically important suppliers in New York City where no less than 42 percent of the blood in hospitals came from paid donors. By 1962 the city's blood systems had proved to be among the nation's most chaotic and wasteful. More than 150 blood banks—commercial and nonprofit—operated in New York City without a uniform policy or centralized control.[12]

Across the nation, voluntary blood largely came from nonprofit blood banks affiliated with the American Red Cross or from various community blood banks. Hospitals—both private and public—also operated a large number of blood banks. They preferred voluntary blood for their patients and did not themselves pay donors. However, hospitals routinely discarded thousands of units of outdated blood when they could not use them in house. Thus, when their supplies of volunteer blood ran short (as often happened), hospitals relied on the smaller number of private blood centers whose supplies and profitability derived exclusively from paying donors. Because of these shortages, many commercial blood bankers were able to charge higher rates.

New York City's voluntary systems of blood banking were, by some accounts, being set up for failure by for-profit blood bankers. Waste, confusion, and poor standards in the citywide system exacerbated blood shortages, and critics of the commercial blood banks argued by 1962 that New Yorkers were experiencing such problems more acutely than other places because the city had too many "going concerns" in the blood business.[13] The assumption shared by many critics was that for-profit blood bankers had little incentive to improve coordination or standards precisely because they benefited from the haphazard, inefficient character of the existing system. In fact, some hemophilia advocates familiar with the situation in New York City reasoned that such problems were inherent to the practice of paying donors for blood or plasma because such problems were not endemic in Los Angeles, Rochester, and the state of Connecticut where voluntary systems still prevailed.[14]

Despite the unusual depth of New York City's blood shortage in 1962, the crisis there was not entirely unique. Blood profiteering, by many accounts, was emerging as a national problem that arose from faults in America's uncoordinated and increasingly neglected voluntary blood donation system. In 1964 such profiteering came before the U.S. Congress and was framed as an antitrust issue before the Senate Judiciary Committee, in part because the Federal Trade Commission (FTC) had drawn the scorn of Senator Edward V. Long (D-MO) for charging the Kansas City Hospital Association, the community blood bank of Kansas City, and several prominent pathologists for conspiracy to prevent the sale of blood by two commercial blood banks operating in Kansas City. Senator Long maintained that the "FTC was neither established to tamper with vital community services in the field of medicine, nor were the antitrust laws written to harass those nonprofit organizations that today supply most of the blood used in transfusions in the United States." He therefore proposed a bill (S. 2560) that exempted nonprofit blood bankers from the jurisdiction of federal antitrust laws. Consequently, much of the expert testimony during this congressional hearing on "Blood Banks and Antitrust Laws" valorized the nonprofit organization that promoted voluntary blood donation while highlighting the worst abuses of the for-profit blood trade. Long and his allies entered into the congressional record an array of reports from the American media suggesting that blood from paid donors was more likely to be tainted by hepatitis or other blood-borne diseases (although the issue of blood quality had no bearing on whether the activities of community blood banks should be exempted from the antitrust laws). The commercial blood banks were also accused of selling American hospitals outdated and mislabeled blood while simultaneously asserting their right to not accept the return of unused, blood from their consumers on the grounds that it was "outdated."[15] Long's bill did not make it out of committee. The testimony of blood bankers crumbled under interrogation by proponents of strong antitrust laws. Yet, in bringing the issue of blood profiteering before

Congress for the first time, the critics of commercial blood banks were making headway with their arguments that for-profit enterprises contributed to blood shortages by encouraging waste.[16]

News of blood shortages, poor blood quality, and failed efforts to remedy such problems in the early 1960s only served to heighten anxieties among patients and families about the adequacy of the nation's blood delivery system to meet their needs. Earlier, in the 1950s, blood bankers had implemented a blood credit system in many parts of the United States to help combat the problem of local blood shortages, but this remedy created problems of its own, especially for people with hemophilia. Blood credits prevented waste by redistributing supplies from overstocked blood banks to those with critical shortages. In theory, any blood bank—whether commercial or nonprofit—could receive credits for giving blood to another operation. Yet, by 1962, the system was encountering serious problems in many parts of the country. Without adequate coordination or oversight, it proved difficult for blood banks and hospitals to balance their books. There were frequent runs on the bank in New York City, for instance. As one blood bank administrator said, "Everyone wants to get paid off and then there isn't enough blood to go around."[17] Hemophilia patients and families were acutely aware of the faults in the blood system because they were asked to pay for its inefficiencies. Hospitals usually asked hemophilia patients to either pay a replacement fee for the blood they had "borrowed" or find donors for each unit of blood they had consumed. Because so many hemophilia patients were children, it usually was the task of their parents to round up family members, friends, co-workers, and even strangers to donate blood on behalf of their sons.

Robert Massie's 1963 hemophilia feature for the *Saturday Evening Post* described the burden of the existing blood economy on families with bleeding disorders, as well as innovative efforts among local NHF chapters to combat the problem. "The chapters," he said, "vary greatly in size and effectiveness, but their common bond is an overwhelming need for blood." He then described how the NHF's Metropolitan chapter (in New York City) was collecting five thousand blood donations a year to help make up for the nine thousand units of plasma its members used in 1962 and then paying cash directly to hospitals and blood banks for the units they could not collect themselves. Bernard Segal, the chapter's director, told Massie: "We expect all our hemophilia families to pay us back in blood or money, but we advance unlimited credit." The NHF did so because hospitals and blood banks did not extend unlimited credit to either the foundation or the patients and families that used their blood services. In extending blood credits to its members, therefore, the NHF was providing a critical service for patients whose blood plasma treatments were not guaranteed in this capitalist system.[18]

Even with the NHF working on their behalf, most hemophilia patients struggled to balance their blood accounts with their local hospitals in the early 1960s. Blood banks and hospitals were demanding more than ever. In their efforts to break even or make profits, blood bankers increasingly required patients to replace blood units in ratios of two, three, or even five to one. Although the Red Cross and other voluntary organizations pressed for the blood sector to adopt a one-to-one replacement ratio, hemophilia patients and their families in New York City increasingly found themselves at the mercy of a booming and increasingly commercialized blood economy.

The problems associated with this commercializing blood economy were exacerbated by the fact that many hemophilia patients lacked adequate health insurance during this era. Many health insurers did not cover blood or plasma, or they put caps on how much they would reimburse. Getting health insurance at all was also a problem. As Robert Massie knew from experience, "None of the medical insurance plans will pick up coverage of a hemophiliac unless the parent is in a company group."[19] In effect, these trends reinforced long-standing images of the hemophilia patient as both a poor financial risk and a burdensome charity case.

Thus, in the early 1960s, public discussions of hemophilia turned to the peculiar fate of chronic bleeders in the current blood supply system. For the first time, the "hemophiliac" was widely portrayed as an individual whose experience exemplified what problems ordinary citizens could expect if they utilized the nation's blood banking system. Binder's 1962 story for the *New York Times* was part of a wave of journalistic critiques of the blood economy that would be a catalyst for significant reforms in the 1970s.[20] Like later journalists and investigators, Binder drew on the experiences of the hemophilia community to explain to the public that any transfusion recipient could fall victim to this system that had burdened hemophilia patients with insurmountable debts. With the encouragement of advocates of improved hemophilia care, the media's discussion of blood shortages began highlighting the special burdens of the hemophiliac as a cautionary tale for anyone who might one day need transfusion services. For many advocates, such stories also became an occasion for them to remind the public that hemophilia patients were deserving of the nation's blood donation services; people with hemophilia were hard-working Americans and model citizens who invested in their communities, they argued.[21] Thus, in recounting the efforts of the Metropolitan chapter of the NHF to round up more than one hundred units of blood for one hemophilia patient, Bernard Segal wrote: "The National Hemophilia Foundation knows of other cities where the community takes responsibility for collecting and making available to all its members the blood and plasma that they may require."[22] Who, Segal implicitly asked, should be responsible for collecting blood for the community?

The apparent inability of American society to meet the expressed needs of people with chronic bleeding disorders was difficult for hemophilia patients and families to accept. Historians of the United States have sometimes characterized the late 1950s as an era in which national prosperity bred complacence among many Americans about their social responsibilities and duties as citizens. Hemophilia patients and their families had difficulty accepting any hints of civic disengagement because their own struggles for adequate blood supplies demanded more, not less civic-mindedness on the part of the American public. When John F. Kennedy rose to the presidency in 1960, he challenged Americans to affirm their social responsibilities and civic duties, to do more for their country.[23] The hemophilia community, like many other groups, had reason to take hope from this message. Yet, as it became clear by 1960 that voluntary blood donation was not keeping pace with demand, the sentiment among many hemophilia patients and their advocates was to value social responsibility, civic virtue, and the rights of citizenship all the more.

Hemophilia patients and their advocates had another problem besides decreased levels of voluntary blood donation in the early 1960s: the hemophilia community's continuous requests for blood plasma were having the unfortunate effect of highlighting the hemophilia patient's chronic dependency rather than his capacity for autonomy. Even sympathetic journalists such as Massie recounted stories of "panic-stricken" hemophiliac families begging to be allowed to keep extra plasma in their home freezers during the Cuban missile crisis.[24] Unfortunately, in the eyes of many Americans, such images of desperation usually made hemophilia patients and families seem more like victims in a rarely seen tragedy than otherwise creditable, "normal" subjects capable of autonomous pursuits. With growing demands for blood and shrinking donor rolls, patients and their advocates were being constantly reminded that American apathy for voluntary blood donation set people with hemophilia apart from the rest of society.

For people with hemophilia, blood supply problems therefore highlighted the problem of stigma as well as the need for a more robust commitment from Americans to civic virtues. Culturally speaking, hemophiliacs were still not considered "fit." Nothing drove this home as much as the fact that men with bleeding disorders were categorized as 4-F, unfit for military service. The government's rationale in excluding such men was to avoid the risks associated with bleeding disorders, especially the high cost of transfusion therapy. Even in cases where a man was visibly healthy and had no known history of bleeding, the Selective Service system called upon doctors to mark him 4-F when his blood test indicated even a mild or subclinical clotting abnormality. In times of war, these young men were fortunate sons perhaps, but the characterization of hemophiliacs as "unfit" made it easier for the public to think that people with hemophilia led diminished lives that were less worthy of social and economic investment. Thus, in the hemophilia community's calls for greater civic action and voluntary blood donation, advocates stressed that hemophilia patients were otherwise normal boys and men who deserved public support in their aspirations for normalcy.

Because hemophilia advocates embraced the empowering norms of American identity and citizenship that were the legacy of World War II's patriotic blood drives, they justifiably concluded amid the blood crises of the early 1960s that the effectiveness of hemophilia management would remain limited without sufficient public support for voluntary blood donation in the United States. Hemophilia advocates therefore began to play active roles in publicizing the unfairness and potential pitfalls of the current system. For example, as commercial blood banks and other for-profit enterprises flourished in the early 1960s, it became increasingly common to see hemophilia patients and their families and advocates exhorting their fellow Americans to consider the plight of the chronic bleeder as no different from that of the average blood consumer, if not citizen. More often than not, hemophilia patients and their families merely wanted John and Jane Public to give more freely of their blood.

Even as advocates were arguing for more robust voluntary blood donation in the 1960s, blood bankers and pharmaceutical companies invested successfully in technological solutions to the current blood shortages. Much of the innovation hinged, as it had immediately after World War II, on ways to use blood more efficiently, to break whole blood into its components so that the red cells, white cells, platelets, and plasma in each unit could be exploited for their particular therapeutic properties. Edwin Cohn's midcentury vision of blood component therapy would be fully realized in the mid-1960s. Not only were plasma fraction technologies fueling innovation in the area of experimental clotting factor concentrates, but physicians and surgeons were embracing plasma-derived resources of all kinds. Moreover, as evidenced by growing demand among hemophilia patients for plasma transfusions, medicine's increasing uses for blood and plasma was driving some of the blood shortages seen in the late 1950s and early 1960s. Blood bankers turned to a technology called plasmapheresis to help them meet the ever-increasing demand for plasma.

The use of plasmapheresis to increase supplies of source plasma for both medical and research uses was a novel, nontherapeutic use of an older therapeutic technique. Originally conceived in 1914 before transfusions were widely practicable, plasmapheresis allowed physicians to draw blood plasma from a patient for later therapeutic use on that same patient.[25] Later in the 1950s, experimental clinicians began successfully using it for the treatment of a variety of maladies. Then, in the 1960s, experimental hematologists adapted the technique to facilitate the availability of plasma and plasma products. The nontherapeutic application of plasmapheresis involved drawing whole blood from the donor, centrifuging it to separate the plasma, and reinfusing the red cells back into the donor. The drawn plasma could then be frozen, and later used for research, for the production of commercial plasma products, or to treat any patient who needed a plasma transfusion.

By 1965, innovative blood bankers and plasma fractionation companies were employing the then cumbersome process to meet their demands for raw plasma and plasma products because the real economic advantage of plasmapheresis was the frequency with which donors could give. Because plasma donors retained their red cells, they were not at immediate risk for anemia as donors of whole blood were. Without the risk of anemia, donors could now give as frequently as twice a week (rather than every two months): 104 times a year rather than 6.[26] Plasma donors were usually paid, ostensibly, for their inconvenience (because the process was uncomfortable and lasted approximately two hours). However, where plasmapheresis was available, family members and friends of hemophiliacs could now donate more frequently. If the plasma was not immediately used for their loved one, these friends and family members could help balance the patient's "blood credit" accounts and did so presumably without remuneration.[27]

The phrase "paid donor" nevertheless requires some explanation. After all, people who took payments in exchange for their plasma were not—in the strict sense—donors. There seems to have been a preference among nonprofit blood bankers and the for-profit plasma industry to retain the pretense of a "gift exchange" when it came to paying blood and plasma donors. In doing so, blood bankers built on the goodwill that people had acquired toward voluntary systems of blood donation. Yet there were no visible campaigns, in the 1960s or later, to inform the American public about the difference between paid and voluntary systems of "donation." Whether plasmapheresis centers operated for profit or as part of a nonprofit organization such as the American Red Cross, they advertised regularly in newspapers and other media for "plasma donors." Thus, those "donors" who subjected themselves to plasmapheresis regularly not only received payment but could maintain the illusion that their paid "work" was giftlike insofar as it benefited some patient or researcher.

Of course, the introduction of plasmapheresis as a technique for increasing source plasma was absolutely critical to the sustainability as well as profitability of the growing blood plasma industry. The pharmaceutical firms that engaged in the production of Cohn plasma fraction I in the 1940s and 1950s never profited from this investment. These companies produced plasma fractions for bleeding episodes on a small scale. They were supplying a limited amount of Cohn fraction I (rich in fibrinogen as well as factor VIII) at a very high cost to desperate patients with bleeding disorders. Single doses, for instance, cost fifty dollars or more. As Robert Cutter, president of Cutter Pharmaceuticals put it: "In the final analysis, we reached the only possible conclusion, deciding that because it was truly a life-saving product we could not in good conscience withhold it from those who needed it. . . . it was not up to us to decide that $50.00, $100.00, $200.00, or even more is too high a price for a man to pay to save his life or that of his wife or child."[28] Some product was also being sent to experimental physicians and biochemists, who in turn utilized it as a research tool in the hope that their investigations would reveal how to make a safe, effective, and truly profitable plasma concentrate for hemophilia and other bleeding disorders. Indeed, most of the research on plasma concentrates before 1964 took place in universities, largely at public expense. Then, as blood researchers outside of industry began to demonstrate the promise of new concentrates, these companies sought ways of securing large amounts of source plasma to ensure that concentrates could be delivered to consumers. Thus, for the pharmaceutical firms that were investing in the plasma fractionation industry, the application of plasmapheresis to the general problem of collecting and distributing plasma was an innovation that opened the way to plasma being the truly profitable commodity that Cohn foretold.

The blood economy grew dramatically after 1964 as clotting factor concentrates, plasmapheresis, and other innovations facilitated a split in how the blood business conducted its affairs. Hospitals and blood banks continued collecting whole blood as they had since World War II, but plasma, as Douglas Starr has eloquently described, suddenly "became an industrial affair." The collection business boomed as plasma centers appeared overnight to meet the demands of a pharmaceutical industry that was now investing heavily in what was now being called the *biologics* industry. Some of these plasma centers belonged to Armour, Cutter, and other drug firms that Cohn had enrolled in the 1940s to pioneer plasma fractionation and related ventures, but there were new companies as well that collected and sold raw plasma to the nation's biologics manufacturers. As Starr put it, "Like drilling rigs at an oil field, [plasma centers] sprouted wherever the resources seemed promising—around army bases and college campuses, in downtrodden neighborhoods, and along the Mexican-American border."[29]

Key barriers to a steady supply of plasma products now seemed surmountable, and the growing availability of source plasma in the late 1960s gave some potency to the commercial blood industry's claim that the way to solve blood shortages was to invest not only in technological innovation but also in commercial enterprises aimed at recruiting large numbers of plasma donors. Buttressing existing voluntary blood distribution systems, the argument went, was a lofty ideal that would certainly benefit the industry as well as consumers, but it had never proved sufficient to make plasma and its therapeutic derivatives widely available to the public. The credibility of this argument, despite growing claims of blood profiteering in the late 1960s, convinced Americans involved in the delivery of transfusion services that commercialism in the blood plasma economy was necessary, if not preferable. Indeed, as would become clear in the coming decade, the supply and consumption of plasma were increasingly subject to different rules from the handling of whole blood, despite the fact that Americans continued to view them as they had in the immediate post–World War II years: as a gift more than a commodity.

"Normal Lives Possible": The Social Origins of a Technological Revolution

As the media introduced clotting factor VIII concentrate to Americans (beginning in 1966 with the claim that this experimental therapy made "normal lives possible"), this innovation began to embody the promise of modern medicine for many people in the American hemophilia community.[30] However, this promising new treatment was only the most visible in a string of technological developments that would help empower efforts to manage hemophilia during the 1960s. If we are to understand the integral relationship between calls for normalcy, autonomy, and the embrace of clotting factor concentrates, the growing promise of hemophilia management must be understood in terms of the larger social and political economy of which this therapeutic enterprise was a part.

Hemophilia specialists, for example, were increasingly optimistic after 1965 about the community's ability to overcome persistent problems as they embraced the most recent fruits of hematological innovation. By 1970, even the blood shortage crises of the early 1960s were seen in a different light because most estimates now put total blood donation—paid and voluntary—above six million units a year, surpassing the previous peak collection years in World War II.[31] Commercial and voluntary efforts to boost blood and plasma donation in the late 1960s did a better job of alleviating the shortages that appeared from time to time. Plasma, in particular, was more readily available, as plasmapheresis facilitated the growth of the plasma industry. But the first commercial clotting factor concentrate and plasmapheresis were only two of three hematological innovations that facilitated radical change in how physicians managed hemophilia and patients experienced their medical condition. The first of these innovations to signal imminent progress in managing hemophilia was cryoprecipitate.

In the early 1960s, observers readily acknowledged that advances in treatment facilitated positive demographic changes within the hemophilia population, but few would have said that they expected the vast majority of hemophilia patients to live into middle and old age. Beginning in the 1965, however, experts as well as patients and their families began to embrace the likelihood that even boys with severe hemophilia could mature and grow old in the new therapeutic climate. The difference, by firsthand accounts, was the appearance of cryoprecipitate on the therapeutic scene. Cryoprecipitate rapidly accelerated the pace of medical progress in the next decade and made it abundantly clear that the life prospects for hemophilia patients would dramatically improve.

Cryoprecipitate was the 1964 invention of Stanford physiologist and coagulation specialist Judith Graham Pool.[32] She described cryoprecipitate as "an entirely new approach to the production of a concentrate" of antihemophilic clotting factor.[33] The novelty of Pool's approach grew out of her serendipitous observation in 1959 that frozen plasma when slowly thawed leaves behind a residue—"a cold-insoluble precipitate"—that is saturated with the clotting protein that most hemophilic plasma lacks (namely, factor VIII).[34] Pool was not the first clotting researcher to observe the phenomenon.[35] She was, however, the first to translate this observation into a simple and inexpensive technique for producing an effective plasma-derived concentrate (rich in factor VIII, fibrinogen, von Willebrand factor, and factor XIII) for the treatment of classical hemophilia and related bleeding disorders.[36] By 1964, many clotting researchers had found frozen plasma left behind a residue rich in clotting factor VIII when thawed. Pool's genius, then, was in transforming a known but largely understudied phenomenon into an effective therapy—the first truly potent plasma concentrate that could consistently halt bleeding in patients with severe hemophilia A.

The therapeutic concentrate made by Pool's cryoprecipitation technique became popularly known as cryo. As Pool envisioned it, virtually any health professional could make cryo from donated whole blood using items that were commonly found in most American hospitals and blood banks in the 1960s. All that was needed was the standard double plastic bag set for collecting and storing donated blood, a sodium citrate solution to keep the blood from clotting, a refrigerated centrifuge to spin the bags (and thereby separate the blood plasma from the red cells), a dry ice solution to freeze the plasma bag, a refrigerator to thaw the frozen plasma (and thereby collect the cold-insoluble precipitate in one of the sterile plastic bags), and a freezer to store the sterile bag containing the cryoprecipitate. Cryo could be stored for weeks (months even), then thawed and mixed with a citrated saline solution for transfusion into the patient. More importantly, cryo effectively arrested bleeding episodes in most hemophilia patients as it usually proved to be ten to fifteen times more potent than fresh plasma in treating classic hemophilia.[37]

The processing technique that Pool devised in 1964 also provided an elegant solution to a series of problems that had plagued hemophilia treatment since World War II. In the 1940s and 1950s, clinicians were frequently unable to arrest the bleeding of the hemophilia patient after transfusing what they hoped were adequate amounts of blood or plasma. As such, clinicians were often compelled to transfuse high volumes of plasma into the hemophilia patient, which risked overloading his circulatory system. In the postwar era, hemophilia patients succumbed to this complication relatively frequently. Like the less potent Cohn plasma fractions before it, cryo allowed patients to receive adequate amounts of antihemophilic clotting factor in a low-volume transfusion. The adoption of cryo as a routine treatment for hemophilia thus marked the end of risky high-volume transfusions for hemophilia patients. Cryo's measurable potency also ensured its use as a prophylactic measure on those occasions—such as a tooth extraction—when the hemophilia patient was expected to bleed. Only after 1965, for instance, did surgery on hemophilia patients become a widely practicable enterprise. Cryo therefore delivered a level of control over hemophilic bleeding that had long eluded clinicians.

The adaptability of Pool's technique to existing blood product delivery systems also ensured its rapid adoption as a standard hemophilia treatment. Cryo was typically made by blood banks because it could be constituted from single units of blood—unlike the traditional Cohn plasma fractions, which required multiple units of blood plasma and larger-scale production. Moreover, if a blood bank required large amounts of antihemophilic clotting factor (factor VIII), cryo could also be produced in larger—or "pooled"—batches using multiple bags of plasma. Indeed, as Pool had envisioned, blood banks profited from the by-products of her cryo-precipitation technique because it offered them a practical means for producing sterile bags full of packed red cells as well as plasma poor in certain clotting factors. That is, other therapeutic products such as red cells, albumin, and gamma globulin could be produced using the components of whole blood that were leftover from the cryoprecipitation process. It promised to reduce waste from spoilage even as it helped hematologists control hemophilic bleeds.

Given the delivery systems that were in place for hemophilia treatment in the mid-1960s, it became obvious to hematologists that Pool's cryoprecipitation technique was the simplest, most adaptable, and least expensive procedure for making a concentrated form of plasma rich in antihemophilic clotting factor. As such, Pool's cryoprecipitate discovery not only provided hemophilia doctors with a new and powerful way to control bleeding but also accelerated the ongoing efforts in universities, pharmaceutical firms, and the American Red Cross to develop even more potent clotting concentrates for hemophilia and other bleeding disorders. It was a technical innovation that made possible the commercial clotting factor concentrates that soon followed.

In fact, Pool's cryoprecipitate discovery was adaptable to each side of the evolving blood business. For the blood bankers whose plasma sources came entirely from whole blood donors (voluntary and paid), the breakthrough provided a truly effective concentrate for stopping hemophilic bleeding. For the pharmaceutical firms and commercial plasma centers that were just beginning to employ plasmapheresis and paid donors to raise the supply of plasma, Pool's innovation facilitated the industrial production of clotting factor concentrates by overcoming the problems that plagued older fractionation methods and clarifying the process by which new, more potent plasma products would be made.

Blood bankers became the main suppliers of cryo for patients because the therapeutic product could be produced on site using the donor blood that they acquired through their standard channels. And though commercial plasma centers sometimes acted as suppliers of source plasma to hospital and independent blood banks, the pharmaceutical industry chose not to invest in the manufacture of cryo for therapeutic use by patients. Economies of scale, along with the perishable nature of blood plasma, dictated that only products made from extremely large pools of plasma would be profitable. The industry adapted Pool's cryoprecipitation method to scale up the manufacture of its forthcoming AHF concentrates, but consumers of cryo were not considered a sufficiently profitable market to divert source plasma to the widespread production of both therapeutic products. As such, cryo—treatments made locally by blood and plasma bankers—did not become an "industrial" product in the sense that later concentrates of clotting factor would be. Even where it was made from pooled plasma, the scale of cryo-precipitate production was too small to generate much profit for its maker. Because of this economic rationale, the patient's experience of using cryo would be different from the experience of using the commercially manu-factured concentrates that began to appear on the market in the late 1960s.

Among hemophilia doctors, blood bankers, and plasma brokers, the per-ceived benefits of cryo paled in comparison to what hemophilia patients and families thought of this new treatment. Many hemophilia patients im-mediately recognized that cryo's capacity to control their bleeds provided them with a concrete opportunity for greater autonomy. Patients, parents, and guardians could administer it at home or school rather than always relying on hospitals or doctors for treatment. Moreover, just as the avail-ability of blood and plasma transfusions affected patients in the immedi-ate postwar era, cryo's advantages over older treatments also encouraged patients to embrace civic consciousness and activism. The experience of "Adam H.," a hemophilic college student in the 1960s, attests to this fact. As Adam told Susan Resnick, the discovery of cryo led to his participation in the NHF and his working out of the New York Blood Center to bring in donors in exchange for cryo: "I made a decision," he said, "that my future was too important to leave in the hands of others . . . and it [cryo] was a means of knowing what was going on and being able to be somewhat in control."[38] Cryo, Adam realized, would deliver him the kind of autonomy he desired only if he and other advocates transformed this technique for controlling bleeds into an occasion for a new, freer lifestyle. Yet, despite its limitations, cryo was definitely a breakthrough that he and other patients could capitalize upon.

For all of its wonders and genuine therapeutic advances, cryoprecipitate ultimately came to be seen by patients as well as hematologists as a tem-porary solution to the hemophiliac's problems, a mere "stepping-stone" on the way to developing a more satisfying therapeutic product, the commercial clotting factor concentrate.[39] Cryo delivered greater potency and reduced risk of complications from high-volume transfusion. And while cryo could be stored in a freezer or refrigerator in ways that allowed patients and families a great deal more mobility, it still had significant disadvantages. Most physicians in the 1960s proved unwilling to allow their patients or their parents to administer cryo outside the clinic. Patients in the middle of a bleed sometimes had to endure excruciating pain while waiting for this frozen plasma concentrate to be thawed and reconstituted for transfusion. More critically, consumers of cryo continued to face many of the same challenges they had when they relied wholly on blood banks for their whole blood and plasma transfusions, including dwindling numbers of voluntary blood donors and rising costs related to inefficiencies, poor standards, and shortages in the blood business.

Cryo was not yet the "insulin shot" that people with hemophilia and their physicians had occasionally dreamed of. It undoubtedly provided better control of bleeding and a freer lifestyle, but it did not deliver the degrees of autonomy that many patients and families ultimately sought in their aspiration for "normal lives." Indeed, leading hemophilia specialists were optimistic that they could do better by their patients by treating cryo as a critical step on the path toward a better concentrate. Clotting factor concentrates, as Brinkhous and other hematologists reportedly envisioned in the mid- to late 1960s, would one day soon be "so safe and stable" and so "convenient" that people with hemophilia "will be able to carry it around and inject themselves, into muscle, just as diabetics now do with insulin."[40]

The promise of clotting factor concentrates was embedded, of course, in an evolving therapeutic landscape that stretched back to the years immediately after World War II—the first time that plasma fractions were widely promoted as promising new treatments for hemophilia patients.[41] In proclaiming the appearance of Hyland's new factor VIII concentrate in March 1968, the *Wall Street Journal* pointed out that there had been two decades of "painstaking progress" that occasioned the current "step forward" and that ongoing research ensured that more potent concentrates were on the way. The only potential problems noted for the new treatment were supply and expense, because "the concentrates, which are in short supply now . . ., may cost a hemophilia patient about $6,000 a year."[42] Investors assumed, in other words, that hemophilia patients, advocates, and therapists would all embrace the new factor VIII concentrate despite its limitations or costs.

The public announcement of Hyland's concentrate in 1968 marked the first time in the United States that hemophilia patients were visibly treated as a truly promising consumer market. This excitement was manifest on Monday, March 26, as unexpectedly active and possibly insider trading of Baxter's stock occurred following unofficial reports that the company would soon introduce its concentrate. The New York Stock Exchange shut down trading on the stock until the following day, when Baxter formally announced federal approval to market Hyland's factor VIII concentrate nationally.[43] Although Baxter representatives declined to estimate the size of the potential market, the *Wall Street Journal* unofficially targeted potential sales of $3 million to $4 million within two years, with eventual annual sales of $15 million. Wall Street investors were obviously thrilled by the prospects of an "insulin-like" drug for hemophilia patients. Baxter's stock price enjoyed a healthy bump that week, and the company was enjoying record profits—including a 20 percent net increase in revenue in the second quarter of 1968—on the strength of sales of its three newest products: its AHF concentrates as well as an artificial kidney machine and a cholesterol-lowering drug.[44] Hemophilia had suddenly joined a growing number of chronic conditions that investors could view as a profit center. Consumers of clotting factor concentrates were now on the way to becoming a captive market.

The March 1968 announcement of the forthcoming availability of high-potency factor VIII concentrates raised the stakes of hemophilia management across the United States. Hyland/Baxter would soon have competition, as Cutter Laboratories, Abbott Laboratories, and other pharmaceutical firms won approval to sell their own clotting factor concentrates.[45] In 1970 Courtland Scientific Products (a division of Abbott Laboratories) claimed its new factor VIII concentrate was "packaged with all the necessary components for reconstitution and administration" and thus offered the hemophilia patient the "portability and convenience . . . to move about and enjoy a more normal life." It was sold, in short, as the "the hemophiliac's passport to freedom" (fig. 5.2).[46] Manufacturers planned to market the concentrate as a single-dose treatment that could be delivered intravenously by syringe on an outpatient, office, or emergency home treatment basis.[47] Yet Hyland

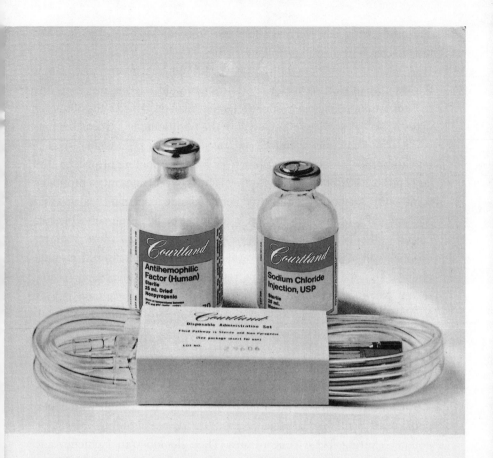

PASSPORT TO FREEDOM for the hemophiliac

Courtland's Antihemophilic Factor (Human), packaged with all the necessary components for reconstitution and administration, offers the hemophiliac the chance to travel with the assurance of care. The portability and convenience of Courtland's AHF allows him to move about and enjoy a more normal life.

For the physician, Courtland's AHF provides the specific advantages of a known assay, conserving the amount of AHF needed and providing optimum treatment. It assures rapid reduction of bleeding episodes and even allows the hemophiliac to be treated on an out-patient basis.

Cautions: Prepared from fresh pooled plasma. Despite careful selection of donors, plasma may contain the causative agent of viral hepatitis.
Contraindications: There are no known contraindications to Courtland Antihemophilic Factor (Human).
Package circular available on request.

Courtland Scientific Products,
Division of Abbott Laboratories.

Courtland

FIGURE 5.2. "Passport to Freedom," 1970 Advertisement for Courtland's Factor VIII Concentrate (pamphlet interior). Ad identifies both the promise of factor VIII concentrate ("a more normal life") and the peril (the risk of "viral hepatitis").

and other firms also worried about the "unpredictable" character of the raw materials needed to manufacture their new biologicals.

What many outsiders did not know, and industry insiders did, is that the viability of clotting factor concentrates would rely on increasing the scale of commercial plasma donation rather than drawing on the nonprofit plasmapheresis services offered within the traditional blood banking networks. The companies therefore embraced for-profit plasmapheresis centers and other less advertised practices (such as pooling of plasma into large production lots) to make clotting factor concentrates into a profitable commodity. Advocates of improved hemophilia management realized that the availability of the concentrates would hinge on large sources of plasma, but they initially assumed that source plasma would come more from traditional, voluntary supply lines rather than from the for-profit plasmapheresis centers on which plasma fractionation companies soon became reliant. Not knowing fully how blood bankers and the plasma industry were going to handle the need for an ever greater supply of "donor" plasma, advocates felt compelled in the late 1960s to redouble their efforts to promote voluntary donation.

Understandably, then, it was with heightened measures of both excitement and anxiety that the U.S. hemophilia community embraced clotting factor concentrates in the late 1960s. On the one hand, people with hemophilia were justifiably enthusiastic about the potential of these new high-potency clotting factor concentrates. Their demonstrated potency and promised convenience provided reasonable evidence that they could empower hemophilia patients in their search for greater autonomy. On the other hand, many participants and observers recognized that any effort to manage hemophilia using a plasma-derived product would encounter the blood shortages that now seemed inextricably woven into the fabric of American society.

News of Hyland's new factor VIII concentrate spread rapidly through the U.S. hemophilia community in the spring of 1968. The NHF, for example, obtained permission to reprint the *Wall Street Journal* story and promptly notified its chapters to "make maximum use of this excellent reprint by sending it to medical and professional individuals, community service agencies, medical institutions, major contributors, city, county and state officials, related agencies and, of course, individual members of the chapter."[48] Attached to its chapter bulletin was a press release and an additional statement prepared by Martin Rosenthal, the longtime medical director of the NHF. Both of these documents referred to Hyland's new product as a "superconcentrate."[49]

Rosenthal's press release announced the NHF's intention to pledge its resources and manpower to the task of expanded advocacy, "so that the benefits of a recently announced 'superconcentrate' of the AHF factor (factor VIII) . . . can be made available to all who require this therapy." His assessment of the new concentrate was even more blunt: "While the advent of this truly high potency therapy makes the future seem even brighter for the hemophilia patient, paradoxically it does impose new burdens upon all those who are involved in providing care for the hemophilia patient." Rosenthal warned, "An even greater effort will now have to go into blood donor recruitment in order to supply the raw material necessary for the manufacturer of this product." He was calling for "greater educational efforts" to facilitate blood and plasma collection and "proper usage" of the concentrates themselves.[50]

The "new burdens" described by Rosenthal in March 1968 were quite familiar to hemophilia patients and their advocates in the United States. Indeed, as I have been arguing, blood supply problems had first facilitated the need for such advocacy in the immediate postwar years. What was novel in 1968 did not derive from what the sudden availability of commercial concentrates required of chapter members but rather from that technology-driven logic that translated the appearance of Hyland's "superconcentrate" into a moral justification for its widespread use among hemophilia patients. It now "becomes imperative," as Rosenthal put it, "that nothing shall interrupt the future supply of this new material, as well as the materials of the future that may be even better."[51]

Sixties-era hematological innovations were undoubtedly the catalyst for a revolution in the management of hemophilia, but much of the meaningful change was actually transpiring on social and economic fronts. For instance, the availability of the first commercial factor VIII concentrate in 1968 did not immediately offer a solution for all hemophilia patients—an estimated 20 percent of the hemophilia population had to wait a couple of years longer for a commercial concentrate rich in clotting factor IX to appear on the market.[52] But most importantly, the emerging lifestyles for hemophilia patients associated with cryo, on the one hand, and commercial concentrates, on the other, represented different potential relationships to the evolving political economy of health surrounding consumers of blood and plasma.

It was hardly accidental, given this rapidly evolving political economy, that patients, therapists, and advocates expressed even greater optimism in the late 1960s about high-potency clotting factor concentrates than they did about cryo. Even though cryoprecipitate was a tremendous therapeutic advance beyond the traditional fresh plasma transfusions of the 1950s and early 1960s, plasma sources for cryo still largely came from the voluntary sources that blood banks preferred. As such, patients using cryo were still subject to many of the problems that had plagued the blood economy since World War II. Thus, even though cryo actually offered unprecedented levels of health and autonomy when it first appeared in 1965, it still tended to reinforce the old dependencies experienced by chronic consumers of blood and plasma products. In contrast to cryo, the widespread availability of commercial plasma products—along with the new industrializing economy that produced them—promised to alleviate the old problems even if they did not solve them per se.

Even though it was not immediately apparent to consumers, the future health of the hemophilia patient, circa 1968–70, was no longer as critically dependent on the health of the voluntary blood donation system as it had been. As clotting factor concentrates began to emerge on the market, patients could plausibly purchase their treatments from commercial suppliers. Above all, this meant that patients no longer had to rely solely on the civic-mindedness and goodwill of others to guarantee their path toward greater autonomy. A free-market solution was emerging that would make the viability of improving hemophilia care a largely commercial enterprise.

Hemophilia patients had been consumers of blood and plasma products since the late 1930s, but they had never been taken seriously as creditable blood consumers until various interests in American medicine and society capitalized on this array of hematological technologies. Thus, as the 1960s came to a close, hemophilia patients were being characterized as valuable customers for the first time (even though investors recognized that insurance companies and Medicaid, rather than the patients themselves, would foot the bill for many of these treatments). It was no longer assumed, as it had been since the advent of mass transfusion services, that hemophiliacs were essentially a losing financial proposition when it came to their chronic consumption of blood or plasma. In fact, as hinted by the evolution of the nation's blood economy (and particularly with the conversion of plasma products into an industrial affair), the hemophilia patient's status as a consumer rose dramatically with the viability of plasma as a profitable commodity.

Commercialization would have another, largely unarticulated benefit; it freed the chronic consumers of plasma products from much of the direct psychological and social trauma of finding their own blood supplies. Of course, consumers paid higher prices for the privilege of having private companies produce their plasma treatments. But the hidden virtue of commercial concentrates was that they simplified the problem of access to effective treatments for hemophilic bleeding by reducing the complex burden that hemophilia patients and families had long faced into a seemingly simple one of financial cost. Thus, it was no accident that the question that began to dominate discussions of hemophilia treatment with the announcement of the first commercial factor VIII concentrate was whether patients could afford such life-changing treatments.

The Emergence of Comprehensive Care

If melioristic rhetoric continued to valorize scientific and technological know-how in the 1960s, the more immediate progress experienced by hemophilia patients at the time came from physicians and experts whose perspectives on medical innovation had a decidedly social focus. Despite their differences, both cryo and concentrates offered a radical and decidedly positive transformation in the lifestyles that patients could engage. Yet, the hemophilia patient's life prospects hinged as much on the emergence of comprehensive care in this same era as it did from technological innovation. The positive changes promised by cryo and commercial concentrates could be realized only by making these therapies an integral part of the patient's lifestyle. And such integration required the intervention of experts and skilled care givers to provide patients and their families with the knowledge and resources they needed to render cryo and commercial concentrates into truly liberating, normalizing treatments. Most importantly, the comprehensive care movement for hemophilia patients recognized the changing demographics of the hemophilia community and embodied the social character of the changes that both physicians and patients would witness as the 1960s gave way to the 1970s.

Pediatrician Shelby Dietrich founded the first of many treatment clinics that devoted their resources to managing the comprehensive effects of hemophilia in patients at Los Angeles' Orthopaedic Hospital in the early 1960s. Dietrich had been introduced to the treatment of hemophilic boys when the small clinic she worked at in Los Angeles reached an agreement with the California Hemophilia Society to provide care to the local hemophilia patients (all of whom where children). She found the experience difficult, particularly because what little she initially knew about hemophilia was based on a few lessons in medical school and a movie she had seen about Rasputin. The therapeutic results were often dismal, blood products were difficult to acquire, and finances were always a problem. In 1962 Dietrich moved her practice to Orthopaedic Hospital at the recommendation of an orthopedist friend. Once there, she found that the hospital had a "top-notch" physical therapy program. She began to seek funding for her hemophilia patients through the U.S. Division of Vocational Rehabilitation, and in 1963 she received a grant. The rehabilitation program that she created featured a diversely trained staff, including another pediatrician, an orthopedist, a physical therapist, a social worker, a vocational counselor, a psychologist, and a dentist, all of whom consulted with one another as a "team" when treating the pediatric hemophilia patients at their clinic.[53]

By 1966, Dietrich had two hundred hemophilia patients from ages two to sixty years under her care, and they were being encouraged to "lead lives of normal physical activity." As she told a reporter for the *Los Angeles Times*, "the popular idea of what a hemophilia patient's life must be like—living in constant fear of bleeding to death from even a minor cut or bruise—is not true even without the new concentrated anti-hemophilic factor." At the time of her conversation with the reporter, Dietrich was testing one of Hyland's experimental batches of AHF concentrate. Yet, for Dietrich, these concentrates were not magic bullets to be used in isolation. Rather, she envisioned them as part of a comprehensive, ongoing treatment program that could realize the promise of commercial concentrates when they did became widely available. With both, she argued, "the contrast between the lives of a hemophilia patient and those of other people . . . will be non-existent."[54]

Dietrich's multidisciplinary team approach was innovative for another reason: it provided the hemophilic boy with every opportunity to grow into a normal man. As she told the reporter, "90% of hemophilic children grow to adulthood . . . and many doctors are as unaware of what advances are being made as is the general public. . . . hemophilia patients can do practically any kind of work anybody else can do." Dietrich noted that adult hemophilia patients in her clinic included "clerks, grocers, a physician, two physicists, salesmen and one or more examples of almost any kind of job one can think of." She added, "There are even motorcyclists and hot-rodders."[55] Her comments captured a more general demographic truth: the "adult hemophiliac" community was now emerging. At University Hospital in Cleveland, for example, Oscar Ratnoff and his colleagues had elevated the median life expectancy of their severe hemophilia patients to nearly forty years of age by 1960.[56] Patients with moderate and milder bleeding disorders were living well beyond that.

The rising visibility of the adult hemophilia patient was due, of course, to the fact that transfusion medicine had made it increasingly likely since World War II that people with severe bleeding disorders would survive childhood and adolescence. But additional progress in the 1960s was also due, in part, to the emergence of psychosocial perspectives on hemophilia. Social workers and psychiatrists had become increasingly interested in helping hemophilia patients achieve some normalcy in their lives, and their engagement with patients led them to question many of the common assumptions about hemophilia and its effects. During the late 1950s, for example, most people—including most physicians—assumed that adult hemophilia patients were unable to have a stable occupation because of severe physical limitations and impairments that these patients had accumulated over their lifetime. Therapists who worked closely with hemophilia patients began to scrutinize such assumptions and even question their normative status.

In the late 1950s, Alfred Katz, a social worker, served as the executive director of the New York Hemophilia Foundation, one of the larger chapters in the growing NHF; this leadership role exposed him to the full array of problems faced by people with hemophilia in the United States. His position in the NHF allowed him to articulate how the rehabilitation and vocational possibilities of the nation's hemophilia patients might best be realized. As Katz explained, the current model of management not only ignored how hemophilia affected the social and psychological well-being of families but also failed to address the critical fact that "the most general and pervasive psychosocial problem for . . . parents is to give their [hemophilic] child physical protection and, at the same time, avoid making him overdependent and eventually a psychological invalid."[57]

In 1959 Katz published "Some Psychosocial Problems in Hemophilia," an article aimed at professional social workers who "might encounter persons with this illness in the course of their work." As Katz saw it, the medical problems of the hemophilia patient were far better understood than its social and psychological aspects. During this era, a competent physician could pursue an effective course of action to control bleeding in the hemophilia patient, yet Katz found no comparable approach for treating the "severe problems" and "psychosocial stress" that the medical management of hemophilia imposed upon the patient and his family. The latter problem, he advised, "must be considered a serious health problem for those affected and for the community."[58]

Katz's emphasis on "psychosocial stress" brought the problems of the adult hemophilia patient into view for the growing community of hemophilia specialists. Katz's focus was on the life course of the typical hemophilia patient because he—like other advocates of the psychosocial approach—believed that this was the only way to ensure effective treatment for a chronic disease across the patient's lifetime. For instance, Katz observed that social service assistance was "rarely sought by or extended to adult [hemophilia] patients in hospitals or attending clinics." Instead, hospital social services for hemophilia patients were focusing their efforts on the problems of chronically ill children, measuring their overall fitness for "normal" childhood activities such as school or summer camp as well as their individual eligibility for assistance under Crippled Children's programs. "What has been lacking," he argued, "has been an approach to the hemophilia patient through a program of counseling and advisement that would start at an early age, and that would tend to forestall the development of some of the special problems that hemophilic adolescents and young men encounter." Katz reasoned that even though adult hemophilia patients oftentimes lacked stable employment, "the possibilities of their becoming self-maintaining were . . . excellent" when rehabilitative and vocational services were extended to them.[59]

The therapeutic concern for overdependency was not new. By the late 1950s, treatment specialists were consciously trying to combat invalidism by turning hemophilic boys into adolescents and men who had "learned to live with their affliction and protect their bodies."[60] However, as pioneers of the psychosocial perspective argued, medical specialists would never be able to succeed in their efforts without the aid of social services that could address the specific developmental needs of hemophilia patients and families. In support of this argument, Katz gave extensive attention to the case of Harry B., an adult hemophilia patient, whose "chronic passive dependency" was "not realistically related to his actual medical condition" but was rather the all-too-common outcome of an adolescence in which development had been arrested by this hemophilia patient's "awareness that he is afflicted by a chronic disease . . . that has multiple implications for marriage and parenthood roles and for the highly valued role of worker in our culture."[61] Such psychosocial perspectives on the hemophilia patient articulated the needs of the hemophilic boy-child in terms of the varied life experiences and outcomes of adult hemophilia patients.

Katz's psychosocial studies of hemophilia in the late 1950s and 1960s constitute a valuable source for understanding how the illness experience was evolving for people with bleeding disorders, particularly in relation to the patient's efforts to manage stigma. In 1958 Katz left his work at the New York chapter of the NHF and joined the faculty at the University of California in Los Angeles. Three years later, with support from UCLA and substantial outside funding from the Vocational Rehabilitation Administration of the U.S. Department of Health, Education, and Welfare, Katz began interviewing adult hemophilia patients across North America in a sweeping effort to determine how well adjusted (i.e., "normalized") adult hemophilia patients were and what factors promoted or limited their adjustment to society. The Katz study on the "Social and Vocational Adaptation of the Hemophiliac Adult," appeared in January 1965. Its findings were based on a cohort of 1,055 adult hemophilia patients in the United States and Canada; its stated purpose was "to present data on the vocational experience, vocational attitudes and adjustment of the adult hemophilia patient."[62] However, Katz's evidence went far beyond issues of vocational adaptation. It spoke to hemophilia's status in America as a "form of social deviance" and outlined the detrimental effects of its stigma on the life course of hemophilia patients. Through the eyes of America's adult hemophilia patients, Katz documented the social factors that would need to be overcome to ensure that younger generations of hemophilic boys could pass into manhood without suffering the disabling effects of hemophilia's stigmatization in American society.

The findings of this groundbreaking psychosocial study contained some well-known truths about the social circumstances among hemophilia patients as well as some surprising new ones, among them:

1. Most hemophilia patients now survive into at least middle age.
2. Hemophilia is not specific to any race, ethnic, or socioeconomic group.
3. Many hemophilia patients marry and have children.
4. Most hemophilia patients live with families.
5. Hemophilia patients have a broad range of educational achievement.
6. Many hemophilia patients can and do work steadily.
7. Small groups of hemophilia patients are sociopsychologically disabled.
8. Many hemophilia patients have active personal and social lives.[63]

Most critically, many of these basic truths of the hemophilia experience came not from Katz but from patients.

People with hemophilia valued normality. "What advice would you give to parents whose child has hemophilia?" was among the ninety-nine questions asked of patients. Most adult patients surveyed wanted parents to encourage "normality" above all else. When the majority of adult hemophilia patients expressed a preference for normality, they were undoubtedly saying that the "hemophilic child should be permitted great freedom of activity with few or no restrictions on his behavior."[64] This call for normality was consistent with what many parents and advocates had been stressing for the past decade. However, patients had their own take on the meanings of normality that revealed a generational divide between parents and patients. As one thirty-one-year-old patient and university graduate student wrote:

> The parents should learn proper care but protectiveness should be kept at an absolute minimum. Unfortunately present knowledge does not permit as casual an approach to the problem as say heart disease—yet we should strive for something like this—it is a fact to be lived with and

adjusted to. . . . The child has special needs due to hemophilia but he still has the ordinary human physical and emotional requirements and these should be cared for first.

Katz called this young man's remarks a "representative excerpt" that incorporated "many of the ideas most frequently expressed by respondents." Among the critical ideas expressed by this patient was his assertion of a need to be treated normally (as having "ordinary" as well as "special" needs). The man also asserted his "right" to manage information about himself that would be potentially stigmatizing and, tellingly, voiced significant skepticism of those parents and advocates in the NHF who presumed to speak for the needs of patients.

Parents should be cautioned against telling everybody about the child's condition—he has a right to his privacy as a person even as a child. I doubt much good is really accomplished by the parent telling everyone about their child's disease—in reality it probably satisfies parental needs for recognition. Certainly it doesn't contribute to the child's integrity or healthy individuation. I would also warn parents away from the hemophilia assocs. It's jargon but to the point to say they are "sob sisters." . . . I feel that the hemophilia patient needs help in working to an adult life that may or may not come otherwise. The results are rather obvious—the individual arrives at adulthood with nothing.

Such testimony by adult males with hemophilia challenged the existing therapeutic climate surrounding younger patients and began to shape therapeutic ideas and practices during the late 1960s and 1970s.[65] Normalcy, from this perspective, was meaningful to patients only if it was put in the service of the patient's autonomy.

The growth and maturation of North America's hemophilia population would command significant attention in the coming years, in part because of psychosocial studies of hemophilia patients as well as the spread of the comprehensive care model pioneered by Shelby Dietrich and others. In fact, the emerging literature on the psychosocial dimensions of hemophilia provides a particularly useful window into the evolving needs of a maturing population and the overall trajectory of hemophilia management. Psychosocial studies purportedly gave patients and advocates vital information on how to combat the stigma of hemophilia in American society. Such information facilitated the efforts of parents, therapists, and other advocates in shaping hemophilic boys into well-adjusted and productive men.

The Possibility of a "Daredevil Gesture"

Hematologist Martin Rosenthal had it right when he told the American hemophilia community in 1968 that concentrates made "the future seem even brighter" for people with hemophilia. Even before concentrates were widely available, the demographics of the American hemophilia population were changing for the better. By the late 1960s, the voice of the hemophilia community was no longer limited to parents speaking for their fragile sons; patients with hemophilia were increasingly teenagers or adults who could speak for themselves. Furthermore, the excitement and hype surrounding clotting factor concentrates promised that Americans in the coming generations would see no dramatic difference between the life of a hemophiliac and that of a healthy person. Thus, boys and men who experienced hemophilia in the transformative 1960s increasingly experienced themselves not as charity cases or dependents but as credibly normal people.

As if to alleviate any doubt that a hemophiliac could pass as credibly normal as concentrates became available in 1969–70, the American Broadcasting Corporation devoted an episode of its new television medical drama, *Marcus Welby, M.D.*, to the story of a wholesome, normal-looking teenager who proved relatively successful at hiding his hemophilia from his classmates in the new community where he has just moved. While sharing several themes in common with *Medic*'s portrait of hemophilia of 1954, this prime-time drama downplayed the details of state-of-the-art achievements in hemophilia treatment in order to highlight the psychosocial dynamics between patients, families, doctors, and friends that medical progress had occasioned by late 1960s. The episode, titled "The Daredevil Gesture" and directed by Steven Spielberg, showcased just how close boys and adolescents with hemophilia were to fulfilling their aspirations for both normalcy and autonomy. The tension in this medical drama issued from a simple truth: while treatment advances gave "bleeders" the appearance of normalcy, hemophilia was still a serious condition that required vigilance and maturity to negotiate.

The climactic scene in "The Daredevil Gesture" takes place on a geological field trip where the seventeen-year-old protagonist, Larry Bellows (Frank Webb), puts himself at risk for serious trauma. Typical of the episode's focus, the interpersonal dynamics leading up to this crucial scene are highlighted more than the technological medicine. Larry's mother initially forbids Larry to attend; then feeling guilty for always saying no, she tells Larry that he can go if Dr. Welby (Robert Young) approves. Welby, in turn, refuses to endorse Larry's participation, telling Larry that he is nearly an adult and thus leaving it up to the teenager to decide whether the risk of this field trip is worth it. Larry decides it is; but knowing his mom will disapprove, he forges her signature on a permission slip. Of course, when hiking the hills with his classmates the next day, Larry encounters trouble. His "daredevil gesture" is made fully apparent when a classmate falls into a ravine. Larry must climb down a precipitous cliff to save his friend. Larry gets there safely but initiates a knee bleed while carrying his mate back to the group's meeting point. Larry's heroism and injury together reveal his secret. Circumstances have forced him to self-identify as a "bleeder." In the closing scene after Larry's bleed is treated (a concentrate "injection" followed by a plasma transfusion), Dr. Welby reasserts his prescription to his young patient that everything will turn out well as long as Larry takes responsibility for himself and exercises good judgment when deciding which actions are reasonable risks and which are foolhardy. The treatment of hemophilia in this *Marcus Welby, M.D.* episode is thus a coming-of-age story on a couple of levels; it explicitly tells the tale of Larry's passage into a normal adult while implicitly relating the recent transformation of hemophilia into a chronic but manageable condition.[66]

Aspirations for personal autonomy as well as normality were blossoming not only among fictional hemophiliacs on television but among actual boys and adolescents with hemophilia in the late 1960s. In fact, the perspectives of adolescent and adult hemophilia patients who had grown up in the age of transfusions were extremely important in shaping the character of the American hemophilia community as new, more potent treatments for controlling bleeding became available after 1964. A different tone and style of advocacy were emerging as hemophilia patients increasingly began to contribute to debates about bleeding disorders and their management. Parents, who had long been the vocal center of the hemophilia community, were still dominant; but their attention was increasingly focused on the demands of their maturing sons by 1970. "Normality" was being advanced in terms of an autonomy that increasingly was being achieved by the rising number of adolescents and young adults with hemophilia: the freedom to travel, play sports, grow up, attend college, get married, have children and careers, and grow old. Finally, a growing variety of medical specialists were being enrolled into the cause. The hemophilia treatment community expanded beyond hematologists and orthopedists in the 1960s to include specialized nurses, psychiatrists, dentists, pediatricians, physical therapists, social workers, and a growing number of experts devoted to the social and vocational well-being of the hemophilia patient. Certainly, cryo and concentrate were critical to the maturation of the therapeutic landscape as well as the maturation of hemophilic boys into men, but for these boys and men the everyday focus was on lifestyle transformations that were presenting such diverse challenges to the patients themselves, their families, and their physicians.

Like the fictional Larry Bellows, adolescent and adult hemophiliacs were acutely aware that their place within American society was still a precarious one. Promises of normality, and the autonomy that presumably accompanied it, were still the ideal in 1969–70 rather than a reality for all patients. To be sure, the gap between the ideal and the real was closing, but it was still very evident on two fronts. First, people with hemophilia widely recognized that their situation had historically been one of dependence on parents and doctors and that their productivity and standing within society relied on both the ability of communities to accommodate their specific needs and their own capacity to conform to recognizable norms within their communities. While these features of the hemophilia patient's experience were not often made explicit in public discussions about hemophilia, the actions of adult hemophilia patients would increasingly impact the course of hemophilia advocacy in the coming decades. This is what "The Daredevil Gesture" made so clear; normalcy, argued Dr. Welby, was contingent on Larry's capacity to act maturely and honestly; it meant fitting into his community as well as taking well-calculated risks. The message was highlighted in the final scene of the television episode. Larry's two closest friends are visiting him at Dr. Welby's office to see if he is okay. Their presence tells Larry that they are not running away now that they know he is a hemophiliac. His friends tell him: "A bunch of us got together and decided we will try to help. . . . If ever you need it, we want to volunteer our blood." Larry gets the message: where gift-exchanges thrive, there will be no repeat of the childhood isolation that drove him to move to a new community and a new school in the first place. At least, that is how it played on television. In the real world, of course, commercialization was overtaking voluntary networks as clotting factor concentrates promised to become the hemophiliac's passport to freedom.

Second, the sense in which clotting factor concentrates made the future seem bright for real-life hematologists like Martin Rosenthal was briefly highlighted at the very end of "The Daredevil Gesture," again from the mouth of Dr. Welby. When one of Larry's classmates asks Dr. Welby if Larry needs to go to hospital, Welby says it won't be necessary. When she asks if Larry will be out of school for a while, the response is "He'll be there in the morning." It is at this point that Welby announces to Larry, friends, and family: "No, it look's like Larry's going to be one of the lucky ones. We're just waiting for word to start you on a new program . . . a kind of do-it-yourself deal. When we get the details, we'll talk about it. . . . We think it's going to mean a whole new life, for all of you." Here, the script was subtly referring to the prospects of hemophilia patients self-administering their own clotting factor concentrates—an allusion to an opportunity for ever-greater degrees of autonomy. The catch, of course, was that Larry would be "one of the lucky ones" who had access both to concentrates and to physicians who promoted self-administration. In 1969–70, the reality was that most hemophilia patients still had limited access to such resources; private insurance and existing government health services rarely, if ever, covered the direct costs of hemophilia care. The income of the Bellows family was never mentioned in "The Daredevil Gesture," yet the familial dynamics were. Larry's mother was raising him with the help of his older sister, and his father had abandoned the family after Larry's diagnosis; neither circumstance suggests the type of household that would actually qualify Larry as a "lucky" hemophiliac in 1970.

The gap between the ideal and reality of recent progress was acutely visible for many patients and families as the 1960s gave way to the 1970s. As a result, NHF leaders wanted members "poised and ready for a vigorous move forward" so that the organization could "crystallize the progress of the past and energize all future progress." The NHF even titled its annual report of 1970–71, *The Irony of Growth and Progress*, to break with "the tradition of rosy optimism and pie-in-the-sky-bye-'n-bye" found in the typical annual report. Advocates were stressing "a curious anomaly—

an irony—about the progress of the 1960's." Money and blood were in such short supply, they argued, that no amount of scientific progress would translate into real change for patients without strengthening the advocacy movement as whole.[67]

In fact, hemophilia was no longer just a concern for afflicted families, their physicians, and a few specialists as the sixties came to a close. With the introduction of increasingly potent plasma treatments for bleeding disorders, hemophilia attracted the growing interest of the pharmaceutical industry, insurance companies, and the government. These stakeholders in hemophilia management generated their own perspectives on how to ensure people with hemophilia got the treatments they needed. Yet, for everyone with a stake in improved hemophilia care, recent advances were beginning to highlight the limits and potential trade-offs of the long-promised revolution in hematological management of bleeding disorders. By 1970 the new freedoms embodied in concentrates posed hidden as well as visible challenges for patients, families, doctors, drug companies, and health providers. New risks as well as unprecedented opportunities were emerging. The potential rewards were higher, and no one wanted to look back.

CHAPTER SIX

Autonomy and Other Imperatives
of the Health Consumer

B etween 1969 and 1973, television stations in New York City and other
major markets regularly broadcast minute-long advertisements on
behalf of the National Hemophilia Foundation. In one award-winning
spot, a teenage boy named Eric Friedland stared into the camera and introduced himself: "I'm a hemophiliac. You know, the people who can't stop
bleeding." Eric then exclaimed, "Watch," as he pricked his finger, allowing
a drop of blood to emerge.

> Don't worry; it's nothing serious, but a year ago this could have put me
> in the hospital. Now my bleeding is under control because of a thing
> called clotting factor. I was lucky. They picked me to test it out on, and
> for a year I've been living and bleeding like a normal person. But get-
> ting it to the thousands of other people who need it is another story. It's
> very expensive.

The television ads pointed to the existence of clotting factor concentrates,
their high costs, and the fact that most hemophilia patients could not afford it. According to one ad, "100 hemophiliacs can afford the clotting factor, 100,000 can't." Each spot asked for donations and concluded with the
NHF's new campaign slogan, "We're so close, yet so far." Amazingly, the
foundation arranged for such television ads to run 150 times per month in
New York City over the span of four years. By comparison, ads publicizing
cancer awareness in the same market ran an average of six times per month.

To varying degrees, the NHF had always promoted awareness about the hemophilia patient's condition in the United States. Between 1969 and 1973, however, the foundation enacted a resolute commitment to publicity. It hired the state-of-the-art advertising firm Della Femina, Travisano & Partners (perhaps best known today for its 1972 singing cat Meow Mix commercial). In addition to the high-profile television ads, the NHF campaign slogan was prominently "featured on car cards, billboard posters, newspaper mats, radio . . . and all door-to-door drive materials." In fact, the "so close, yet so far" publicity campaign was the most visible sign yet that health for the hemophilia patient was a purchasable commodity that most patients could not afford.[1]

During the early 1970s, advocates turned to the high financial cost of commercial clotting factor concentrates and sought help from the federal government to make advanced hemophilia care more widely available to patients. They did this by arguing that hemophilia patients—despite their chronic dependency on plasma treatments—were a creditable group of health consumers, boys and men who were wholly capable of being productive Americans when given access to state-of-the-art medicine. Many hemophilia advocates initially interpreted the potency of clotting factor concentrates as justification that their high cost should be borne by the federal government; that people with hemophilia were especially deserving of public investment. Nathan Smith thought it appropriate in 1973 to describe the NHF as a "'consumers union' for hemophiliacs" and explained that the NHF's efforts to address the "economic implications" of hemophilia treatment required the advancement of legal protections as well as federal legislation. Citing a recent suit against the federal government that sought "equal protection under the law" for hemophiliacs, Smith argued that "financial inadequacy should not subject hemophiliacs, any more than heroin addicts (who presently receive methadone and other therapy without charge) to pain, misery, suffering, and permanent joint damage."[2] Smith was not alone in his outspoken advocacy efforts. He was among a group of leading adults with hemophilia who sought to transform clotting factor concentrates from a purchasable commodity into a "right."

As the hemophilia community struggled to publicize the dilemmas posed by the existence of clotting factor concentrates in the early 1970s, it joined a growing number of Americans who were concerned about the exploding costs of medical care and the necessity to distribute the fruits of medical innovation fairly. In this sense, the hemophilia patient's emergence as a health consumer allowed the disease to function as a site where concerned Americans could debate the role of the federal government in ensuring the health of its citizenry.

This chapter thus examines how hemophilia advocates in the 1970s capitalized on recent medical and social innovations in disease management and identifies the new opportunities and risks that emerged with the NHF's main political achievement. Although the NHF ultimately found it politically unwise to press the federal government to cover the direct costs of commercial clotting factor, leading advocates won a remarkable political victory in 1975 when the U.S. Congress approved a hemophilia bill that publicly subsidized comprehensive care programs for people with hemophilia across the nation. Here, the NHF's successful entrance into formal politics in the 1970s illustrates how advocates were able to leverage medical progress in managing bleeding disorders into concrete benefits that helped ensure greater health and autonomy for hemophilia patients. This success, I argue, hinged on the rising credibility of the claim that people with hemophilia were capable—through access to modern treatments—of leading "normal" lives. Thus, where advocates successfully argued the merit of public investments in people with hemophilia in the 1970s, they effectively convinced leading Americans that hemophilia patients were credibly normal people whose "inalienable" rights to life, liberty, and the pursuit of happiness should be affirmed by subsidizing hemophilia treatment centers across the nation.

Persons with hemophilia were certainly not alone in discovering that there was purchasing—and therefore political—power to be found in their status as health consumers. Many groups of Americans were discovering the implications of being health consumers in the 1970s. To a certain degree, then, hemophilia was one among several diseases that allowed Americans to grasp the politics of health consumption. Breast cancer, sickle cell disease, and end-stage kidney disease were other notable diseases that functioned as microcosms of the nation's political economy of health during this same time period.[3] However, what was unique about hemophilia was the way that this disease crystallized how physicians, policy experts, and politicians thought about blood's status as a public good. Nowhere was blood's ambiguous status as simultaneous commodity and gift more obvious. Everyone agreed that blood and its plasma derivatives were a national resource. Yet there was no consensus about how best to treat these resources or those who depended on them for their health.

In fact, as advocates portrayed access to modern hemophilia management as necessary for realizing their dreams of greater health and autonomy, they tied the plight of the hemophilia patient to concerns about the state of the nation's blood supply as well as to broader debates about funding medical care for all Americans. This strategy situated concerns about the availability of blood and plasma beside not only the hemophilia patient's long quest for greater health and autonomy but also a range of difficult governance issues. Thus, the question of the hemophiliac's right to normalcy sat alongside larger questions facing leading Americans about how to guarantee citizens access to modern medical care as well as how to ensure that everyone received prompt and effective blood services when they needed them.

Hemophilia as Microcosm: The Politics of Blood Consumption

The federal government had long overlooked people with hemophilia when, in the early 1970s, the American hemophilia community suddenly became the beneficiary of two political realities that the federal government could no longer ignore. First and foremost, people with hemophilia found some encouragement in the fact that prominent political leaders were taking the nation's "health care crisis" seriously. That crisis centered upon the problem of rising medical costs and the fact that many Americans—especially people with chronic illnesses—did not have adequate health insurance to cover their medical needs. Alongside calls for a national health care plan, the state of the U.S. blood supply was also emerging as a source of increased public concern. Blood and health policy experts identified the American hemophilia population as a critical bellwether for improving the nation's blood delivery system. This fact, coupled with the national debate about expanding the role of the federal government in delivering health care, put people with hemophilia in an unprecedented position—one that gave hemophilia advocates some leverage for advancing hemophilia care across the nation.

The NHF's publicity campaigns of the early 1970s therefore sought to capitalize on the hemophilia patient's new status as a creditable health consumer at a time when a growing number of Americans viewed access to modern medicine as a national priority. In the late 1960s, liberals and conservatives across the United States were employing the rhetoric of "crisis" when speaking about health care.[4] In their efforts to convince Americans that reforms beyond Medicare and Medicaid (which was established in 1965) were necessary, politicians as far removed from one another as Republican president Richard Nixon and Democratic senator Edward Kennedy acknowledged that the price of health care was skyrocketing beyond the reach of many Americans.

Growing numbers of Americans were in favor of some kind of national health insurance program by 1970; not surprisingly, there was considerable support for a national health insurance program among people with hemophilia. The appeal of universal health care was believed to be its capacity to cut costs while ensuring that most Americans—beyond just the elderly and the poor—would have access to existing medical care. Although President Nixon opposed national health insurance, he agreed that the nation faced a "massive crisis" in the area of health.[5] This position did not necessarily put Nixon at odds with those in his own party. Significant elements within both the Republican and Democratic parties wanted the nation to confront the rapidly escalating costs of Medicare and Medicaid, although some disagreed about the roles to be played by the public and private sectors in reforming the system. In fact, as Paul Starr has noted, traditional oppositions to a national health insurance plan were "so frail" by 1970 that even hospitals, the American Medical Association, and the insurance industry were making their own proposals for a national plan.[6] Indeed, the climate surrounding the health care "crisis" was characterized by widespread optimism and opportunism in the early 1970s. Despite suspicions on the right about unnecessary expansions in the role of the federal government, Americans largely assumed that reforms to the health care system were both politically necessary and achievable. Hemophilia patients and their advocates were among those Americans sharing this hopeful attitude.[7]

Between 1969 and 1973, advocates at the NHF operated on the assumption that the most pressing health problem confronting the nation's hemophilia patients was one with which most Americans could now identify: rising costs. Higher health care costs limited Americans' access to otherwise available treatment services. Moreover, now that Americans seemed interested in addressing health care problems on a national scale, there was a growing consensus within the American hemophilia community by 1969 that the NHF should not only publicize the plight of the nation's hemophilia patients but also "enter politics" on their behalf.[8]

Given the claims surrounding commercial clotting factor in the early 1970s, people with hemophilia were no longer content with just getting by. Not only did they see themselves as deserving of medical treatment as any other sick American, but they now had a potent means of "normalization" that argued for their inclusion into any federal effort to guarantee health care to its healthiest, most creditable citizens. Simply put, with the emergence of effective clotting factor replacement therapies, leading advocates reasoned that they were now in a position to persuade the federal government that it should provide hemophilia patients with the standard of care they needed to become autonomous and productive Americans.

Hemophilia was not the only disease gaining visibility. In the early 1970s, President Nixon initiated America's "war on cancer" and also devoted significant resources to research on sickle cell anemia in an effort to address charges that the federal government was ignoring the health care needs of African Americans. As described by Keith Wailoo, this focus on cancer and sickle cell anemia "reflected the Republican president's pragmatism and his often-used strategy of pre-empting liberal domestic initiatives by co-opting aspects of the left's agenda into his own, while also appeasing conservatives and speaking for the concerns of the 'silent majority.'" Nixon thus implemented a politically effective strategy of reducing the federal government's overall commitment to health, while establishing himself as a leader on the health care front.[9]

The Nixon administration's health policy proved paradoxical in its implications for many Americans confronting chronic illness, including the hemophilia community. On the one hand, it was committed to less overall funding for health and disease, with the resource pie becoming smaller for patients, physicians, and researchers alike; and, on the other hand, it gave the appearance that the federal government was willing to provide direct support to those diseases and conditions whose treatment could be proved meritorious. In supporting research for cancer and sickle cell anemia, the Nixon administration laid out the possibility that substantial federal support was still available for the research and treatment of politically creditable disease problems. Of course, in the interest of controlling costs and limiting government's involvement in "private" matters, the Nixon administration was more interested in delimiting such possibilities rather than realizing them. For advocacy groups such as the NHF, the practical effect of Nixon's health policy was that it promised a hearing of their plight while simultaneously ensuring that they would face intense competition for any government support they might seek. The burden was therefore placed on specific groups of health consumers to prove that their problems were worthy of federal support. In the 1970s, the hemophilia community thus found itself competing with other so-called categorical illness groups. They were pitted in a battle for recognition and federal support against people with diabetes, heart disease, muscular dystrophy, and cystic fibrosis (to name just a few).[10]

The NHF proved itself to be up to the challenge set forth by the Nixon administration. According to Susan Resnick, the foundation's ability to adapt to the era's political climate was the "hallmark" of its successful advocacy for comprehensive hemophilia treatment centers in the 1970s. Success blossomed from the awareness among NHF leaders of "what would sell and what would work" once Nixon emphasized health education as a way of cutting health care costs. Nixon's "philosophy of encouraging individual Americans to take responsibility for their own health," reasoned Resnick, ultimately "influence[d] the politically astute medical leaders of the hemophilia community as they planned for the future."[11]

Advocates of improved hemophilia management were primed for success in this fiscally conservative environment because they already had a ready-made argument in response to Nixon's calls for personal responsibility: they were now able to argue that Americans with hemophilia were capable of leading normal lives. In the 1970s, then, advocates effectively embraced the aspirations for normality that characterized the postwar hemophilia community in the United States to make the argument that they were a meritorious group of American citizens who took responsibility for their health and were productive members of society. The NHF thereby transformed an existing ethic among patients and their advocates into a potent rhetorical strategy for arguing that Americans with hemophilia deserved public support. In other words, the NHF's forays into politics yielded fruit in the 1970s precisely because advocates were working on fertile ground that proponents of hemophilia management had been cultivating for nearly two decades.

The hemophilia community also benefited in the early 1970s from another economic reality that the federal government could no longer ignore—they were being recognized as important consumers of plasma products at a time when the federal government was forced to address the unsustainable condition of the nation's blood supply. While the nation's health care crisis centered upon the problem of rising costs and their effect on health consumers in America, the blood supply crisis illustrated to observant Americans how rising costs could have a detrimental impact on the quality of medical services that everyone received. Here, the abnormality of the "hemophiliac"—in the form of his heavy reliance on plasma products—helped situate people with hemophilia as a significant constituency in any efforts to reform the nation's blood services complex.

The problems with the nation's blood resources had a long history by the early 1970s. We have seen how the voluntary donor system that supplied blood to many Americans during World War II had proved inadequate to rising demands in peacetime. Thus, when the commercial blood industry emerged in the United States in the late 1950s and early 1960s to meet growing demand, it generated considerable problems and controversy. Blood collected by commercial enterprises not only was more costly (because of low supply, high demand, and the expense of collection) but was also proving to be less safe. Especially after 1962, apprehensiveness about profiteering in the blood industry prompted expanded media coverage of questionable donor recruitment. Both commercial blood bankers and the maturing plasma fractionation industry were turning to paid donors, who reportedly had higher rates of hepatitis and other blood-borne infections than mainstream Americans who voluntarily donated their blood did.[12] By 1971 there was considerable public concern that government should do more to protect the nation's blood consumers from unreasonable costs and preventable risks. Intensifying media focus, growing public concern, and rising numbers of liability and tort cases surrounding blood banking and transfusion services required federal and state governments to confront the blood supply problem.

Beginning in the late 1960s, probing media coverage that highlighted the questionable quality of paid blood and plasma donors put people with hemophilia in a precarious position, even though the broader public discussion did not focus on them explicitly. Media exposés of "skid row" and incarcerated "donors" suggested to hemophilia specialists, blood bankers, government agencies, and pharmaceutical companies that heavy users of commercial blood or plasma were at higher risk for transfusion-related infections, yet shutting down such operations threatened to cut off the supplies of blood and plasma that were so essential to making hemophilia treatments.[13] Within the hemophilia community itself, the question of blood quality received little to no attention. The focus there was entirely consumed by the pressing need to make hemophilia care more effective and less burdensome by facilitating access to plasma treatments and bringing down the high costs of commercial concentrates.

Given the political climate surrounding both health care and blood in the early 1970s, the federal government could no longer effectively ignore the plight of Americans with hemophilia. In 1971 the Nixon administration responded to public concerns about the blood supply by turning to the expertise of the National Heart and Lung Institute (NHLI). Within the federal government, it was the responsibility of the National Blood Resources Program at the NHLI to make sure that adequate supplies of blood were available to meet the needs of the American people. Yet the government still lacked reliable information about blood banking activities in the United States. Describing the problem, hematologist Douglas Surgenor observed that all existing information about the nation's blood banking complex was "fragmentary, anecdotal and confused." In fact, the nation's blood economy had become so diverse and decentralized by the late 1960s that no one could say for sure how much blood was being collected, let alone what was being done with it.[14] To address the blood supply problem in a way that fit with the priorities of Nixon's health agenda, the NHLI devised a cost-effective strategy for dealing with the problem that situated the "hemophiliac" as a test of how well the blood delivery system was serving all Americans.

The NHLI's strategy thus placed hemophilia at the center of the nation's blood crisis. In the spring of 1971, the NHLI distributed a request for proposals (RFP) to conduct a "pilot study of blood banking and blood resources" in the United States.[15] That RFP asked specifically for proposals that could develop information about the blood needs of hemophilia patients. An advisory committee at the NHLI had decided, in other words, that knowledge about the treatment needs of the American hemophilia population would provide the government with actionable intelligence to address the nation's larger blood supply crisis.[16] The hematologists on the NHLI's advisory board focused their attention on the U.S. hemophilia community because they were well aware that hemophilia patients consumed more blood on average than any other kind of patient. The experts at the NHLI also knew that the Nixon administration would not tolerate a "long-term study conducted in isolation from the real or perceived program urgencies of today." A focused and short-term study of the hemophilia population therefore emerged as a politically wise investment for NHLI. As Surgenor put it, this approach averted the danger of becoming "an almost boundless enterprise in both time and expense."[17]

These political decisions had the immediate effect of transforming the hemophilia patient into a representative blood consumer. It did not matter that the hemophilia patient's consumption of blood was atypical, both in his reliance on plasma rather than whole blood and in the amounts he consumed. For NHLI, the uniquely high demand and usage of plasma by hemophiliacs highlighted both the strengths and weakness of the current blood services complex. Moreover, the NHLI's political decision to frame the treatment needs of the hemophilia population as a microcosm of the condition of the American blood consumer gave the hemophiliac's reputation as a chronic plasma user an unprecedented level of social and political significance.[18]

The NHLI published its three-volume *Blood Resource Studies* on June 30, 1972, thereby providing hemophilia patients, specialists, and other advocates with an empowering array of new information about their community and the blood economy on which they thrived. The first volume looked at blood supply and use, the second examined the regulatory issues surrounding blood, and the third focused specifically on the therapeutic climate surrounding hemophilia.[19] The NLHI's report promised to deliver an overview of the major participants in the "blood services complex," including the American National Red Cross, the American Association of Blood Banks, various commercial enterprises, and regulatory agencies. Additionally, it assessed the functional capacities of these organizations (for collecting, processing, and distributing blood) and accounted for how blood products, credits, and dollars "flowed" through this complex system.[20]

The expressed purpose of the NHLI's third volume, *Pilot Study of Hemophilia Treatment*, was to provide the federal government with a resource for understanding the supply and demand problems placed on the nation's blood services by a representative group of blood consumers, but hemophilia advocates found uses of their own for it—including the doctors among them. The *Pilot Study* became an authoritative source in the early 1970s for understanding the prevalence of hemophilia in the United States, the kinds of physicians treating hemophilia patients, and the therapeutic preferences and practices of physicians, treatment centers, and patients. Among the findings was confirmation that hemophilia patients were geographically concentrated in areas of the United States where specialized treatment was available. The Middle Atlantic region, which included New York, New Jersey, and Pennsylvania, thus accounted for about 26 percent of the nation's total hemophilia population. Concentrations of patients in California and New England correlated with the presence of treatment centers.[21] The study also documented that hemophilia patients whose condition was undertreated had difficulty attending school or holding jobs. Lastly, the study suggested that hemophilia patients with severe bleeding tendencies were prospering from access to cryoprecipitate and the newer commercial clotting factor concentrates. Such findings were extremely valuable to advocates at the NHF when they actively began lobbying for federal funding of hemophilia treatment in 1973.

But if these results were what leaders at the NHF might have expected, the NHLI *Pilot Study* also turned up more surprising results. The most interesting of these was the fact that among the 10,780 physicians treating hemophilia in 1970 and 1971, 60 percent had treated only one hemophilia patient. By contrast, 7 physicians who were associated with a handful of specialized hemophilia clinics reported treating more than one hundred patients each. The data clearly showed that even though most hemophilia patients received their treatment from physicians working in private practice, as much as 42 percent of the hemophilia population was being treated by a few specialists at hospitals that had devoted attention to comprehensive hemophilia care.

Equally stunning was the statistic that only 7 percent of treating physicians were trained as hematologists. It was widely assumed that the hematologists were playing a more prominent role in day-to-day hemophilia treatment, yet they ranked far behind internists and pediatricians, who together still represented 80 percent of the physicians treating the nation's hemophilia patients in 1970 and 1971.[22] This finding was politically relevant for many leading hemophilia specialists because they were less than enthused by the idea that most physicians learned what they knew about hemophilia from their residency training or continuing education;

it signified the need to secure greater resources for clinical training of hemophilia doctors.

A third surprise for many people in the hemophilia treatment community derived from the NHLI report's prevalence studies. Before 1972, estimates of the U.S. hemophilia population were generally said to range between 40,000 and 100,000 persons. In contrast, the *Pilot Study* found that there were only 25,499 persons in the United States who were treated between 1970 and 1971 as patients with a severe or moderate form of hemophilia. Among these hemophilia patients, 80 percent suffered from hemophilia A (factor VIII deficiency) while the other 20 percent suffered from hemophilia B (factor IX deficiency).[23] Moreover, although the data showed that there were considerably fewer hemophilia patients in the United States than expected, it also demonstrated that treatment of this population of chronic blood users would be financially burdensome given the fact that the vast majority of physicians were using cryoprecipitate or commercial clotting concentrates. Among its most important findings, then, the 1972 study concluded that the cost of episodic care for the nation's 25,000 hemophilia patients would range from a minimum of $31 million to as much as $80 million per year. The cost of prophylactic care—which called for regular infusions of plasma products to prevent any bleeding—was even higher, ranging from $58 million to $300 million.[24]

Finally, the NHLI *Pilot Study* unexpectedly reported a median age of 11.5 years for hemophilia patients (as compared to 26.8 years for normal males in the United States). As the report put it, "It is generally believed that the life expectancy of hemophilia patients has increased and that, with the advent of improved replacement therapy, the hemophilia patient [also] has [an] increased opportunity to lead a more normal life." Yet, on its surface, the study results suggested otherwise. A full 88 percent of the hemophilia patients treated in 1970 and 1971 were under the age of twenty-five. The NHLI report noted, however, that while shorter life-span might be a factor, the present numbers more likely reflected the fact that younger hemophilia patients might be seeking treatment to a greater extent than older patients. As the report explained further,

> Within the past 25 years, habits of seeking medical care in the U.S.
> have altered significantly, with more persons seeking medical care at
> a younger age. Younger persons tend to be more likely to actively seek

care, and are less content to simply live with illness or disability. Among the older generations, the norm of seeking medical attention is generally less well established. This may be particularly true among hemophiliacs, for whom effective treatment is a relatively recent development.[25]

Much of the information produced by the NHLI's study of hemophilia treatment was preliminary or ambiguous; it did not, for example, have adequate data on health insurance or the annual costs of plasma treatments to allow clear analysis of the financial burden on patients and families. The report nevertheless proved to be a critical resource for hemophilia care advocates as they argued for expanded public support after 1972.

The NHLI's *Pilot Study* was a telling snapshot of the U.S. hemophilia population in the early 1970s, one that allowed advocates to understand not only the current state of hemophilia management in America but also the possibilities for effective management if sufficient public resources were allocated. Unwittingly, the study also pointed beyond the hemophilia patient's status as a "representative" blood consumer to highlight the unusual demands that hemophilia patients placed on both the nation's health care delivery system and its blood services. Advocates had played a critical role in gathering information for the study and often read it as highlighting the unique needs of people with chronic bleeding disorders.

Although the NHLI commissioned its *Pilot Study* as a critical bellwether of the nation's blood resources and services, neither the authors of the report nor its readers brought attention to the fact that there was a growing and meaningful difference between the systems for delivering plasma and whole blood to American consumers. This omission is important, given that the NHLI *Pilot Study* actually showed how atypical these consumers of blood were. Unlike most blood transfusion recipients, hemophilia patients were almost exclusively using plasma products. In fact, among patients with classic hemophilia, treatment in the early 1970s was still equally divided between those using cryoprecipitate and those using the much heralded but more expensive dry concentrate of commercial factor VIII. Thus, a telling fact about hemophilia care—namely, that hemophilia patients were consuming increasingly large amounts of plasma from commercial rather than voluntary sources—remained largely invisible in the early 1970s.

In retrospect, there is great irony in the fact that the NHLI report neglected to investigate differences between chronic use of plasma products and occasional use of whole blood transfusions. After all, the Nixon administration commissioned the NHLI's *Blood Resource Studies* in response to persistent media coverage in the United States of the "bad blood" flowing through commercial blood banks and plasma farms, Richard Titmuss's controversial book *The Gift Relationship*, and growing concerns from public health advocates about high rates of post-transfusion hepatitis. The study was supposed to provide the federal government and the American public with information that would be helpful not only for assessing the nation's blood supply lines but also for evaluating the quality and safety of the nation's blood services. So it later proved quite unfortunate that the NHLI's *Blood Resources Studies* did not make information about post-transfusion complications and disease the subject of a more inquiry.

Thus, with respect to hemophilia treatment, the NHLI report did not seek out information on the relative risks of using pooled plasma products vis-à-vis the occasional plasma or whole blood transfusion or give any attention to cases of transfusion-related hepatitis among hemophiliacs. In the context of the times, these can be interpreted as reasonable oversights by hematologists because hemophilia specialists were focused on preventing deaths and debility from bleeding while post-transfusion hepatitis (where detected) was not usually considered an imminent threat to the patient. That said, the science of post-transfusion hepatitis was also advancing very quickly in the late 1960s and 1970s, in part, because hepatitis researchers made good use of the fact that blood serum drawn from hemophilia patients was very often loaded with hepatitis antibodies. The assumption among these hepatitis researchers was that exposure to blood-borne viruses was common among multiple-transfusion recipients—making the blood of hemophiliac a relatively unique research tool.[26]

Yet, public discussion of hemophilia in the 1970s continued to cast patients with bleeding disorders as it had since the late 1950s and early 1960s: as heavy users of the nation's overburdened voluntary blood delivery system. Thus, despite significant oversights in the NHLI's investigation of hemophilia treatment, the proximity of the hemophilia patient to debates about managing the nation's blood supply brought novel and seemingly positive attention to the hemophilia community at the very moment that many Americans were debating whether citizens had a "right" to medical care in the United States.

The existence of the NHLI *Pilot Study* helped advocates frame their arguments to the government and the public, as hope for a national health insurance program eventually collapsed between 1972 and 1974.[27] In effect, the NHLI blood studies gave hemophilia advocates an "independent" assessment of the state of hemophilia care in the United States, one that became an important tool in the NHF's efforts between 1973 and 1975 to convince the federal government and public to provide people with hemophilia some special consideration. This snapshot of America's hemophilia demographic thus confirmed for many observers that, where blood resources and modern management were made available, people with hemophilia were living credibly normal lives.

From "Home Care" to "Total Care"

The dramatic changes in hemophilia management that followed the introduction of cryoprecipitate and clotting factor concentrates have frequently been described as a therapeutic revolution. Physicians and the media have often cited concentrates themselves as the critical breakthrough. Yet comprehensive care deserves more credit for the dramatic improvements in the quality of life for people with hemophilia than any particular therapeutic product that emerged between 1964 and 1972. The new forms of normalcy and autonomy that cryo and commercial concentrates made possible could be realized only with attention to their integration into lives of patients and their families. Indeed, during the early 1970s there was significant debate about how pooled plasma products might best be used to achieve the goals of the hemophilia community. That debate centered, in many ways, on the practice of home transfusion care and the extent to which it was the best means for promoting normalcy for people with hemophilia. Moreover, the perceived successes of home care would increasingly influence efforts by the NHF to garner public and federal support for people with hemophilia.

The debate over home transfusion care began to garner greater attention outside the hemophilia treatment community with the release of NHLI's *Pilot Study* in 1972. To the surprise and chagrin of many hemophilia specialists, the report unearthed evidence that physicians had limited influence over the patients' behavior once the doctor extended the privilege of home transfusion care to them. Only 10 percent of the surveyed hemophilia population engaged in a "family infusion" or "self-administration" program that allowed it to use plasma products outside the clinic.[28] Most hemophilia doctors still had not widely endorsed home care because they wanted greater control of over treatment than what products and modes of administration patients should use. Yet, among the 10 percent of patients who did engage in home use, 74 percent believed they could "decide themselves if infusion is needed," and 72 percent acknowledged that they did not consult a physician "prior to infusion." These facts contrasted markedly with the assumptions of the pioneering hemophilia doctors who endorsed home care, most of whom said that their patients regularly consulted them (by phone) before and after any home infusion.[29] Thus, the NHLI study revealed that the proponents of home transfusion care apparently had less control over their patients' treatment than they had previously thought.

The portrait of home care that emerged from the NHLI's study suggested its limited significance for the nation's hemophilia patients (because only 10 percent of the patient population engaged in the practice by 1972), but home transfusion care would grow dramatically in the next decade as most hemophilia patients embraced the freedom to decide for themselves when to infuse their plasma concentrates.[30] The NHLI study did not explain why the experiences of hemophilia doctors and patients differed so markedly or have much to say about the diversity of experiences that underlay many of its findings. For instance, the study made little of the fact that almost all of the hemophilia patients who practiced home transfusion care in the early 1970s were adults. Nor did the study comment on the fact that home care was overwhelmingly preferred by that minority of experienced hemophilia specialists who treated large numbers of hemophilia patients. In short, the NHLI *Pilot Study* on hemophilia treatment assumed that home care was important to some doctors and patients, yet it failed to emphasize the profound and growing significance of this practice in the U.S. community.

In 1972 the practice of home care was gaining considerable momentum at major treatment centers in the United States. Home care was already available in Los Angeles, Boston, Chicago, Fort Worth, Nashville, the San

Francisco Bay area, and much of New York State and Pennsylvania.[31] Patients or their families were being trained by medical professionals in these areas to administer pooled plasma products at home. Thus, as long as the patient had a supply of cryoprecipitate or clotting factor concentrates at home in the freezer or refrigerator, it was only necessary for the patient to consult a physician by phone before treating a bleeding episode. This therapeutic approach had two noticeable advantages over the more typical outpatient treatments: the patient could avoid numerous trips to the clinic or hospital, and bleeds usually stopped before the secondary effects of bleeding manifested. For patients and families, home care meant not only greater independence from doctors and fewer costly visits to the hospital but also quick relief from the pain and crippling that accompanied bleeding episodes.

Doctors who promoted home transfusion care endorsed the practice because they believed that self-administration by the patient or a family member increased opportunities to treat bleeds early and often—reducing pain and the longer-term crippling effects of repeated joint bleeds. But a few aggressive hemophilia specialists in the early 1970s also saw home care as a bridge toward instituting programs for prophylactic treatment. Since the mid-1950s, experimental hematologists had envisioned therapeutic prophylaxis as the ultimate application of any concentrated clotting factor. The idea was that hemophilic bleeding could be entirely prevented if therapeutic levels of clotting factor could be maintained in the patient's circulation at all times. With the availability of cryo and concentrate in the late 1960s, a few enterprising hemophilia specialists began testing the concept in their patients—allowing their patients to infuse cryo or concentrate on a regular basis at home, independent of any actual bleeding symptoms. Home transfusion care was essential, in other words, to realizing the prophylactic ideal. The patients who enjoyed such aggressive episodic treatment in the home were still small in number in 1972 (only 4 percent of the patient population), yet their physicians claimed better outcomes than those found among patients with less aggressive home care, and far superior results to those seen in the 90 percent of patients who still received episodic treatment at their local hospital or doctor's office. The main problem, however, was that prophylactic treatment was incredibly expensive. The high cost of concentrate made it prohibitively expensive for patients to infuse when they were not experiencing actual symptoms.[32]

Pediatrician Jack Lazerson of Stanford Medical School was among those hemophilia doctors who believed that the era of prophylactic treatment had already arrived—despite the high cost of prophylaxis. The need to prevent bleeds before they became a problem was just too great. Lazerson saw, in other words, that hemophilia patients who needed physical therapy for lack of regular infusions became trapped in a vicious cycle: "When they bled, their joints were immobilized, muscle atrophy occurred as well as fibrosis and scarring of the joint. Physical therapy to overcome these problems in turn led to recurrence of bleeding. Eventually the boy with hemophilia became an orthopaedic patient whose cases or braces only increased muscle atrophy."[33] To break the cycle, Lazerson and other enthusiasts of aggressive home transfusion care advocated strategic uses of prophylaxis. Cryoprecipitate or clotting factor concentrate should be given before any physical therapy, they said, so that the patient could tolerate spells of relatively strenuous activity. Such treatment regimens improved the patient's range of motion, maintained muscle mass, and increased the chances that any necessary orthopedic surgery on the patient would be successful (because the patient would now have sufficient muscle mass to support reconstructed joints). Moreover, Lazerson recognized that patients with severe bleeding conditions often experienced extended periods of health over the course of their life. They therefore advised episodic care during these healthy periods (thus saving on the cost of treatment) and prophylactic care when the patient was expecting trauma or experiencing spells of illness or disability. Within the context of a home care setting, this strategy worked beautifully, he argued, for the majority of patients and families that could not also cover the full costs of their blood products. Yet, even for those specialists who promoted home care, they could not reasonably expect their patients to commit financially to prophylactic use of cryo or concentrate. The practicability of prophylactic care—like all forms of home transfusion care—entailed that the cost burden of plasma concentrates be shifted away from patients and their families.

Despite evidence in the early 1970s that home transfusion care was gaining popularity in the U.S. hemophilia community, there was still some considerable resistance to the practice from physicians who wanted to control the terms of treatment. When it became clear in 1972 that most patients using home care were not consulting their physicians before and after infusions, critics of home care had confirmation that patients could not be trusted to act in their own interest. Physicians, they argued, were best positioned to advise patients on the appropriate use of cryo or concentrate.

Proponents of home care, on the other hand, endorsed greater trust of patients by their physicians. One of the earliest and most outspoken proponents of home care was Anthony Britten, who in 1970 was a hematologist at Tufts University and president of the New England Hemophilia Association. In an editorial for the *New England Journal of Medicine*, entitled "A Little Freedom for the Hemophiliac," Britten explained that physicians would be well advised to trust the patient's own clinical judgment. He related the following anecdote.

A hemophilic patient of mine, 24 years old, recently told an interviewer, "I have for many years been able to discern quite accurately the severity of a hemorrhage and to determine whether or not an infusion will be necessary. The development of this skill has enabled me to function as an active partner to the physician." . . . This is not vain arrogance. It is true. In addition, he can infuse himself skillfully and without help. He knows exactly when he needs medical advice, which is rarely. With a supply of factor VIII and without a doctor, he can maintain good health.[34]

For Britten, hemophilia patients were "often better judges of their bleeding than physicians."[35]

The prompt for Britten's editorializing on the promise of home transfusion care was a peer-reviewed clinical study published in 1970 by Fred Rabiner and Margaret Telfer of Chicago's Michael Reese Hospital. This study, by two leading hemophilia specialists, lent support to the claim that home transfusion was already being successfully practiced. Rabiner and Telfer monitored the health status of eleven boys between the ages of two and sixteen and three adults with hemophilia A after the patients or their parents were taught how to administer concentrates for bleeding episodes. The study lasted eighteen months, during which time the group experienced 317 episodes of bleeding. Among the positive findings was the fact that these patients made a combined total of only sixteen visits to the clinic because of a bleed. Not surprisingly, these Chicago physicians observed that patients and their relatives were "enthusiastic because of the time saved, rapid relief of pain and opportunity of helping the patient within the family unit." The doctors also concluded that home transfusions were a "reasonable substitute" until the day when prophylactic therapy proved feasible. But most revealing, Rabiner and Telfer's article noted that they pursued their study only because of patient demands.[36]

Michael Reese Hospital served a group of about one hundred patients spread over a 150-mile radius. "Although Chicago has an excellent highway system," Rabiner and Telfer noted, "the necessity of traveling long distances with a bleeding patient, frequently in congested traffic," presented both patients and physicians with a real problem. As a remedy, these Chicago specialists asked physicians nearer to the patients to share the responsibility for their care. This turned out to be an impracticable solution because, as the authors noted, "physicians in small communities see very few such patients . . . have great difficulty maintaining the necessary 24-hour emergency service . . . [and many] do not appreciate the necessity for prompt [plasma] replacement therapy." They even found cases of local physicians withholding treatment "for a variety of fallacious and outmoded reasons." Then, Rabiner and Telfer noted that patients and families had little tolerance for uninformed physicians because they "know the value of adequate therapy, and will go to any lengths to get it."[37] There seemed little hope of relief until Rabiner heard about the ongoing practice of home transfusion care among families.

Rabiner learned about home care from an unusual family that had already become accustomed to the practice. As related in the article, "the solution was suggested to us from the experiences of a family with two hemophilic boys who had to move from a community, where the boys received good care, to an area with no hemophilia center." The story continued:

> After many frustrations they consulted their previous physician and described their plight. He taught the parents to transfuse their children with fresh-frozen plasma at home, and arranged to keep them supplied with sufficient plasma. When the family moved to Chicago, they joined the Michael Reese Hospital Clinic but continued home transfusion because of its many advantages. They finally told us their story, with great trepidation, fearing that we would ask them to discontinue what had become a way of life to them.

In fact, Rabiner and Telfer admitted that they had initially opposed the proposal. Only after a "cautious appraisal" of the idea did they ultimately conclude that a home transfusion program might work.

In their final summary, Rabiner and Telfer reasoned that home care worked effectively if five conditions were met. The patient and his family needed to be clearly informed of the risks involved. The transfusionist needed to demonstrate an ability to prepare the medication correctly and administer it intravenously. The patient should consult a physician by telephone before each transfusion and allow him to perform a follow-up examination. Finally, they demanded that the physician have "full control" of plasma products issued to patients. Even though the legal consultant at Michael Reese Hospital informed them that practitioners of experimental home dialysis had set a legal precedent for home transfusion care, Rabiner and Telfer still decided to exert as much control over self-administration of plasma products as possible.[38] The effect of their caution was more than rhetorical and was important to doctors who were initially skeptical about the practice of home transfusion care in the 1970s.

There was more to the story than Rabiner and Telfer admitted in their published article. Charles Abilgaard, a hemophilia specialist at Chicago's Children's Memorial Hospital, recalls that Rabiner first heard about home treatment via a network of mothers who secretly practiced it in Illinois. A nurse and mother of two hemophilic boys named Mrs. O'Brien initially told Rabiner. O'Brien had learned about the practice from a Mrs. J. Green, a mother of three hemophilic boys and five carrier daughters. Although Abilgaard was previously familiar with these families, he did not learn of their grass-roots promotion of self-transfusion until Rabiner and Telfer's 1970s study prompted a vivid memory. Abilgaard first met Mrs. Green in the mid-1960s while conducting a clinical study of one of Hyland's experimental concentrates at Children's Memorial. The Green boys were enrolled in his study and had always been something of a mystery to Abilgaard after he discovered that they had higher levels of factor VIII in their bloodstream than expected. Knowing that Mrs. Green's husband worked for the railroad and appeared to be absent much of the time, Abilgaard wondered how she managed to handle three sick sons along with five healthy daughters. He did not connect the boys' higher factor VIII levels with Mrs. Green's remarkable coping powers. On reading Rabiner and Telfer's paper, however, Abilgaard suddenly knew why the Greens fared so well. Mrs. Green not only had been treating her own sons at home with transfusions of fresh-frozen plasma but had also been teaching other patients and families how to do home transfusion care.[39]

While it is hard to say who "invented" home transfusion care, an open-minded physician at the Carter Blood Center in Fort Worth, Texas, appears to have been pivotal in promoting it.[40] During the late 1950s, Mrs. Green's sons were patients of Richard Halden Jr. at the Carter Center. Halden encouraged parents of his pediatric patients to learn how to administer plasma transfusions on their own beginning in 1960. He defied established medical convention, which prohibited parents and patients from self-administration of blood, because he felt it was a good way for these beleaguered parents to keep their hemophilic sons out of the hospital. When the Greens moved to Chicago in 1961, Mrs. Green complained to Halden that her sons could not get the same kind of care there. Because Mrs. Green's burden was particularly heavy and because she had long ago demonstrated her expertise at handling blood products, Halden agreed to supply her with the transfusion materials. As told by Susan Resnick, "Mrs. Green would take the long railroad trip back and forth to Texas to get the necessary supplies and would secretly infuse her sons in the back bedroom."[41] The secrecy continued until Mrs. Green began to share her knowledge with a few other mothers in the Chicago area. By 1969, Richard Halden was openly publicizing his previously hidden advocacy of home transfusion care.[42]

Between 1968 and 1972, the practice of home transfusions began to grow, largely driven by patient demands. Among those physicians who initially opposed it were some who worried that home care would undermine their authority as well as the quality of their patients' care. When presented with evidence of the significant advantages offered by home care, opponents attempted to explain them away. In November 1972 the respected blood clotting expert Oscar Ratnoff listened to Margaret Telfer give a conference paper on home care. After Dr. Telfer noted that two-thirds of her patients faced a minimum drive of thirty minutes to get to Michael Reese Hospital, Ratnoff countered that home care may be suitable in some regions of the country but not others. He wryly noted:

> This is an important sociologic difference from one community to the next, which may explain the popularity of home treatment in different areas. For example, in California where Dr. Kasper's patients get home transfusions, they'd practically die of old age before getting to the Los Angeles Orthopedic Hospital. In Cleveland [where he worked], most

patients live within 30 minutes of the hospital. There is a feeling of comfort on the part of the mothers to know that every episode is looked at by a physician. . . . Dr. Britten raises the issue [in his *New England Journal* editorial] that patients have something emotional to gain by assuming control, but sometimes we must balance that with an innate conservatism; in certain situations, perhaps the doctor should retain control.[43]

In the late 1950s, Oscar Ratnoff was among the most open-minded and progressive hemophilia doctors in the United States. At that time, his approach to treatment was considered liberal. Fifteen years later, his advocacy of the same practice could be labeled "innate conservatism." Such was the shifting landscape of hemophilia management that by the mid-1970s even the most conservative of hemophilia specialists would acclimate themselves to the advantages of home transfusion care.

Home care of hemophilia was more widely embraced between 1973 and 1975 when more physicians realized that it might mean expanded resources for them and their patients. In 1973 the NHF was lobbying aggressively in the U.S. Congress for federal support of modern hemophilia treatment. In this context, a small group of hemophilia treatment experts working through the NHF devised a plan that envisioned home care as part of a multidisciplinary "team" approach, the goal of which was to provide for the "total care of the hemophilia patient."[44] Louis Aledort, one of the new co-medical directors of the NHF, embraced the concept of home transfusion care monitored by a nationwide system of hemophilia treatment centers, each having a team of diversely trained health professionals who were devoted to seeing hemophilia as a disease deserving comprehensive care. This vision of hemophilia care, which reflected the demands of patients and families (as leading hemophilia doctors understood it), proved useful in advancing the NHF's demands for public recognition and support.

The NHF's Lobbying Experience and Legislative Success

In ways that both helped and hindered the advocacy of improved hemophilia management, the forces constituting the political climate surrounding health and disease in the early 1970s often expanded far beyond what the Nixon administration, the Democratic majority in Congress, or any politician recognized. The 1960s had witnessed numerous advances in medicine that were changing how society managed disease problems and that called on policy makers and politicians to make tough decisions with far-reaching but uncertain impact. In fact, the politics of chronic disease management underwent a radical change in the United States on October 30, 1972, when President Nixon signed a congressional bill extending Medicare coverage to patients who suffered from chronic kidney failure. In effect, the new law provided these chronically ill patients with coverage for their hemodialysis treatments, in both the clinic and the home. This kidney disease legislation was a historic entitlement in that it represented the first time that the federal government agreed to fund treatment for Americans with a specific medical diagnosis. To borrow a phrase from nephrologist and historian Steven Peitzman, this federal legislation transformed the experience of chronic renal disease into a wholly new kind of entity. For dialysis patients and their doctors, kidney failure became a "disease of entitlement" known by the administrative term "end-stage renal disease" (ESRD).[45] This development had serious implications for the lobbying efforts of hemophilia care advocates in the United States because its passage heightened awareness on Capitol Hill that Congress had opened the door to the various disease and patient advocacy groups.

Those patients, physicians, and politicians who supported the Medicare entitlement for ESRD in 1972 declared it a great success. It did not take long, however, before Washington insiders realized that the cost of this kidney dialysis program was going to be burdensome to the federal government. When the bill became law, the attention of both pundits and public was focused on the presidential election of 1972. In the rush to garner the goodwill of voters, neither Nixon nor Congress had waited until accurate assessments of the program's costs were available. The size and growth of the dialysis patient population had been grossly underestimated, prompting the *New York Times* to run an editorial in January 1973 about the burdensome costs of the ESRD entitlement. The editorial was titled "Medicarelessness" and brought significant public and political scrutiny to the imprudence of federal support for the treatment of particular medical diagnoses.[46]

In autumn 1973, ten months after Washington insiders had digested the news of the government's "medicarelessness" regarding dialysis treatments, the NHF was preparing to lobby the U.S. Congress for legislation that would provide some much-needed relief to American hemophilia patients. Advocates at the NHF faced the difficult task of convincing a Congress that was now reluctant to entitle anyone else to a specific form of treatment. The political climate was not open, in other words, to arguments from the hemophilia community that called upon the government to pay directly for clotting factor concentrates. Still, NHF lobbyists recognized the dialysis hearings as a model for their own lobbying effort. One of most memorable events of the ESRD deliberations was the testimony of Shep Glazer, a forty-three-year-old chronic renal patient who underwent dialysis on the floor of the House. While Glazer's staged treatment may not have proved critical to the actual passing of the bill, it set a cultural precedent for emotionally charged medical testimony within the halls of Congress.[47] Hemophilia care advocates would soon exploit this opening.

On November 15, 1973, a diverse group of advocates met before the Senate Committee on Labor and Public Welfare to provide testimony in favor of legislation that would fund programs for diagnosis and treatment of hemophilia in the United States. Eric and Louis Friedland were among those testifying before Congress. Eric was one of the two hemophilic boys featured in the NHF's television spots during the early 1970s introduced at the beginning of this chapter. Lou Friedland was not only Eric's father but also the driving force behind the NHF's publicity campaigns of the era. As NHF chairman, Lou Friedland was spending much of his free time advocating for hemophilia patients. His position within the media—as president of MCA-TV in New York City—gave him considerable pull and influence. Over time, he had become friends with Senator Harrison Williams, a Democrat from New Jersey who was also chair of the Senate's Committee on Labor and Public Welfare.

In 1973 Senator Williams proposed a bill that sought to fund hemophilia treatment on a nationwide basis through an amendment to the Public Health Service Act. Jacob Javits, the well-known Republican senator from New York, co-sponsored the bill. The language of the bill noted the significant number of Americans "who suffer from hemophilia," the existence of "the technology and the skill to enable such individuals to lead productive lives," and "the high cost of such technology and skills [that] are in most cases denying the benefits of such advances to individuals suffering from hemophilia."[48] The technological ethos that had long driven progress in hemophilia care was making its first public appearance before the U.S. Congress, here cast by advocates as an imperative for public support of their treatments.

The public testimony for the hemophilia bill before the Senate Committee on Labor and Public Welfare was highly organized and well orchestrated. Between the introduction of Senator Williams's hemophilia bill on March 23 and the hearing on November 15, the NHF had already approached a number of key senators using a professional lobbyist as well as a grass-roots campaign by many hemophilia patients, families, doctors, and nurses. As planned, the hemophilia community's testimony before congressional lawmakers would make a favorable impression.

The hearing itself opened with an apology. The NHF had arranged for a large group of patients, families, and supporters to attend the event. The Senate Subcommittee was taken by surprise at the crowded room. "We apologize," said Senator Williams. "We frankly did not know that that we should have engaged the auditorium for this hearing."[49] After submitting prepared statements by himself and Senator Robert Dole of Kansas, Williams turned to the first of three panels. The first panel included personal testimony from Roy Heavner (NHF president and an adult hemophilia patient), Louis Friedland (NHF chairman), Louis Aledort (NHF medical director and hematologist at New York's Mount Sinai Hospital), Kathryn Earnshaw (NHF executive director who formerly worked for the Cystic Fibrosis Foundation), and Elizabeth Wincott (a social worker from Mount Sinai Hospital).[50] There was even testimony from Sam Huff (a former professional football player for the Washington Redskins) whose interest in raising awareness about hemophilia stretched back to childhood nosebleeds that doctors had misdiagnosed as hemophilia.

Of these testimonies, the most memorable was that of Lou Friedland, who spoke on behalf of "fathers of hemophilia patients, and especially for those fathers whose sons have not escaped the chains of this disease as my son has done." This father's testimony left little doubt that the hemophilic boy's life could become "normal" if the proper resources were mobilized on his behalf. Lou Friedland began by describing the crippling effects of hemophilia on his son, how Eric had to live "in leather braces day and night, never . . . [taking] them off." Then, to demonstrate the transformed nature of Eric's disability, Lou produced a golf bag along with the leather and metal braces that Eric had worn during his first seventeen years.

> You can barely lift these braces [indicating] when you put them all into a golf bag. Nothing moves. The joints do not move. Sometimes they do if you are lucky. The muscle and everything else deteriorate pretty badly. Eric wore these on his legs much of his young life. He wore these on his arms. He wore this on his hand very often. Eric is a hell of a pianist now and doesn't need any of this.

Lou Friedland spoke of the amazing changes that occurred in Eric's life once his son became "one of the first kids to be put on a daily routine of self-infusion."

> Every day of his life he gives himself an infusion of a white substance about the size of a quarter cube of sugar and makes an injection into the vein. He protects himself for that day so he can live a very normal life during that day. I will tell you this for Eric, he has lived one heck of a normal life for the last four and half years. The first year out, he drove 40,000 miles, and as I say "straight up." He went to Europe, traveled all over Europe. He has a girlfriend, and she is a remarkable gal. He also attends Harvard as a student.

Friedland's testimony then turned into that of a wealthy man, one who recognized that his family was fortunate to enjoy the privilege of what medicine could now offer the hemophilic child.

> Here is a boy who . . . now lives a perfectly normal existence, and then some. But it costs us $60 a day. He takes two vials, $30 a vial, and he should really take four or five, but that is another question. It costs up to $22,000 a year.
>
> What about the other kids? How many kids do we know—I pay for it, by the way—how many kids do you know in this world whose parents could give them $22,000 a year, or even the $5,000 or $6,000 a year which on average we think it would take to take care of most of the hemophiliacs.

Senators Williams and Peter Dominick of Colorado immediately questioned Lou Friedland about the braces. They were both amazed to see that

Eric, who had worn these braces until he was seventeen, no longer needed them.[51] Before yielding the floor, Friedland explained in detail how the use of clotting factor concentrates had allowed Eric to build up his physique and become mobile.

For a while, the panel turned to dryer, mostly expert testimony regarding the costs and character of hemophilia treatment. Ever the showman, however, Friedland took the podium before the morning session could end. This time he played the four TV spots, which were the most visible aspect of the NHF's publicity campaign between 1969 and 1973. Friedland described the TV spots as "probably the most widely played ... spots in television history for this type of thing. They brought our cause to thousands of cab drivers and college professors everywhere." More importantly, the TV spots reiterated his point that the potential for transforming the lives of hemophilic boys was already available to "rich kids" like Eric. He pointed to his healthy twenty-two-year-old son at the back of the room, saying "he is prettier now," and then showed the audience a TV spot which depicted Eric four and a half years earlier. On the screen, everyone got a glimpse of a paler, thinner, and noticeably less vibrant young man.[52]

The day's second panel returned to the potential of contemporary technologies to free hemophilic boys in the United States from the tragedy of bleeding and crippling. Orthopedist Marvin Gilbert opened the session with expert testimony describing why hemophilia patients should no longer have to endure damaged joints, weakened muscles, crutches, bulky braces, wheelchairs, or risky surgical procedures. "These complications should not occur," he said, "... and in the future the orthopedic surgeon should not be called upon to treat deformity, but only to set the wrist fracture or tape the sprained ankle of the 'normal hemophiliac' who has biked to school, played ball in the playground, and achieved in the classroom on an equal footing with all his classmates." Gilbert told the audience that Senator Williams's hemophilia bill represented an opportunity to "'straighten the [hemophilic] child' before he is bent." Here, Gilbert was alluding to his earlier definition of orthopedics as the practice of straightening the child. (He counseled the senators on Greek, pointing out that *ortho* means "straight" and *pedia* means "child.")[53]

The testimony then turned again to the patients themselves; this time, there were echoes of Glazer's 1971 dialysis testimony. At the request of Senator Williams, Eric Friedland approached the podium carrying his clotting factor concentrate and transfusion apparatus. The teenager's expertise at self-administration was evident to everyone in the room as he infused the clotting factor while speaking about changes in his life, the ease and simplicity of the procedure, and his hope that "no hemophiliac will ever have to be deprived of the treatment." Eric's comments lasted less than three minutes, during which time he completed his transfusion.[54] Another father-and-son team, Frank Backer and Frank Jr., then explained what life was like for the hemophilic family before home care was possible. Frank Sr. emphasized the "miraculous results" that followed his son's treatment following ninety-four consecutive days of treatment at New York City's Mount Sinai Hospital: "The greatest thrill of my life was when I saw him upright after about 9½ years in wheelchairs."[55] Home care and prophylaxis expert Jack Lazerson followed that testimony. The rest of the day witnessed testimony from an alternating series of patients, long-embattled parents, and treatment and blood experts. One of the experts was Warren Jewett, a biomedical engineer whose company, Bio-Gant Corp., was working to improve the yield of active clotting factor in plasma fractionation processes. Jewett was not only a leading advocate but a healthy and accomplished adult with hemophilia. Such testimony provided further evidence that hemophilic boys could develop into productive men and citizens if they received good care and were encouraged to flourish. In short, this 1973 public hearing was a wildly successful, historic event for hemophilia patients in the United States. To this day, federal lawmakers in Congress regard hemophilia advocates as one of the best-organized "categorical illness" groups in the country.

As evidenced at the hearing, the days of braced and wheelchair-bound hemophilic boys were being replaced in the 1970s with images of "normal," healthy-looking boys. Images of adolescent and adult hemophilia patients were also becoming more common. The NHF's "poster children" looked noticeably different in the 1970s than they did in the 1950s and early 1960s. There were fewer atrophied or "bent" limbs, and adolescent patients no longer looked like "cripples." In fact, in many cases, it was not evident from images alone that the boys and young men were sick or disabled at all.[56]

It was 1975 before Americans with hemophilia began to see the actual benefits of the NHF's well-orchestrated political campaign. Despite the success of the November 1973 hearing, Congress did not pass its hemophilia bill subsidizing hemophilia care until December 1974.[57] Despite significant support for the legislation in Congress, President Gerald Ford twice vetoed bills that contained provisions for grants to the nation's growing network of hemophilia treatment centers (HTCs) before signing it into law on July 29, 1975. Ford was not opposed to hemophilia treatment per se; he objected to costly health programs more generally, and the hemophilia legislation had been folded into a larger bill containing formula grants for "expensive" health services that included community mental health services, family planning programs, and home health services, disease control, and rape prevention. In its first opportunity to contest Ford's decision, the U.S. Congress overturned his veto by comfortable margins, in part so that HTCs throughout the country could receive the federal funding sought by the NHF.

Reflecting hemophilia's reputation as an affliction of boys, the Office of Maternal and Child Health administered the new federal resources for hemophilia care by building upon existing program resources for "crippled children." The new hemophilia law also provided grants to HTCs to hire support staff and facilitate comprehensive care programs, but it did not subsidize the costs of treatment directly. Following the backlash against the earlier ESRD entitlement, hemophilia advocates had wisely chosen not to push for a direct entitlement to clotting factor concentrates. But the new federal support was undoubtedly an unprecedented victory for hemophilia advocacy. In the form of new or expanded hemophilia treatment centers, patients gained access to comprehensive care services that had been previously scarce. Moreover (as some advocates soon realized), these federally funded treatment centers could themselves act as brokers for getting pharmaceutical firms to provide their patients with concentrate at a lower cost.[58] So even though federal support did not extend to direct payments for treatment, the new federal resources gave hemophilia treatment specialists and their institutions the capacity to lower the financial as well as physical and emotional burdens on their patients.

The political climate after 1972 was not one in which funding for "categorical illnesses" was easily obtained. The hemophilia community's legislative success was in large part due to the organizational skill and political acumen of the leaders of the NHF, especially their foresight in portraying the needs of persons with hemophilia in a way that Americans could appreciate and support. Yet the NHF also benefited from the increasing visibility of the nation's blood crisis in the 1960s and early 1970s. Many policy and lawmakers could see that hemophilia patients were in a precarious position with respect to the scarcity of plasma resources, even as they were amazed to see what a tremendously positive impact such resources made when patients had access to them. At the same time, any treatment method that promised lower costs would be welcomed.

Quite astutely, NHF leaders sought funding for hemophilia treatment centers using the argument that home transfusion care was less costly than the more prevalent practice of giving transfusions on an outpatient basis. In fact, the case for the cost-effectiveness of comprehensive care programs built upon the work of Dr. Peter Levine, who pioneered a home care program at Tufts–New England Medical Center in Boston. In 1973 Levine's clinic witnessed a 45 percent decrease in total health costs, a 76 percent decrease in outpatient fees, an 89 percent decrease in hospitalization costs, and a 15 percent decrease in moneys spent on concentrated clotting factor. The study also demonstrated, for instance, that home care allowed patients and their families to use only as much product as they needed. In contrast, physicians in private practices and at hospitals often gave patients larger doses than they needed, at higher cost. Under home transfusion care, hemophilia patients and their families proved themselves to be informed health consumers. And as hemophilia care advocates repeatedly argued, informed consumers kept costs low.[59] With such data suggesting the medical and societal benefits of home care, NHF leaders argued that the costs of hemophilia care were controllable. What they lacked, however, were good comparative data. There was no visible effort, for instance, to compare the costs of hemophilia care vis-à-vis the expense of dialysis care (which was beginning to spiral out of control following Congress's ESRD entitlement). Nor did advocates advance an explicit cost-effectiveness equation that detailed how much more productive hemophilic adults could be if their disability were prevented despite their interest in being able to determine the long-term cost of "crippling" and "lost income."[60] But hemophilia doctors and advocates were nonetheless persuasive at pointing out the obvious: access to clotting factor concentrates, comprehensive care, and home treatment programs visibly transformed the lives (and bodies) of hemophilic boys and men.

Above all, the NHF and its medical advisers were able to communicate the groundswell of grass-roots support for home care transfusion services that persons with hemophilia and their families had lobbied their doctors for in the late 1960s and early 1970s. Parents like Louis Friedland and patients like Eric Friedland and Warren Jewett played critical and high-profile roles in convincing politicians and the public alike that hemophilia patients deserved programs to facilitate their transition into normal, productive citizens. To deploy a phrase coined in relation to diabetes advocacy, the normalizing power of home transfusion care gave hemophilia patients, families, and their physician-advocates powerful motivation to make sure that their hopes were not "buried in the categorical illness graveyard."[61]

A telling cultural moment in the rising status of hemophilia occurred in the spring of 1975 when Robert and Suzanne Massie published *Journey*, an engaging memoir about their experience raising their hemophilic son, Bobby (Robert Jr.).[62] In the late 1960s Robert Massie had published a best-selling history *Nicholas and Alexandra* that detailed the tragic implications of hemophilia on imperial Russia as well as the Romanov family. In 1971 the film version of *Nicholas and Alexandra* appeared on the big screen, garnering two academy awards as well as bringing significant public attention to hemophilia.[63] *Journey* was the Massie family's effort to keep hemophilia in the public eye by emphasizing the "democratic" character of this hereditary bleeding disorder more than its reputation as a "royal malady." And the Massie family's memoir was successful in that regard. As one critic noted, *Journey* was not the story of a "disease of kings," but one that was "democratic in its attack."[64] The Massie's memoir effectively captured the challenges of raising a child with hemophilia in an era of significant medical progress and made the subject of hemophilia a less romantic, less distant problem than it had been when most educated Americans associated it with European royalty or the deceased monarchies of Russia and Spain.

Yet, as other critics observed in 1975, the book sounded notes of caution about spiraling costs and limited access to these promising treatments.[65] *Journey*, which the Massies completed during the same time frame that the NHF was successfully lobbying for public funding of hemophilia care, effectively conveyed how the plight of hemophilic boys was being both transformed and neglected. Like Eric Friedland, Bobby Massie had enjoyed the privilege of access to concentrates. He had thrived after 1968 and was attending Princeton University in the mid-1970s.[66] Yet, as Robert Sr. pointed out in the book, their family moved to France in the late 1960s so that Bobby could receive clotting factor at no cost through the French national health system. In the words of one hospital administrator, the book provided eloquent testimony to the fact that Americans "leave catastrophic illness to be handled by those who can least handle it."[67]

Yet, even as many Americans were learning through the Massies about the burdens of hemophilia by reading *Journey* or reviews of it, advocacy was changing the landscape of hemophilia care. In fact, the day after the *Los Angeles Times* published a critical reflection on the Massie's memoir, entitled "U.S. Neglect of the Chronically Ill," President Ford helped alleviate the problem by signing the hemophilia act that Congress had recently passed. Overnight, it seemed, Americans with hemophilia were no longer destined for the categorical illness graveyard. In July 1975 hemophilia care advocates and the federal government had seemingly transformed this catastrophic bleeding disorder into a socially meritorious condition deserving of public support.

The Risks beyond the Categorical Illness Graveyard

With greater access to comprehensive hemophilia care after 1975, hemophilia patients achieved greater degrees of health and autonomy in greater numbers, but they were soon confronting the limits of medical management as the adolescents and adults among them began to see evidence that there were trade-offs to state-of-the-art hemophilia care. The lives of patients were increasingly "normal." Commercial clotting factor concentrates in particular came into wider use. Cryo use diminished significantly; most patients saw it as a less convenient, less potent treatment that did not fit their ideal of an autonomous lifestyle, but also supplies of cryo disappeared as blood banks and commercial plasma interests labeled it a financially burdensome product to handle. Yet, as more hemophilia patients turned to hemophilia treatment centers for their expertise and home use of commercial clotting factors for the obvious benefits they afforded, significant numbers of patients experienced complications from their plasma-derived concentrates that made it difficult for some of them to thrive as hoped.

The complexity of medically managed hemophilia—its complications and risks—thus became a critical focus for many treatment specialists after 1975. At this time, specialists were beginning to witness hemophilia's emergence as a full-blown pathology of progress, an experience that included the much-heralded positive effects of comprehensive medical care as well as the persistence of certain disabling complications that were not yet widely publicized—even among patients. In March 1976, for instance, the NHF co-sponsored a workshop for the hemophilia experts with the Bureau of Biologics at the U.S. Food and Drug Administration and the Division of Blood Diseases and Resources at the National Heart Lung and Blood Institute (formerly NHLI). Titled "Unsolved Therapeutic Problems in Hemophilia," the conference focused on a range of problems confronting the hemophilia community that reflected the limits of recent progress. The complications of therapy included liver abnormalities, hypertension, loss of kidney function, and immunological problems. What the workshop revealed was a striking set of persistent problems and what the organizers called a "lack of broad based data from which to draw conclusions."[68]

Despite the limited data, many of the invited hemophilia treatment specialists drew on the roughly ten years of experience they did have treating hemophilia with cryo or clotting factor concentrates. It had long been known that a significant minority of patients receiving plasma products developed antibodies to the clotting factor protein (either factor VIII or factor IX), but the age of concentrates witnessed the emergence of patients whose immune response to infusions of concentrated clotting factor was sufficient to negate the therapeutic benefit of the product. Specialists spoke of antibodies to concentrated clotting factor as an inhibitor to hemophilia treatment, and patients who acquired these inhibitors were at risk for intractable and potentially fatal bleeding episodes. The late 1970s witnessed a rising concern with so-called inhibitor hemophilia as one of the most serious complications of treatment.

Another complication that drew the attention of hemophilia experts in the mid-1970s was the increase of hypertension and serious heart and kidney disease in the adult hemophilia population. As more patients survived to adulthood, physicians were seeing more disability among hemophilia patients related to circulatory problems. As in earlier eras, chronic reliance on transfusions put the bodies of hemophilia patients under repeated stress. The dramatically lower volumes of plasma products that came with cryo and concentrates was less taxing on the circulatory system (and initially promised to reduce mortality among hemophiliacs from heart disease), but the cumulative effects of even low-volume transfusions were still a strain on hemophilic bodies over the long term. Thus, as more hemophilia patients lived into middle and even old age, heart disease remained a serious complication to be managed.

However, the one complication that truly dominated expert discussions of hemophilia treatment in the 1970s was the high rate of liver abnormalities found in hemophilia patients following the widespread change to clotting factor concentrates manufactured using large pools of human plasma. Between 1970 and 1972, as commercial clotting factor concentrates began to enjoy widespread use, various hemophilia experts were noting an increase in abnormal liver tests and symptoms of post-transfusion hepatitis in patients using these products. Suspected as a cause for the rising incidence of hepatitis was the pooling of plasma products. Cutter Pharmaceuticals' new factor IX concentrate, which had entered the market in 1969 for the treatment of hemophilia B patients, was a particular subject of scrutiny. By 1976, hemophilia specialists were struggling to make sense of the increasingly high rates of hepatitis B antibodies and elevated transaminase levels that could be found in all hemophilia patients. A critical concern and uncertainty was whether such abnormal blood tests were a precursor to increased rates of "chronic active hepatitis with or without postnecrotic cirrhosis." In fact, by 1976, more than 50 percent of hemophilia patients in the United States had blood tests that indicated abnormal liver function and/or hepatitis B antibodies, which in turn led hemophilia treatment specialists to worry whether these patients would ultimately develop fatal liver disease or cancer.[69]

Because cryo and clotting factor concentrates were both blood products that are manufactured using pools of human plasma, hemophilia treatment specialists suspected no later than 1970 that patients using these pooled plasma products were at higher risk for post-transfusion hepatitis. Indeed, plasma fractionation experts had been aware as early as the late 1940s that larger pool sizes theoretically entailed greater risk that recipients of plasma products could acquire post-transfusion hepatitis. Specifically, the greater the number of donors involved, the greater the chance that the recipient would contract a case of serum hepatitis. With their widespread appearance on the market in the early 1970s, commercial plasma concentrates were manufactured in substantially larger pool sizes than cryoprecipitate. A single lot of commercial concentrate often contained the plasma of ten thousand to twenty thousand donors, whereas a lot of cryo usually contained as few as six to twenty donors, and sometimes as little as one to five. In theory, the risk of post-transfusion hepatitis was dramatically higher for consumers of concentrates because it took only one donor carrying hepatitis virus to infect the whole lot. In addition to transforming blood plasma into its functional components, plasma fractionation therefore had an unwanted capacity—what would later become known as a "revenge effect"—of being able to efficiently disseminate blood-borne pathogens from one tainted unit of plasma to the whole lot. No recipient of a plasma product had ever been completely safe from post-transfusion hepatitis, but products made from single donor plasma or smaller plasma pools were exponentially safer. Those products, by definition, involved little to no pooling of blood plasma. Thus, when the 1972 NHLI *Pilot Study of Hemophilia Treatment* revealed that physicians were using concentrates more and more, it did note that as many as 15 percent of physicians ranked risk of serum hepatitis as a major reason for choosing one blood product over another.[70]

Hepatitis experts, moreover, had begun to categorize hemophilia patients at increased risk not only for hepatitis B antibodies, elevated transaminase levels, and asymptomatic liver disease but also for full-blown liver disease itself. Hepatitis specialists Leonard Seeff and Jay Hoofnagle, reporting from the Veterans Administration Hospital and Georgetown University's School of Medicine in Washington, D.C., related to participants of the 1976 Workshop on "Unsolved Problems" that the "individual with hemophilia is at high risk of developing acute viral hepatitis" because of repeated use of plasma products. "Indeed it is for this reason that hemophiliac serum was chosen in which to perform the original immunological investigations designed to identify the hepatitis virus, with the ultimate discovery of the hepatitis B surface antigen (HbsAg, Australian Antigen) and antibody." Seeff and Hoofnagle were pointing out that Baruch Blumberg's role in the discovery of hepatitis B virus—which won the Nobel Prize in Medicine that year (1976)—hinged not only on identification of the hepatitis B surface antigen in blood serum samples drawn from a leukemia patient of aboriginal Australian descent but also on his use of blood serum drawn from a hemophilia patient in New York City. Blumberg and Harvey Alter chose serum from a hemophilia patient on the correct assumption that this man had acquired the requisite titer of hepatitis antibodies to initiate a reaction with their suspected antigen. Thus, in 1976 Seeff and

Hoofnagle appeared eager to infer that higher rates of acute liver disease should be expected among hemophilia patients, even if most forms of chronic active hepatitis currently seen in these patients "may be a benign or an only slowly progressive disease." These hepatitis experts called for mandatory surveillance of the hemophilia population in concluding their talk before hemophilia experts and even opined that "it is conceivable that future study of hepatitis in the hemophiliac may prove to be as fruitful in the search for the virus of non-A, non-B hepatitis [today called hepatitis C] as it was for the virus of type B hepatitis."[71]

While the possibility of such blood-borne infections was certainly a concern in every hematologist's mind during the 1970s, they were usually not considered a good reason to withhold cryoprecipitate or commercial concentrate from hemophilia patients with moderate to severe forms of the disease. After evaluating the cause of death of 122 American patients and 206 patients abroad, Louis Aledort reported to the 1976 "Unsolved Therapeutic Problems in Hemophilia" workshop, "They die young." "Inhibitors did not appear to contribute to death," he said. "Spontaneous bleeding was the major cause of demise, with trauma following closely behind." Death from liver disease and other complications of post-transfusion hepatitis did not appear to be a significant cause of mortality among patients in 1976. Although the data were limited, such results prompted hemophilia treatment specialists to emphasize the dangers of untreated or under-treated hemophilia more than express their worries about the complications of intensive management like inhibitor development or post-transfusion hepatitis.[72]

The decisions about treatment that hemophilia specialists made in the late 1970s typically revolved more around convenience and cost rather than the hidden complications or uncertain risks of clotting factor replacement therapy that began to trouble hemophilia specialists as they scaled up their hemophilia treatment centers following the summer of 1975. Since the mid-1960s, convenience and efficacy—in the form of greater "freedom" or autonomy—was what concentrate manufacturers promised and patients and families persistently demanded. It is not surprising, then, that hemophilia specialists most often cited convenience as their reason for recommending pooled plasma products—and especially concentrates—over other treatment options. Moreover, cost was the only frequent obstacle that prevented physicians from prescribing what they otherwise "considered to be ideal treatments for their patients."[73] Susan Resnick has called these findings "harbingers" and argued that cost was the "key determinant" in making decisions about patient treatment and hemophilia policy in the United States.[74] Lacking sufficient data on the hemophilia population to determine what the true scale of complication and risk was in the late 1970s, most leading hemophilia specialists focused on the business of realizing the promise of hemophilia treatment centers. Thus, they continued to stress the problem of cost as the most serious impediment to the long-term as well as immediate benefit of their patients. Cost remained the big threat because most adults with hemophilia lacked health insurance and federal subsidies from the new hemophilia law were never sufficient to meet the needs of the growing numbers of patients with bleeding disorders who relied on the expanding number of hemophilia treatment centers.

Hemophilia experts in the late 1970s were acutely aware that post-transfusion infections—primarily in the form of hepatitis B—were a major problem for clinical management, but it was largely considered an intractable problem that leading specialists did not represent as an immediate threat to patients with severe to moderate bleeding disorders. Generally speaking, most hemophilia experts in the 1970s did not fully disclose the risks of inhibitor development, heart disease, or post-transfusion hepatitis to their patients. Typically, patients learned of hepatitis after they had acquired a transfusion-related infection, when doctors needed them to know about the condition in order to better manage this "complication." The real threat to patients—as highlighted in the NHLI's study of the blood supply and most of the medical literature—was lack of access to commercial plasma concentrates. Thus, when hemophilia doctors or researchers turned up safety issues related to heavy use of concentrates, they perceived these problems as unfortunate but manageable side effects of a largely melioristic enterprise.

The views of the hemophilia treatment community reflected, in many ways, blood experts' attitudes in the 1970s toward safety issues. In 1972 the federal government shifted oversight of blood and its derivatives from the National Institutes of Health to the Food and Drug Administration, drawing in part on the NHLI blood study that gave support to that idea that greater oversight of blood and plasma brokers was necessary. But the NHLI study did not speak directly to the issue of ridding the blood supply of donors at high risk for transmitting hepatitis, syphilis, and other blood-borne infections. In fact, in the NHLI's *Pilot Study* of hemophilia, the focus was entirely on the treatment needs of hemophilia patients, the scale of the supply of source blood and plasma, and the costs of care. This focus reflected the concerns of the hemophilia treatment community itself. Leading hematologists did not commit themselves to understanding the scale of the problem at this time, and the NHLI study did not seek answers on the matter.

Thus, as comprehensive care spread with the growth of federally funded hemophilia treatment centers after 1975, advocates focused their attention on maintaining the supplies of source plasma that were so critical to the enterprise of hemophilia management. Thus, taking the lead from its medical advisers, NHF officials believed that their position on matters concerning the blood supply in the 1970s was to protect the hemophilia patient's "right" of access to source plasma. This policy was stated concisely in a 1970 amicus curiae brief submitted to the Supreme Court of Illinois on behalf of one hospital blood bank. A woman who had contracted hepatitis from a blood transfusion was suing the hospital. The NHF's lawyer believed that the hospital should not be accountable because blood was by its nature a risky product. Consumers know blood is "unavoidably unsafe," he argued. And even if they did not, public policy regarding blood should not make it so costly (through litigation) that the "few who contract hepatitis have a right and privilege to affect those who are less fortunate." Regarding the blood "consumer," that brief then said:

> The consumer needs the blood that is given. Without adequate amounts of blood death will result regardless of the nature of the condition necessitating the transfusion. With few exceptions, no patient would refuse a transfusion if they were informed that there was a chance that they might contract hepatitis, when also informed that the alternative might mean their death. . . . The consumer is willing to accept the blood given them as long as there is no inconvenience. The danger and risk of hepatitis is sufficiently small that they cannot be motivated to action on their own behalf.[75]

The NHF's official views on blood policy did generate a lot of controversy in the 1970s among the experts engaged in reform of the nation's blood services complex. For activists who were fighting for a more robust voluntary blood system in the United States, the views and the growing political clout of the NHF were troublesome. Such activists often emphasized blood safety over cost and availability. Indeed, one of the strongest proponents of blood safety was Stanford surgeon J. Garrott Allen, who once wrote privately of the NHF that "the tendency of hemophilic organizations to be directed by hemophiliacs or their families corrupts this organization from the beginning."[76] Like many doctors surveyed in the 1972 NHLI report, Allen seemed to think that the hemophilia patients lacked the capacity for understanding and informed action on matters of blood safety. Unfortunately, Allen's criticism was misdirected. Here, he identified the NHF's focus on supply over safety as a reflection of the beliefs of patients and families, when (in fact) it was leading hemophilia doctors in the advocacy movement who were framing supply as the pressing danger rather than the risk of post-transfusion hepatitis.

As an advocacy group for hemophilia patients and their families, the NHF drew criticism because some blood policy reformers viewed the organization's priorities and actions as an impediment to the work of organizations and actors who sought to balance safety issues with the problems of supply. Allen's seemingly harsh critique of the NHF was informed by his recent reading of Robert and Suzanne Massie's book, *Journey*. He told Dr. Ian Mitchell, who headed the U.S. Department of Health's efforts to forge a national blood policy in the 1970s, "It would be infinitely better if hemophilia would be forgotten as a separate disease or entity and were a genuine part of the ABC [American Blood Commission]. This is one of the major factors limiting their collection of cryo or of concentrates."[77] The criticism was that the NHF was not even acting in the best interest of hemophilia patients, much less that of the American public. It was a harsh assessment of an organization whose official policy on the American Blood Commission and the forging of a national blood policy was that "the Federal Government move expeditiously to an all volunteer blood system, but not so rapidly as to develop shortages."[78]

Criticism of the NHF's advocacy on blood supply and safety issues was hidden from public view in 1970s. No one was willing to attack the NHF publicly, and there was even some reticence among reformers to attack the pharmaceutical companies that, in Allen's opinion, were promoting unsafe products. In fact, Allen's distrust of the NHF as well as the pharmaceutical industry grew dramatically after the summer of 1974 as he sought to publicize a finding in the journal *Transfusion* that Cutter's factor IX concentrate (Konyne) was produced from blood drawn "100 percent from Skid-Row derelicts" and "has proved extraordinarily hazardous, a 50 to 90 percent rate of icteric hepatitis developing from it," with about half of the cases proving fatal.[79]

In reporting Konyne's possible "mortality rate of 40 percent," Allen explained to Ian Mitchell that Cutter had recently won a court case in a 9-to-3 jury decision in which the attorney for an injured patient was unable to counter the "emotional appeal to the jury of the clinical photos of children bleeding from factor VIII deficiency, presented as identical to factor IX deficiency." Allen continued, "Cutter's attorneys have gone over this ground so many times in trials that a plaintiff's attorney can not possibly prepare himself adequately to come off well. The attorneys who defend these pharmaceutical houses, again and again and again, put the one-time plaintiff's attorney into the same position that the Boston Globe Trotters [sic] would put a high school basketball team!" The only solution, opined Allen, was to control the pharmaceutical industry through appropriate legislation. "Nothing else will change their ways of doing business."[80] In fact, Allen's reading *Journey* fueled his disbelief that "the Private Sector can redeeme [sic] itself."[81]

The debate over the safety of the nation's blood supply raged unresolved for most of the decade. Not until 1978 did the FDA arrive at what Douglas Starr has rightly dubbed a "prescient compromise," when the federal agency began requiring blood banks and plasma collectors to label donor blood as "paid" or "volunteer" on the assumption that "the marketplace [would] accomplish the rest."[82] That rule worked marvelously because hospitals and physicians refused to trade in blood that was suspect. As a result, the practice of paying blood donors immediately disappeared in the United States. However, the FDA did not extend the labeling requirement to plasma in recognition of the commercial plasma industry's claims that it would be unable to have adequate plasma for making clotting factor concentrates and other products if it did not pay its "donors." The practice of paying plasma donors therefore continued, and problematic rates of post-transfusion hepatitis continued rising among recipients of plasma products after 1978 just as they had since the mid-1960s.

The NHF's successful strategy for empowerment in the 1970s fulfilled much of the promise of postwar hemophilia management. It not only delivered greater access to comprehensive care for the nation's population of people with bleeding disorders but also facilitated the normalcy and autonomy that patients and families had long desired. Hemophilia care advocacy earned perhaps its greatest victory in the 1970s; yet this victory— built on greater public recognition of hemophilia's manageability—failed to highlight the uncertainty and risks that recent medical progress embodied for hemophilia patients and their families.

CHAPTER SEVEN

The Mismanagement of Hemophilia and AIDS

B lood and sex had long been intertwined with hemophilia but never more visibly or with such devastating effect than during the first two decades of the AIDS pandemic. Of the twenty thousand or so Americans with hemophilia in the early 1980s, most of them acquired HIV through contaminated blood plasma products that they routinely used to treat their bleeding disorder. Hardest hit were the nation's "severe hemophiliacs," the group of more than eight thousand patients who routinely used clotting factor concentrates. Of this predominantly male population, nine out of ten would acquire HIV before public and private authorities implemented effective donor screening, HIV testing, and viral inactivation methods for plasma products in the United States.[1] The tragic irony of these events was obvious. The treatments that were supposed to facilitate normalcy for the hemophiliac suddenly became vectors for a new and virulent pathology.

More than any other event of the past three decades, the transfusion-related AIDS tragedy of the 1980s has shaped contemporary American perceptions of hemophilia and the people affected by it. Most treatment specialists have sought to learn from the experience and have incorporated its lessons into their renewed efforts to render hemophilia manageable. Some within the community, however, still resist an understanding of the event that recognizes what went wrong and who might have been responsible for tragic paths taken. As recently as 2007, Louis Aledort, a leading hemophilia specialist, chastised Bruce Evatt, a former blood expert at the

Centers for Disease Control and Prevention, in the pages of a respected hematology journal. Evatt had made an earnest effort to document how knowledge of AIDS and the blood supply evolved in relation to the American hemophilia community in the early 1980s. Aledort's questionable advice to Evatt and other would-be historians is telling: "Now is the time for healing, not finger-pointing."[2]

The story of hemophilia in the 1980s is fundamentally a story of biomedical progress gone awry. Without modern medicine's heavy reliance of blood transfusion technologies, AIDS would have manifested itself in society very differently—likely sparing the "hemophiliac" all together. Beyond this fact, what happened in the hemophilia-AIDS tragedy remains contested by those who experienced it because there were no winners, nearly everyone made mistakes, and there is little incentive for the individuals involved to dwell on the history to the extent that an accurate accounting of their actions (or inactions) would require.[3]

The nation's hemophilia population was poorly served in the 1980s by the federal government, the blood industry, and even voluntary health organizations such as the National Hemophilia Foundation and the American Red Cross. All of these institutions deserve some blame. None has fully confronted its role in the making of the crisis—despite some notable attempts in the 1990s within the courts, the U.S. Congress, and the Institute of Medicine of the National Academy of Sciences (IOM). In 2001, for example, one group of Harvard physicians went so far as to argue that the IOM's 1995 hearing on the matter of transfusion-related AIDS "failed to address the hemophilia community's demands for accountability and justice" even as it "indicated necessary improvements to the management of the blood supply." There is considerable truth here. However, these well-intentioned physicians also concluded that efforts to understand what happened to the American hemophilia community had been "framed as a failure of management and oversight rather than a moral failure of the for-profit health-care system."[4] Such assessments deserve comment, particularly if we are to write the history of such events in ways that promote healing.

As the media has consistently pointed out over the years, corporate greed combined with institutional inertia and all-too-human denial to bring about this AIDS catastrophe for people with hemophilia. However, if we leave aside the question of whether for-profit enterprises should be indicted for what happened to people with hemophilia, it should be said that the majority has not been wrong to frame transfusion-related AIDS as a failure of management or oversight. Thus, for those who think that greed played a determining role here, I urge them to question whether their interpretation is really at odds with the idea that failures in management are fundamental to this story.

The goal, as I see it, is to understand that we will never really understand the extent to which greed, sloth, pride, or any other base motive explains this catastrophic event in recent medical history unless we deal first with the more fundamental question of what management of hemophilia entails in the first place. After all, it is hardly clear that America's post-transfusion AIDS epidemic would have been averted had the biomedical companies done more to protect their consumers' health, or had government regulators put the interests of public health and safety at the top of their agendas, or had physicians been less paternalistic and more forthright with patients about the risks involved. Certainly, the suffering and loss of life would have been lessened had one or more of these groups lived up to their responsibilities. But can anyone justifiably say that the transfusion-related AIDS epidemic would have been prevented had everybody's intent and actions been pure? What is most compelling in this story is not the fact that people made mistakes or the possibility that the marketplace allegedly bred systemic "moral failure." More critical is the fact that most everyone involved in these events genuinely believed that they were acting in the best interests of patients and families. So to interpret this tragic event in all its profundity, one must necessarily interrogate what the "management" of hemophilia meant to the people involved.

If we take the long view, the story of hemophilia's transformation from a chronic, manageable disease in the 1970s into the iatrogenic, or medically induced, tragedy it became in the 1980s is a cautionary tale about relying so heavily on medical experts and their technologies to deliver historically elusive goals like "normalcy," autonomy, or even improved health. There are clearly limits to what biomedicine can do to deliver health, and the recent intersection of hemophilia and AIDS offers some lessons on where those limits lie.

To comprehend the tragedy that befell people with hemophilia, it is therefore critical to see how the hemophilia community's traditional aspirations for normality led to complications in the AIDS era. Many thoughtful people in the hemophilia community—including patients and physicians—remained committed to using commercial clotting factor concentrates despite growing realization that these plasma-derived treatments could transmit AIDS. Why? To understand this disturbing fact, I argue, is to grapple with the decades-old promise in the American hemophilia community that "normal lives" were possible.

There remains a pressing need today to understand why the complex medical and social system for managing bleeding disorders that hemophilia management advocates had promoted from the 1950s to the 1970s ultimately killed most of the patients in the 1980s and 1990s. Understandably, the tainted blood scandals involving people with hemophilia and AIDS have generated controversy, hard feelings, and questionable history. The remedy, I argue, is to recognize that the various realities of the 1980s made it impossible for people with hemophilia to avoid AIDS and highly unlikely that physicians and advocates could act effectively on their behalf. Yet I also explain that some of the worst outcomes of this iatrogenic catastrophe were avoidable.

The Canary in the Coal Mine

Well before physicians recognized HIV as a devastating problem for people with bleeding disorders, experts at the Centers for Disease Control and Prevention (CDC) found in the hemophilia experience important clues about the nature of the emergent AIDS epidemic. Based in Atlanta, Georgia, the CDC is the federal agency charged with promoting public health and safety through the reduction of burdens associated with disease and disease risks. Today, the American medical and public health establishment treats the health of the hemophilia population as an early warning system for tracking the spread of HIV/AIDS, hepatitis B and C, and other blood-borne pathogens. That they do so is a legacy of how the CDC first became acquainted with AIDS in the 1980s.

There is a long-standing rationale for viewing the hemophilia population as the nation's proverbial "canary in the coal mine" when it comes to problems with the nation's blood supply.[5] That rationale predated the emergence of AIDS in the United States. When journalists in the 1960s began analyzing chronic blood shortages in many parts of the country, they documented that people with hemophilia were among those who suffered most. When the media turned in the early 1970s to condemn the alarming rates of post-transfusion hepatitis, policy makers and the federal government not only traced the source of the problem to businesses that paid donors for their blood and plasma but also recognized that transfusion-related disease often manifested in people with hemophilia before anyone else. As journalist Douglas Starr effectively demonstrated in 1998's *Blood: An Epic History of Medicine and Commerce*, efforts in the 1970s to reform the oversight and handling of the "blood services complex" did not translate into a safer or more plentiful blood supply in the United States.[6]

Blood supply reform efforts typically recognized the vulnerability of the hemophilia population to faults within the system while doing little to remedy their situation. Presumably, the blood services complex addressed the needs of all people with bleeding problems. Yet the system was never really designed to serve patients who were in chronic need of blood or plasma; it effectively focused on the needs of patients who required blood in the short term: for surgery, for an injury, or for an acute condition. Where the welfare of hemophilia patients figured explicitly in the governance of blood supplies, the focus in the 1970s was less on guaranteeing safety than it was on securing adequate supplies of blood plasma to meet increased demand by such patients across the nation. There was little incentive within the system, as it had been organized, to treat post-transfusion hepatitis as preventable among hemophilia patients and other heavy blood consumers. By 1980, then, many blood experts viewed the hemophilia patient's vulnerability to hepatitis and other faults within the blood services complex as an intractable problem.

In the early 1980s, and quite unintentionally, the system situated "the hemophiliac" similarly to the miner's caged canary; his radical dependency on a system designed for sustaining him also made him expendable should the going get tough. No one has ever defended this aspect of the system, but efforts to reform it before the outbreak of AIDS were feeble. The late 1970s policy of labeling blood as coming from "paid" donors substantially reduced rates of post-transfusion hepatitis among recipients of whole blood transfusions. However, that labeling policy did not extend to plasma or plasma concentrates, largely out of concern that the commercial plasma industry could not meet the demand for plasma products without paying donors. Thus, in the 1990s, it was with legitimate reason that people with hemophilia often highlighted how the government and even their own doctors had treated them like the miner's canaries in the preceding decade.[7] The doctors objected to such characterizations, and some have rightly questioned the model of intentionality implied by the "canaries" metaphor.[8] However, the analogy is apt in one important way. While doctors certainly did not view or treat their hemophilia patients as personally expendable, the blood services complex that existed in the 1970s and 1980s clearly highlighted the extreme vulnerability of hemophilia patients to blood-borne infections: first hepatitis B, then HIV/AIDS and hepatitis C. Thus, the canary metaphor accentuates what is most paradoxical about the tragic position of people with hemophilia in the era of transfusion-related AIDS: namely, that the hemophilia patient was unintentionally sacrificed by a blood services complex whose agents all purported to have his best interests at heart, but who were unable (and perhaps even unwilling) to fix the system that put him at risk for post-transfusion infections.

Experts at the CDC first learned of a possible connection between hemophilia and the emerging AIDS epidemic in 1982. That January, a physician in Miami phoned the CDC following the death of a sixty-two-year-old hemophiliac a few months earlier. This physician wanted to communicate his belief that this patient had contracted the fatal pneumonia (*Pneumocystis pneumonia* or PCP) from using a factor VIII concentrate. The phone call was quickly referred to Bruce Lee Evatt, the CDC's chief hematologist and resident expert on bleeding disorders. Evatt assured the physician the factor VIII concentrate could not have caused the patient's fatal pneumonia; the purification process for making such concentrates filtered out all pathogenic bacteria and protozoa, including the fungus that causes PCP. Nevertheless, Evatt found this case report deeply troubling because the CDC was actively investigating emergent outbreaks of PCP and Kaposi's sarcoma (KS) in gay men living in San Francisco, Los Angeles, and New York. In fact, the agency's top experts were already entertaining various theories about this sudden rise of maladies that ordinarily did not strike adults in their prime of life unless their immune systems had been severely weakened.[9]

In conjunction with these unusual cases of "opportunistic" PCP or KS, clinicians were also seeing unusual fevers associated with swollen lymph nodes (lymphadenopathy) in gay patients. Working at the UCLA Medical Center, immunologist Michael Gottlieb discovered that these male patients had extremely low counts of critical infection-fighting white blood cells (called CD4-positive lymphocytes or helper T cells). Building on this discovery, frontline clinicians and CDC investigators reasoned that these patients had been exposed to something that was effectively destroying their immune systems.[10] Thus, while no one could say why these gay men were suddenly getting so sick, clinicians began to speak of this new constellation of illnesses as a "syndrome" associated with male homosexuals. After originally referring to the emergent epidemic as "Gay-related immune deficiency" or "GRID," physicians and epidemiologists would begin referring to it as "AIDS" (acquired immune deficiency syndrome) in 1982 at the urging of public health advocates who sought to reduce the stigma to the gay community.

The Miami hemophilia case added a new and foreboding dimension to investigations of this new syndrome, both for what it suggested about the underlying nature of these illnesses and for its potential to "spread" beyond gay men.[11] Until this point, the leading investigators were operating under the assumption that there was something specific to the sex or drug practices of gay men that made them susceptible to the disease. One theory held that patients who had receptive anal intercourse with multiple sex partners might be suffering from immune system overload as their bodies generated a massive antibody response to foreign sperm. Another theory posited drug abuse of amyl nitrate inhalants (or "poppers") as a cause or cofactor of immune system failure. A third was the possibility that the syndrome might be caused by an immune-debilitating agent that spread through sexual contact itself—in other words, AIDS might be a traditional sexually transmitted disease. The appearance of the syndrome in hemophilia patients had implications for all the proposed theories about causation; but most importantly, it complicated the always-problematic assumption that public health officials could contain the epidemic by targeting the reputed behaviors of gay men.[12]

The very idea that symptoms of immune deficiency could appear in a nonhomosexual, hemophilia patient prompted CDC hematologist Bruce Evatt into immediate action. Upon hearing the details of the Miami case in January 1982, Evatt reasoned that if hemophiliacs were contracting PCP or other opportunistic infections, then that was potentially serious evidence in favor of conceptualizing the emergent epidemic as a blood-borne, infectious disease. Hemophilia patients had been widely using commercial factor VIII concentrates for a decade without showing signs that such treatments could compromise their immune systems. Because the blood plasma product itself did not appear to weaken immunity, Evatt made an educated guess that it had been contaminated by the only kind of pathogen small enough to evade the manufacturers' purification processes. The suspect, as he saw it, was likely a blood-borne virus.[13]

Bruce Evatt was particularly disturbed by the idea that the new immune deficiency syndrome might be transmitted through factor VIII concentrates. As the CDC's top blood expert, Evatt not only was familiar with the faults in the blood and plasma delivery systems but also knew that the presence of an imminently lethal blood-borne virus would entail fundamental changes in how physicians, blood bankers, and the commercial plasma industry approached the management of blood as well as hemophilia and other bleeding disorders. Nevertheless, the Miami case provided extremely meager evidence in favor of a link between blood products and the emergent immune deficiency syndrome. In search of other cases, Evatt therefore alerted CDC drug technician Sandra Ford to identify existing pentamidine orders for any PCP patients who might also have a bleeding disorder. Then, as now, physicians used pentamidine, a powerful antimicrobial agent, to treat PCP; the CDC's Division of Host Factors, which Evatt directed, monitored the usage of pentamidine among other "orphan drugs" that physicians used only to treat rare diseases (PCP among them).[14]

The CDC's case for framing the AIDS epidemic as a blood-borne phenomenon emerged in the summer of 1982. On June 11 Ford notified Evatt that a pentamidine order had arrived for a hemophilia-PCP patient in Denver. This information immediately prompted Evatt to send CDC immunologist Dale Lawrence to investigate if the patient had acquired an immune disorder through the use of a blood product. On his arrival at the University of Colorado Medical Center, Lawrence discovered the fifty-nine-year-old patient on a ventilator and was forced to interview the man's wife for any evidence that her husband might have engaged in drug use or sex with men. Lawrence became suitably convinced in his investigations that the patient, a janitor and family man, had contracted his immune disorder through a blood product; he collected three years of data on the different batches of factor VIII concentrates that hemophilia patients in the Denver area had used in conjunction with their care at the university's hemophilia treatment center. Lawrence could find no lot of blood product that appeared to be the culprit, and the evidence for blood transmission of

AIDS remained circumstantial. The investigation nevertheless confirmed Evatt's worst suspicion that more cases were on the horizon.[15]

Additional warnings arrived a couple of weeks later, on July 2, when Evatt was able to confirm a third case in a "previously healthy 27-year-old" from Canton, Ohio. Immediately after the Independence Day weekend, Evatt sent a letter to New York City hematologist Louis Aledort, a medical co-director at the NHF, to notify him that the CDC had documented three cases of immunosuppression in hemophilia patients; included in the letter was the warning, "Hemophiliacs would be prime candidates to develop this syndrome."[16] A week later, Evatt sent similar letters to public health officials across the nation. In his messages, Evatt suggested that the growing incidence of cases involving immune-suppression looked like an epidemic of hepatitis B; the implication of this analogy was that the immune deficiency syndrome—like the hepatitis B virus—could potentially affect anyone who had unprotected sex with a carrier of the hypothetical pathogen, transfused blood from an infected donor, or used syringes contaminated by a victim. There was even the possibility that the condition could be transmitted "vertically" from mother to child during pregnancy or childbirth.

Throughout 1982, CDC investigators lacked even the most basic laboratory evidence to show that the acquired immune deficiency could be transmitted from person to person, yet they became increasingly convinced that they were looking at an epidemic that presented itself as a blood-borne virus. Scientists in North America and Europe were unable to locate any agent responsible for the malady, and therefore knew of no laboratory test that could directly identify who might be infected. Yet, on the basis of reported case histories, the CDC's top investigators (who included STD expert James Curran as well as Bruce Evatt) decided by mid-July that it was time to treat the emergent epidemic as an infectious agent that was likely blood-borne and sexually transmitted. As an additional piece of evidence, the CDC had also documented a large number of cases among intravenous drug users.[17]

By mid-July, the CDC was calling for the entire U.S. Public Health Service (USPHS) to meet with leaders from the blood and plasma industry and their trade associations, the three arms of the nonprofit blood banking community (the American Red Cross, the American Association of Blood Banks, and the Council of Community Blood Centers), the National Hemophilia Foundation, the National Gay Task Force, and other leading activists and health experts from the gay community.[18] CDC investigators hoped that this group of stakeholders would be able to reach a consensus position about the epidemic's relationship to the nation's blood supply and move toward a plan of action.[19]

Medical advisers at the NHF, meanwhile, were pursuing their own course of action. Two days before the committee met, the NHF issued its first hemophilia patient alert on the problem, telling hemophilia treatment centers and NHF chapters that three unusual cases of immune suppression had appeared among hemophiliacs and that the responsible "agent may be a virus transmitted similar to the hepatitis virus by blood." While saying this "hypothesis" was under investigation, the NHF alert repeatedly stressed that "the *risk* of contracting this immunosuppressive agent is *minimal* and CDC is not recommending any change in blood product use at this time." In reference to the upcoming meetings at the USPHS, the patient alert also noted that a "blue ribbon" panel of experts was being established at the Department of Health and Human Services to evaluate this problem, that NHF medical co-director Louis Aledort was serving on the panel, and that the CDC and the NHF were working with hemophilia treatment centers to establish a "carefully planned surveillance and reporting system."[20]

The July 1982 meetings of the USPHS committee were the first major gathering of authorities and community representatives to consider the scale and consequences of the emerging epidemic. While the expressed purpose of the meeting was to review Evatt's evidence of emergent immune deficiencies among hemophilia patients and explain why the CDC thought the epidemic might be blood borne, the CDC was privately urging everyone to consider screening blood donors who fell into one of their "high-risk groups" (gay males with multiple sex partners, intravenous drug users, and recently immigrated Haitians).[21] The evidence for the proposed change in blood policy remained circumstantial, but CDC investigators believed it sufficient to exhort blood bankers, the plasma industry, and even the Food and Drug Administration (FDA) to act on conscience.[22]

Virtually everyone present at the July 27 meeting saw compelling reasons to reject the CDC's proposal. Gay community leaders such as New York physician Roger Enlow argued that it was too early to push guidelines that could restrict the civil liberties of Americans. The NHF opposed any course of action that would limit the use of clotting factor concentrates that were credited with transforming the lives of hemophilia patients. Blood bankers and pharmaceutical representatives resisted the idea that they should move forward voluntarily to screen the blood supplies under their care. The FDA was the only governmental agency with the authority to enforce blood donor policy and monitor blood supplies, and its representatives were denying that an epidemic even existed. At a time when the Reagan administration was slashing budgets in the Department of Health and Human Services, FDA officials privately accused the CDC experts of inventing the epidemic out of unrelated health events so that the CDC could justify its continued funding levels. The CDC's only visible ally for new blood donor guidelines was Dan William, medical director of New York Gay Men's Health Project, who saw this measure as entirely appropriate from a public health standpoint. William, who had been a well-regarded figure in the gay advocacy movement to that point, would lose popularity among many gay activists by supporting the CDC's donor restrictions in the coming months. Instead of endorsing the CDC's blood policy recommendation, almost everyone at the July 1982 meeting agreed on a wait-and-see policy.

Many experts attending this USPHS committee meeting were not only unconvinced that the CDC's findings necessitated sweeping changes in blood policy, but they saw every reason to attack the CDC's approach as contrary to good science. The skeptics described the CDC's evidence as wholly anecdotal: not a single scientific paper had been published that would allow them to evaluate whether the syndrome described by the CDC was blood-borne or sexually transmitted. Evatt, Curran, and other CDC investigators were operating as public health advocates in the midst of a crisis. They were calling on the experts to suspend their normal standards of scientific proof. The skeptics, however, could not fathom treating AIDS as the effect of a transmissible, blood-borne agent without further proof from the CDC, the National Institutes of Health (NIH), or other qualified investigators.[23] Indeed, while the FDA and the majority of experts proved willing to call the problem "acquired immune deficiency syndrome," they took no stand on whether the collection of maladies grouped under this label even counted as a disease. They saw limited evidence in Evatt's data to treat AIDS as an imminent threat to the majority of hemophilia patients, much less to the general public. As one reporter later put it, "How could the government be expected to forge national policy for more than 220 million Americans just because three hemophiliacs got sick?"[24]

If most of the experts present were clinicians and bench scientists who saw no compelling evidence to declare AIDS a public health crisis, Louis Aledort, the NHF's medical co-director, was no exception. He aggressively attacked Evatt's data suggesting that an immune-suppressing virus had contaminated factor VIII supplies. Thus, while casting the CDC's evidence as little more than conjecture, Aledort, like most of the doctors at this USPHS meeting, refused to acknowledge that the AIDS problem amounted to a public health crisis that necessitated suspension of the usual norms of scientific practice. In fact, he insisted that the situation demanded compliance with the strictest standards of proof. He argued for nothing less than full-blown clinical trials to evaluate the risks of clotting factor concentrates before recommending any action that might limit their use within the hemophilia community.

The consensus view of the gathered experts stunned Evatt, Curran, and other CDC investigators. Particularly puzzling were the rigid standards of proof that the majority sought to enforce. Everyone knew that definitive evidence in favor of blood-borne transmission would take months, if not years, to produce. From the CDC vantage point, the consensus would cause unnecessary delay and put lives at risk (especially among hemophiliacs); the available evidence, while admittedly circumstantial, was enough to warrant drawing up a plan of action and taking steps to implement it. However, most experts present saw the CDC position as alarmist, and their own opinions were infused with measures of caution, disbelief, distrust, and even hostility toward the CDC.[25] Nevertheless, everyone agreed that the appearance of AIDS among hemophilia patients was a significant development deserving of further scrutiny. The NHF agreed to monitor hemophilia patients for evidence of possible immune deficiencies (i.e., PCP and other opportunistic infections). This commitment to surveillance, which the NHF moved on immediately, allowed Evatt to extend the CDC's tracking of hemophilia patients beyond the occasional pentamidine request. Moreover, despite misgivings at the FDA about the CDC's AIDS agenda, drug regulators could no longer ignore the dangers to hemophilia patients in their mandated duties to ensure the safety of blood and plasma products.

Over the course of the fall, the CDC gathered more data in favor of the blood-borne hypothesis. Evatt confirmed four more cases, plus another probable case using the surveillance network that he established with the help of the NHF and hemophilia treatment centers. Two of the affected hemophiliacs were children who clearly had no risk behaviors for AIDS other than being consumers of factor VIII concentrates.

The appearance of post-transfusion AIDS in children was the most compelling evidence yet that AIDS was blood-borne. In late October 1982, Harold Jaffe of the CDC began investigating the report of a male toddler who had developed immune problems following multiple blood transfusions. The baby, delivered early at thirty-three weeks in March 1981, developed at birth a life-threatening case of jaundice (hyperbilirubinemia) along with other complications of his prematurity. He received six double-volume exchange transfusions in his first four days of life, and multiple blood products during his first month that included platelets, packed red blood cells, and whole blood drawn from nineteen different donors. At nine months, doctors discovered the infant had a hepatitis infection (non-A, non-B). At fourteen months, his immune system was clearly impaired, and he was suffering from neutropenia, hemolytic anemia, and thrombocytopenia. By seventeen months, the toddler was receiving chemotherapy for an opportunistic mycobacterial infection. The child died in August 1982 while being treated for *Salmonella* sepsis and four other opportunistic infections. Jaffe determined that the child's problems originated on March 11, 1981, with a platelet transfusion. The donated platelets came from an apparently healthy forty-eight-year-old white man from San Francisco, who gave blood at Irwin Memorial Blood Bank on March 10 and only later developed symptoms of AIDS in the fall of 1981.[26] Although the CDC had investigated a few other cases of potential transmission by blood transfusion, the Irwin Memorial infant case was the first indisputable evidence that AIDS could be transmitted by transfusion of a blood product. Along with Jaffe's finding, Evatt's seven confirmed AIDS cases among hemophilia patients constituted substantial evidence in favor of categorizing the syndrome as a blood-borne disease.

In 1982 CDC investigators not only had considerably stronger clinical evidence for blood transmission as fall turned into winter but also had developed a strategy for testing blood for possible contamination on the basis of a study conducted by CDC virologist Thomas Spira. While the viral cause of AIDS remained unknown, Spira found that 88 percent of the blood samples drawn from AIDS patients showed prior exposure of these patients to hepatitis B. The result suggested that (in the absence of a lab test for AIDS) a standard assay for hepatitis B might be used as a surrogate screening test for transfusion-related AIDS and thereby prevent a high percentage of high-risk donors from contributing to the blood supply. Yet CDC experts would continue to meet opposition to their efforts to limit the spread of transfusion-related AIDS through changes to existing blood donation and screening policies. In 1983 that opposition came largely from the blood banking community (which would resist a surrogate test for AIDS) and gay activists (who continued to oppose bans on gay blood donors or explicit questions about sexual orientation), but there was also continued suspicion within the hemophilia treatment community that the CDC's recommendations went too far. The lack of consensus among these stakeholders in the blood policy debate would not only have tragic consequences for people with hemophilia but guarantee that the "hemophiliac" would soon embody for many Americans the dangers of transfusing blood in the AIDS era.[27]

Bad Blood: The Contested Health of the Blood Supply

A lethal mix of corporate interests, ineffective government, fears of stigmatization, as well as AIDS denial among experts, made the health of the nation's blood supply a hotly contested issue from the beginning of 1983 through 1985. Unfortunately, most Americans with hemophilia knew very little about it. As the NHF and its experts grappled with the question of AIDS and the blood supply (and what course of action to take), the vast majority of the hemophilia community remained in the dark between July 1982 and October 1984 as the NHF minimized the risk of AIDS and avoided publicizing the internal debates among blood and hemophilia experts about AIDS.[28] When they did hear talk of blood-borne AIDS in these fateful years, patients were usually assured that no changes in treatment were necessary. In fact, most patients learned little more than what was available through media channels.

As hemophilia patients were left largely unaware of the risks of blood-borne disease, the agencies and experts responsible for ensuring their welfare were engaged in a contentious fight that pitted those seeking costly changes to the nation's blood services complex and those seeking to protect the status quo. By 1982, American hemophilia patients and families had long praised the nation's blood services, even as they suffered through its chronic problems (e.g., blood shortages and the high costs of commercial plasma products). Although the NHF had its own troubles, patients and their families also had a deep reservoir of respect for this national voluntary association, given its decades-old history of helping them negotiate the problems with the system and improve it. When patients learned that AIDS was blood borne, there was little reason for patients and families to question what the NHF, government, or their physicians said about the health of the blood supply.

Delays in the federal government's response to the emergent AIDS epidemic were frequently the result of internal disagreement. The government's delays initially gained notoriety in the mid- to late 1980s as journalists documented how warnings from the CDC, city, and state public health departments and frontline physicians met sharp resistance from the FDA and other agencies. The Reagan administration waited until 1984 before treating AIDS as an issue of national importance, and the president did not publicly utter the word until 1987. Despite the glaring absence of executive leadership on AIDS, the federal government was not ineffectual in its duties to the American public. As is also widely known, C. Everett Koop, the U.S. surgeon general from 1981 to 1989, took a leading role in educating the public as well as the Reagan and Bush administrations about AIDS (and, like officials at the CDC, he took considerable heat for treating AIDS as a critical priority).

Even before Koop challenged Reagan to act on the AIDS issue, CDC and NIH investigators were attentive to key aspects of the crisis. After all, the decision to call the emergent epidemic "AIDS" issued from within the ranks of the Department of Health and Human Services at the July 27 meeting of the USPHS committee. The naming of AIDS at this meeting was a moment whose significance went far beyond the CDC's effort to find a "sexually neutral" term for an epidemic that previously had been characterized as a disease limited to male homosexuals. Still, as journalist Randy Shilts detailed in his 1987 best seller *And the Band Played On*, this fateful meeting should also be remembered as a missed opportunity to curb the spread of transfusion-related AIDS. That is because the meeting's attendees decided that monitoring and studying the claim of a blood-borne pathogen was preferable to following the CDC's expressed preference for refusing blood donors who fell within one of their high-risk groups.[29]

Within a few months of July's USPHS meeting, the consequences of inaction were beginning to dawn on leading treatment specialists in the hemophilia community. In the midst of documenting additional cases of transfusion-related AIDS, Bruce Evatt and Dale Lawrence from the CDC met with the NHF's newly reconstituted Medical and Scientific Advisory Council (MASAC) on October 2 and 3, 1982. This meeting has been portrayed as the "Oh, my God" moment when many of the nation's top hemophilia treaters realized, like Nurse Regina Butler, that "it's going to kill our patients."[30] Although the physicians on MASAC remained cautious and emphasized the need for more data collection, they also passed a resolution calling for the blood industry to exclude plasma donors from populations associated with AIDS (gay men, intravenous drug users, and Haitians). The decision to support restrictions on "high-risk donors" was fraught with danger for the hemophilia community. The peril arose from the uncertainties surrounding AIDS and the known likelihood that any restrictions on blood or plasma donation could negatively impact the supply and cost of plasma products, especially clotting factor concentrates.

Even as MASAC sought to ban "high-risk donors" from donating plasma to fractionation companies, its members initiated another round of reassuring advisories through the NHF's Medical Advisory and Chapter Bulletin communication system to stress that the risk of getting AIDS from clotting factor concentrates was low and that patients should continue with their normal course of treatments. In order not to alarm the broader community of patients and families, the NHF directed the advisories primarily to chapter leaders and physicians. Chapters were advised to put them on file for anyone who inquired. But the advisories were not—in most cases—designated for mass mailings. Many patients did not even know of their existence. By 1983, the advisories did note a certain level of risk where it recommended that physicians avoid using concentrates on hemophilia patients who had not been previously exposed to them (especially newborns). The advisories also recommended that bleeder patients avoid elective surgeries that might use concentrates where they were not immediately required. However, where it got through to patients, the NHF's message was mixed on the safety of the concentrates.[31]

The NHF's schizophrenic response to the CDC's findings reflected a compromise among leading hemophilia treatment specialists that exemplified the psychological as well as material motives behind the initial AIDS skepticism of 1982. On one side of MASAC was a group of specialists led by Louis Aledort, the NHF's medical co-director, who had built New York's Mount Sinai Hospital into one of the nation's first comprehensive care centers in the 1970s. As Douglas Starr has reported, Aledort had formed "a consortium of treatment centers in the New York area to leverage the best prices from the drug companies and provide reliable quantities to patients." Such leverage brought "tens of thousands of dollars in grants" to Mount Sinai Hospital every year while giving New York's hemophilia population access to a less expensive and relatively plentiful supply of clotting factor concentrates.[32] Aledort and his allies argued forcefully for continued use of clotting factor concentrates and diminished the evidence gathered by the CDC. On the other side were equally prominent hemophilia doctors who saw the merit in the CDC's evidence but were no less committed to providing effective comprehensive care for their hemophilia patients. Some of these hematologists considered whether other therapeutic options, especially cryoprecipitate, would reduce the risk of contracting AIDS. But the majority found that it was not enough to say that cryo was safer because it could be made with plasma pools taken from as little as one to ten donors (as opposed to many thousands). In fact, these experts could draw no definitive conclusions from the historically high rates of transfusion-related hepatitis among their patients because no one had adequately studied the relative risks of contracting blood-borne viruses from different plasma products. Finally, because all of the members on MASAC had witnessed the amazing changes wrought by clotting factor concentrates and the total-care approach to hemophilia, they found common ground in a strategy that pressured the plasma fractionation companies to produce and sell safer product without necessitating changes in the existing comprehensive-care system. The NHF's medical advisers all agreed, in essence, that it was counterproductive to diminish the reputation of clotting factor concentrates. As such, the specialists' dependency on clotting factor concentrates not only led to their collective inability to embrace effective hemophilia care without these products but also drove their skepticism regarding AIDS in a direction that put patients in greater danger than necessary.

On January 4, 1983, the CDC hosted the federal government's first public meeting on AIDS at its Atlanta headquarters. A highly contentious discussion ensued as gay leaders and blood bankers openly expressed differing degrees of opposition to the CDC's recommendations for a new blood policy, while leaders from the hemophilia community and plasma fractionation companies now endorsed the CDC's proposal. As Douglas Starr later detailed, the extensive media coverage of this meeting "put everyone on edge," making it difficult to discuss "delicate topics of blood, blood products, and sexual orientation" or to reveal the closely guarded secrets like the reliance of Cutter Laboratories and other manufacturers of clotting factor concentrates on plasma donations from prisons to make their product.[33] The focus of discussion was on the CDC's recommendation to restrict persons within high-risk groups from donating blood and to screen donated blood for AIDS by using the hepatitis B antibody test. The CDC's reasoning, evidence, and motives were all points of contention.

Gay advocates were again vocal in their criticism of the CDC's findings and proposals, and their resistance to any policy that would universally ban homosexual men from giving blood generated visible antagonism between them and the hemophilia advocates present.[34] NHF leadership expressed its official endorsement of the CDC's recommendation for new guidelines that would bar all gay men, intravenous drug users, and Haitians from giving blood or plasma. In contrast, gay leaders remained strongly opposed to such screening as unwarranted discrimination and made clear that they thought segregating high-risk blood donors was really just an effort to scapegoat homosexuals and reassure America's heterosexual majority that AIDS was not a widespread problem. Dr. Bruce Voeller of the openly gay Physicians for Human Rights warned that the proposed donor screening would stigmatize gays in the midst of a major civil rights movement and reasoned that restrictions on gay blood donors could not be effectively enforced because such donors would not self-identify as homosexuals in the first place. Many of the gay advocates particularly resented the sweeping nature of the ban. If any gay men were to be labeled as high risk, Voeller argued, then it should be only that minority of gays who engaged in "fast-lane" lifestyles that included dangerous degrees of sexual promiscuity and/or drug use.[35] From this perspective, most gays were no different from the majority of Americans. Dr. Donald Armstrong of New York's Sloan-Kettering Memorial Cancer Center agreed on ethical grounds:

"I don't think anyone should be screened for donating blood on the basis of sexual preference."[36]

Unintentionally, the CDC's draft recommendation for a new blood donor screening policy pitted gay advocates and hemophilia advocates against one another and created open hostility between these groups as each side saw the other restricting its community's freedom and not allowing its members to lead their lives as they saw fit. NHF held tightly to its view that a universal exclusion on gay blood donors was necessary. The gay advocacy groups granted the need for a certain level of exclusion but resented that they were not being treated like other blood donors. Later in January 1983, the National Gay Task Force joined more than fifty other gay organizations in denouncing the NHF.[37] The gay rights position, in turn, shocked and angered leading hemophilia advocates. Aledort later expressed his vehement opposition to the National Gay Task Force: "They may want to protect their rights, but what about the hemophiliac's right to life?"[38]

Blood bankers and plasma industry representatives benefited from the hostility between gay advocates and the NHF because it allowed them to push forward their own agendas and effectively attack the CDC's recommendation to institute hepatitis core testing of donated blood and plasma. Both the nonprofit and commercial sectors of the blood economy steadfastly opposed the introduction of hepatitis core testing as a prohibitively expensive endeavor that would yield uncertain results.[39] Yet, there were stark differences between the blood bankers and plasma industry on the question of screening out donor groups at high risk for AIDS.

Going into the January 1983 meeting, Evatt knew that the FDA would be unwilling to pressure blood bankers and the plasma industry toward any changes in behavior, so CDC investigators appealed to both groups to act voluntarily in the interest of public health. The evidence in favor of blood-borne transmission in the fall of 1982 had already convinced Alpha Therapeutic Corp. of the blood plasma industry to embrace the CDC's proposed recommendations. In December 1982 Alpha unilaterally began to exclude donors who were "male homosexuals," "drug abusers," or "persons who had been in Haiti." Thus, at the January 1983 meeting, Alpha representatives used the moment to garner some favorable publicity for themselves by explaining that their company would be employing the hepatitis B core antibody test as a surrogate screening tool for AIDS. Seizing the moment in front of the cameras, other representatives from the plasma

industry also endorsed Alpha's plan and indicated their willingness to follow suit.[40] Evatt and others at the CDC welcomed Alpha's readiness to serve
its customer base (the hemophilia treatment centers and their patients) by
implementing measures to reduce the spread of AIDS through transfusions
of plasma products. As Donald Francis later recalled, "Some [of the commercial plasma people] were certainly more receptive [to the CDC's posi-
tion] than the blood bankers." Francis did not presume to know why the
plasma industry was more receptive to blood screening, but he found its
position "interesting because they were always viewed as the low-class
group of blood collecting, because they're commercial and they're seen as
sucking plasma from poor people."[41] In retrospect, the plasma companies'
early willingness to adopt the CDC's recommendations on donor screening
had much to do with liability and the pressure they were getting from NHF.

In contrast, the hematologists in charge of hospital and community
blood banks did not fear legal challenges to the same degree as people in
the commercial plasma industry because existing blood shield laws made
it very difficult for victims of transfusion-related ills to seek and win damages.[42] The main concern of the blood bankers was to keep the blood supply lines functioning, which meant encouraging blood donation. Reflecting
on the events of 1983, Francis opined that the blood bankers seemed
chronically predisposed to inaction: they were "the most status quo, inertia-
seeking people I've ever met in my life." Particularly troubling to the blood
banks were high rate of "false positives" that could be expected from using
a hepatitis B test as a surrogate marker for AIDS. Francis noted that Herbert Perkins, then medical and scientific director of Irwin Memorial Blood
Bank, captured the attitude among the bankers in 1983 saying of the CDC's
plan for screening donors and donated blood, "Well, I think it's a great idea,
except that it cost money, causes trouble, and we have to tell patients—
it causes concern in patients if we have to tell them they're hepatitis B
infected."[43] The blood bankers insisted on having a specific AIDS test,
which—as everyone knew—could be developed only after scientists isolated the cause of AIDS. Whatever their reasons, blood bankers branded
both surrogate AIDS testing and new donor-screening guidelines as an
unwarranted burden that threatened their ability to encourage donation,
operate effectively, and save lives.[44]

Blood bankers felt strongly that they were acting in the interest of public health by protecting medical services necessary to the functioning of the

nation's hospitals and clinics. Whether they were affiliated with the American Association of Blood Banks (AABB), the Council of Community Blood Centers (CCMC), or the American Red Cross (ARC), clinical hematologists had long opposed any changes that would increase the operating costs of blood banks or significantly decrease blood donation. Most blood banks operated for the benefit of their local communities and hospitals, and most were ostensibly a part of the nonprofit sector. Yet, by the late 1970s and early 1980s, blood's growing value as a commodity along with the complex political economy surrounding health care in the United States put tremendous pressure on blood bankers to look at their bottom line. Some blood banks had become moneymaking ventures for the hospitals, universities, or other institutions to which they were affiliated. Others were operating in the red or were chronically on the verge of reducing services. Those that were prospering did not want to cut into their revenues. Those that were not generating enough money did not wish to see their doors close. Blood bankers had strong incentives to promote growth of blood supplies or at least to maintain the status quo.

The considerable competition and infighting between the ARC and the AABB was set aside in 1982 and 1983 when blood bankers realized that AIDS was a threat to the whole enterprise.[45] The imminent threat to responsible blood banking was economic as far as the bankers were concerned. In the tenuous blood economy, the risks of transfusion-related AIDS seemed isolated. A "one in a million" chance of a tainted transfusion was the frequently quoted risk assessment that the AABB and ARC issued in 1983. Blood bankers derived this statistic unadvisedly. They calculated that the risks were small because there were only three confirmed cases of transfusion-related AIDS in 1982 and roughly three million Americans who donated blood that year. Such arithmetic epitomized their wishful thinking.[46]

Consistent with the logic outlined by the blood bankers, NHF representatives worried that supplies of clotting factor concentrates and other plasma products would fall below the requirements of the hemophilia community if federal authorities followed the CDC's advice to exclude gay donors and require hepatitis B testing of donor blood. NHF medical advisers fretted about the extent to which they should threaten the supply lines of blood plasma. Yet these worries were dwarfed by the fear among NHF leaders that AIDS would necessitate restrictions on clotting factor concentrates.

In pitting themselves against gay blood donors (and many blood bankers), NHF leaders were merely playing the odds as they saw them. Realizing that they now had to deal with the reality of hemophiliacs getting AIDS, NHF leaders wished to limit the syndrome's spread "beyond" the gay community while ensuring that the hemophilia community continued to have largely unlimited access to the clotting factor concentrates that most hemophilia treatment specialists and patients credited with rendering hemophilia into a manageable disease. In short, leading hemophilia experts were betting that blood donor restrictions on gays would keep AIDS from mainstreaming into the nation's bloodlines, yet not diminish the supply line of plasma products too severely.

Hemophilia advocates had long framed clotting factor concentrates as the hemophiliac's passport to freedom, thereby making these products synonymous in the minds of most NHF leaders with the pursuit of normalcy, autonomy, and better health. Inadvertently, the mind-set also situated the gay man in oppositional terms to the typical male with hemophilia because it played off the notion that homosexuality was a deviation from "normal" manhood. Regardless of the gay community's stellar reputation for voluntary blood donation or its civic awareness, some leading hemophilia advocates in the 1980s tended to view the gay community's positions as a challenge to the hemophiliac's right to "untainted" clotting factor concentrates.[47] The hemophilia community and the gay community were operating with starkly different ideas about normalcy and autonomy in the blood feud era, a fact that arguably overdetermined how hemophilia advocates and gay activists viewed one another in the first decade of the AIDS epidemic.[48] Also, one cannot discount the prevalence of homophobia in American society during these years. There is little reason to think that hemophilia advocates of the 1980s were radically different from most Americans in holding attitudes that stigmatized homosexuality and that resisted seeing the claims of gay men as deserving equal treatment to their own.

Of course, not everyone in the hemophilia treatment community agreed with the consensus position of the NHF. The minority view was ably represented at this January 4 gathering. Oscar Ratnoff, Cleveland's renowned bleeding disorders expert, broke ranks to suggest that hematologists could prevent AIDS transmission to hemophilia patients by avoiding concentrates and using cryoprecipitate. Cryo was presumably safer because it could be efficiently made on a need-to-treat basis from pools of ten or fewer donors. "Sure it will cost more," he argued, "but not as much as a funeral or the lawsuits we're going to get after more hemophiliac deaths."[49] It was an effort, widely ignored by everyone present, to say that hematologists and blood bankers had more flexibility than people recognized to monitor the source of blood plasma and weed out questionable donors.

The most dramatic moments of the January 1983 meeting came on the heels of the blood bankers' assault on the CDC's evidence and plans, when people began questioning if a blood-borne pathogen was even a likely cause of AIDS. Louis Aledort seized upon the dual themes of scientific skepticism and the small number of transfusion-related AIDS cases to mount his case for embracing clotting factor concentrates. "I'm concerned about the concept that we are convinced is an agent . . .," he said. "We could be doing something through transfusion that causes it . . . or something in the patients' immune complex. Now in another six months we may . . ."[50] Then, infamously, CDC virologist Donald Francis, interrupted Aledort midsentence. Francis was so incensed by the response of the blood bankers and AIDS pathogen skeptics that he reportedly pounded the table and shouted, "How many people have to die? How many deaths do you need? Give us the threshold of death that you need in order to believe that this is happening, and we'll meet at that time and we can start doing something." Other CDC officials were taken aback by Don Francis's forthright but impolitic intervention. Francis, who was unfamiliar with the blood banking community and had only recently arrived as a full-fledged member of the CDC's AIDS task force, went so far in his anger as to suggest that blood bankers were committing "negligent homicide" by diminishing that AIDS was transmissible by blood.[51]

Visibly upset at Francis's allegations, many of the blood bankers held the CDC accountable. A climate of recriminations ensued in the coming days and weeks that generated considerable distrust of the CDC within the hematology community and strong motivation on the part of blood bankers to search out counterevidence that diminished the CDC's warnings of an imminent worsening of the transfusion-related AIDS epidemic. Although the CDC's credibility among blood bankers had been seriously strained by the January meeting, blood bankers had no choice but to work toward consensus for fear of appearing petty and self-serving. Thus, by February, leaders within the American Red Cross felt mounting pressure to consent to some sort of new blood policy guidelines as they recognized that "the extent [to which] the [blood banking] industry (ARC/AABB/CCBC) sticks together against the CDC, it will appear to some segments of the public . . . that we have a self interest which is in conflict with the public interest, unless we can clearly demonstrate that CDC is wrong."[52]

In March 1983, after increasing public pressure for coordinated action, the U.S. Public Health Service finally issued its first official recommendation on blood policy. Nine months had passed since the CDC discovered that hemophilia patients were getting AIDS through their blood plasma products. The new guidelines on blood donation called upon donors at increased risk for AIDS to refrain from giving blood or plasma. Those considered at high risk did not include all gays but only those gay men who were sexually active, had symptoms of AIDS, or had sex with people who did have such symptoms. The new guidelines did not include surrogate testing using the hepatitis B core antibody testing but called for studies into potential screening methods. In effect, the USPHS recommendations were a massively diluted version of the NHF's consensus position.

In the next two years, the CDC's predictions of an expanding epidemic of transfusion-related AIDS would materialize, even though there was evidence by 1985 that the new blood policy guidelines helped mitigate the spread of AIDS among recipients of transfused blood and blood products. The isolation of HIV as the viral cause of AIDS in 1984 facilitated efforts to prevent the spread of AIDS through blood transfusion with the development of an HIV blood test. The U.S. government issued the first license for an ELISA AIDS test on March 2, 1984, to Abbott Laboratories (an American firm that was also one of the major suppliers of plasma concentrates).[53] Blood bank testing for HIV began promptly in April 1985.

The plasma industry did not wait for the HIV test to roll out its own solution to the crisis. Experimental techniques for removing hepatitis viruses from plasma fractions had been around since the early 1970s.[54] Then in 1981 Germany granted a license to the Behringwerke Corporation for the first heat treatment process for factor VIII concentrates. The process killed the lipid coating of the hepatitis B virus, but also reduced the potency of the factor VIII molecule by at least 50 percent. Industry insiders were intrigued but discouraged. Lower potency required the manufacturer to use greater quantities of plasma, producing supply problems and substantially higher costs. A few companies continued to work on the technology, and the FDA received its first application for approval of a heat treatment process from Baxter Healthcare in June 1982, one month before Bruce Evatt announced that AIDS was striking hemophilia patients. The FDA issued the first license to sell a heat-treated clotting factor concentrate in the United States to Baxter in March 1983. Within the next year, Alpha Therapeutics, Armour Pharmaceutical, and Cutter Biological had also received licenses to introduce heat treatment techniques into the pooling process for their own concentrates.[55] While the plasma industry knew before transfusion-related AIDS became visible that heat treatment could eliminate blood-borne hepatitis from donor plasma, industry leaders most certainly delayed implementation because they believed that viral inactivation technologies would worsen the plasma supply issues while driving up the cost of their products. However, the emergence of transfusion-related AIDS made it impractical for the industry to delay any longer. By the end of 1982, leaders in the fractionation industry all knew that the future of their enterprise lay in heat-treated concentrates.

It was fortunate, and not altogether unexpected by hemophilia experts in 1983, that heat treatment killed the newly discovered HIV, given the similar profiles of post-transfusion hepatitis and AIDS. Yet, it was not until December 1983 that MASAC called on the plasma industry to expedite its development of such products, and it was October 1984 before the NHF officially endorsed the use of heat-treated concentrates over the older, vulnerable products.[56] At issue for the treatment experts was the question of whether the heat-treated concentrates were as potent as the old products. As NIH studies of post-transfusion AIDS have shown, it is unlikely that many hemophilia patients in the United States were contracting AIDS after the FDA's 1984 order that all the old unheated clotting factor concentrates be removed from the American market. By its own testimony, the entire plasma fractionation industry was selling only heat-treated product to American consumers in 1985. Unfortunately, these actions by the plasma industry and the NHF did not immediately stop the spread of transfusion-related AIDS to hemophilia patients. The heat-treatment processes were still limited between 1985 and 1988. At least twenty hemophilia patients contracted HIV before plasma fractionators improved their viral inactivation methods to the point that no contaminated product was getting to the market.[57]

Nor did the change to heat-treated clotting factor concentrates immediately change the perception that hemophiliacs were getting AIDS from their products. Many patients and families were beginning to learn of AIDS only in the late 1980s, either as they came down with symptoms of AIDS or as their blood was actually tested for HIV. In fact, even as concentrates became dramatically safer between 1985 and 1989, documented cases of post-transfusion AIDS continued to climb in the United States as hemophilia patients who acquired HIV before 1985 began "sero-converting" in ever-larger numbers. This lived experience of AIDS made it difficult for patients and families to believe the continued claims by the NHF or hemophilia specialists concerning concentrates. As Tom Andrews recalled, "In 1989 the blood supply was safe. I knew it intellectually. The chances of contracting HIV from factor VIII were about one in forty thousand. As a hemophiliac who had raced motorcycles, this was a risk I could accept. But still, it was hard not to suspect misinformation, hard to trust blood companies and hematologists after six years of confusing and contradictory messages."[58] Not until the 1990s did new cases of AIDS among hemophilia patients begin to disappear. By then, only a small minority of hemophilia patients were HIV-free (Tom Andrews among them), but the trust between patients and their advocates had been broken.

"To a Poster Child, Dying Young"

By 1985 the American media was beginning to give relatively steady coverage to the AIDS tragedy among people with hemophilia. Outside of the hemophilia community, diverse groups of Americans found themselves wondering about the significance of hemophilia for the first time, and they did so not through the recent history of hemophilia but through the lens of the emergent AIDS epidemic and transfusion-related HIV. The need to educate the public about AIDS and its impact on the blood supply made hemophilia part of a national conversation. Yet for hemophilia patients and their families, such heightened visibility was a mixed blessing, as popular discussions of hemophilia in the 1980s and 1990s were just as likely to be repressive as they were to be liberating. The AIDS era also signaled the reemergence of older stereotypes about "bleeders" and introduced new stigmas into the lives of people with hemophilia. What was clearly lost was the sense of "normalcy" that hemophilia patients, families, and advocates had seemingly achieved by 1980.

Hemophilia had many faces in the 1980s, but none more recognizable to the American public than that of Ryan White (1971–90). Most Americans knew White not as a "hemophiliac," but rather as an "innocent" victim of AIDS and the epidemic's most identifiable pediatric patient. When White died, *U.S. News and World Report* and other news media framed White's life as the story of "a poster child, dying young."[59]

In the late 1980s, the very idea that AIDS could have a pediatric representative on par with the poster children of the March of Dimes, Easter Seals, and the Muscular Dystrophy Association represented a critical shift in public presentations of AIDS. What journalists, health advocates, and politicians were also saying, of course, is that the image of AIDS embodied by White was not so easily identified with the gay lifestyle, sexual promiscuity, drug addiction, racial and ethnic divides, and the real and imagined problems of urban America. Ryan White's AIDS could potentially afflict anyone. It was a less alien, more manageable portrait of AIDS that helped alleviate some of the fears and stigmas associated with this new and deadly communicable disease.

Just as important was the depiction of White as an "innocent" victim. Until then, most Americans had thought of AIDS largely in terms of volition, as a malady that people brought on themselves through "morally questionable" behaviors, such as sexual promiscuity or illicit drug use.[60] His story exposed some of the faults in the dominant AIDS stereotypes, allowing the public to question the adequacy of a moralizing response that tended to portray anything related to AIDS as tainted, impure.[61] For religious Americans, in particular, the very existence of a "normal" AIDS patient like White countered the pervasive notion that AIDS was a kind of demon scourge on the morally and spiritually suspect.[62] Even former President Ronald Reagan, who avoided public mention of AIDS until 1987, used the occasion of White's death in 1990 to argue for an inclusive attitude to people with AIDS: "We owe it to Ryan to open our hearts and minds to those with AIDS . . . to be compassionate, caring and tolerant."[63] Four months after White's death, the U.S. Congress honored him by passing the Ryan White Comprehensive AIDS Resources Emergency (CARE) Act, the federal government's groundbreaking effort to dedicate resources to the care of persons with AIDS who had no other means of support.[64] It was a fitting tribute that reinforced how Americans' views of AIDS were changing as the epidemic moved into its second decade.

While Ryan White's story has been often told over the years, his hemophilia has been largely absent from the narratives. That oversight is understandable, given that White's fame had everything to do with his status as a persecuted person with AIDS and little to do with his being treated as a "hemophiliac." In the present context, however, his story merits another telling, if only to emphasize that, for people living with hemophilia in the 1980s and 1990s, the meaning and effects of AIDS were inextricably linked to their experience of having a manageable bleeding disorder.

Ryan White's rise to celebrity began in the summer of 1985 when fearful parents in White's hometown of Kokomo, Indiana, pressured local officials into banning the sixth-grader from attending classes in the coming 1985–86 school year. White received an AIDS diagnosis in December 1984 when his T-cell count became dangerously low. He was first barred from attending Kokomo's Western Middle School on July 30, just a few days after actor Rock Hudson announced that he had AIDS. Thus, the Ryan White story broke at a time when Americans still associated the disease entirely with homosexuality and drug use, and the American media began treating Ryan White's situation as a dramatic way to mainstream the AIDS issue. After much debate that August, the Indiana state courts mandated that White be allowed to do his studies by phone when classes commenced. This court decision gave a new twist to a distance-learning practice that hemophilia advocates had encouraged since the early 1950s: a practice that was long used to help mitigate illness-related absenteeism among victims of bleeding disorders was now being employed to protect the community from exposure to an HIV-infected child. It was open to debate whether this practical solution better served the child, the community, or no one at all.

While community involvement and parental input are usually key ingredients in creating a beneficial learning environment, they clearly proved to be a toxic combination for White and other school-age children with HIV/AIDS in the mid- to late 1980s.[65] Some parents who supported the legal case against White cited their fears of the unknown: "We're not saying AIDS is contractible, but we say there is significant doubt, and we're not willing to take risks [with our children]."[66] Others were less vocal about their reasons for keeping White out of school, but their beliefs often emerged in vicious form. When White did happen to encounter other children, for example, it was not uncommon for them to shun him or ridicule him with taunts of being a "fag" or "gay." In November, Indiana's Department of Education ordered the Kokomo school board to admit White; in

December, the school board voted unanimously to appeal. In February 1986 White's situation again seemed to take a turn for the better when public health officials in Howard County ruled that "routine contact" with White would not infect his classmates, a ruling that allowed White to attend classes. But this widely reported "victory" was also short-lived. On the day of White's return to school, 151 of Western Middle School's 360 students remained at home, while a handful transferred to other schools. After this unsettling event, Howard County Circuit Court judge R. Alan Brubaker felt compelled to grant the petition of three concerned families who had previously requested White's permanent removal from school. Describing his decision as a "no-win" situation, Judge Brubaker banned White from the classroom by citing an Indiana state law that prohibited children with communicable diseases from attending school.[67]

Ryan White did eventually return to classes after an April ruling by Howard County Circuit Court judge Jack O'Neill, but the ridicule and hostility that White encountered from other students during the subsequent school year helped contribute to his family's decision to leave Kokomo for good in 1987.[68] The Whites moved to Cicero where administrators, teachers, and students of Hamilton Heights High School welcomed Ryan White following local efforts at AIDS education within the school community.

In the midst of these struggles White became an icon of AIDS awareness, tolerance, and compassion. His celebrity grew tremendously in 1986 and 1987 with television appearances on the *CBS Evening News*, ABC's *Good Morning America*, and NBC's *Today Show* and *Tonight Show* and cover stories in *USA Today* and *People* magazine. World-class diver Greg Louganis, movie star Elizabeth Taylor, and pop icon Elton John were among a long list of notable celebrities who honored White with friendship and gifts, enrolling him in their public efforts to raise awareness and resources for AIDS research and treatment. White's life story was effectively dramatized in a made-for-television movie, *The Ryan White Story*, which aired on ABC in January 1989 to positive reviews. Between 1988 and 1989, White continued to appear regularly on television. His appearances on PBS's *3-2-1 Contact* and Phil Donahue's daytime talk show were explicitly aimed at educating children about AIDS and informing adults about AIDS among children. Yet Ryan White also proved adept in his various public appearances at persuading policy makers and politicians to devote attention and resources to AIDS. Notable here was his testimony to the President's

Commission on AIDS on March 3, 1988, and his linked appearances on ABC's *Nightline* and *CNN* that evening. While his story was born out of repeated tragedy, Ryan White's personal qualities helped transform it into a genuinely heroic saga.

The media often missed the critical significance of hemophilia in White's life story even as they credited White for heroically projecting normalcy in the face of his "death sentence" of AIDS.[69] What journalists overlooked, specifically, was how White's experience as a person with a manageable bleeding disorder frequently shaped his and his family's responses to the AIDS-related events in his life. As White said of his AIDS celebrity in "Growing Up Different," the opening chapter of his autobiography: "Sometimes when I give some speech about AIDS, I say things that sound like an actor on TV. Like, 'I came face to face with death at age thirteen.' Pretty dramatic, huh? To tell you the truth, AIDS didn't seem like such a big deal at first—just another illness. I'd been sick with an incurable disease since the day I was born, and I was used to it."[70] White's approach to AIDS reflected the management culture surrounding hemophilia, including the hemophilia community's attachment to the idea of normality.

White's embrace of this ideal was most apparent when he or his mother stressed that his celebrity was unwanted and that he just wanted a "normal life" for himself. As Jeanne White told one reporter, "I am not comfortable [with television promotion]," and "We are not about buying [or selling] books. . . . [Ryan's autobiography] is an educational tool, about how Ryan wanted to be a normal kid and how he went about doing that while becoming a hero."[71] Ryan himself was frequently blunt about his desire to be a "normal kid."[72] In February 1986, during a brief period when he was allowed to attend Kokomo's Western Middle School, White told one reporter how glad he was that his fellow students treated him "just like everybody else."[73] Or, as Brad Letsinger, one of White's best friends at Hamilton Heights High related: "Ryan . . . didn't want people to feel sorry for him. He hated that. He just wanted to be a regular kid."[74] Such statements—as well as White's tendency to treat AIDS as just another illness—should be understood in terms of his life experience as a child who took the lessons of normalized hemophilia management to heart. In fact, in 1973, long before he became America's most famous pediatric AIDS patient, White was the official poster boy for the Howard County Hemophilia Society.[75] White, like most people with hemophilia, confronted AIDS through the lens of his prior experience of having a treatable bleeding disorder.

The celebrity that Ryan White encountered was unique in many ways, yet his lived experiences as a person with hemophilia also reflected what other boys and men with the bleeding disorder were encountering with the emergence of AIDS in the 1980s. Between 1982 and 1986, hemophilia patients and their families were slow to learn of the risks of AIDS as inaction by various blood interests, failures within government, and poor advocacy by the NHF and other voluntary health organizations made knowledgeable action difficult. By 1987, however, it was clear to most hemophilia patients and families that every person with a bleeding disorder had risked contracting AIDS through his treatments, that most patients who used clotting factor concentrates had contracted HIV at some point in the preceding five years, and that the vast majority of these patients would likely die of complications of their HIV infection rather than their bleeding disorder. Dealing with these facts was difficult enough, but it was only the first in a long series of shocks. AIDS was never limited to homosexuals, but the early, frequent, and pernicious stereotyping of AIDS as a disease of "immorality" and "promiscuity" among gay men posed real dangers to people regardless of their sex or sexuality.

The imagery of innocence surrounding Ryan White was undoubtedly powerful. As attorney Robert Sullivan noted in conjunction with a 1985 case to exclude one seven-year-old from a school in Queens, New York, many children with AIDS come from "parents who are not as responsible as we would like them to be . . . children of an IV drug user or a victim of sexual abuse."[76] When compared to the circumstances of these children, hemophilic children with AIDS seemed pure. In fact, many Americans agreed with the imagery that framed hemophilic children as "normal" (apart from their bleeding disorder). The pervasive imagery of innocence certainly helped mitigate the stigmatizing stereotypes associated with AIDS, but it did not overcome them.

It is easy to overestimate the positive effect that the Ryan White story had in light of the disturbing undercurrents of the "innocent victim" and "poster child dying young" scripts that many Americans embraced in the late 1980s and early 1990s. In fact, the publicity surrounding White and other AIDS poster children was never wholly effective in combating the stigmas associated with AIDS as a "gay" disease or its evolving caricature as a malady of sexual promiscuity or deviance. In 1988, in the midst of Ryan White's celebrity, historian Sander Gilman astutely pointed out that the link between AIDS and various pernicious stereotypes associated with syphilis and other sexually transmitted diseases was "so widespread that it permeated categories of social organization, such as childhood, which would otherwise seem to be generally immune to such stigmatization." Gilman placed White's celebrity against the backdrop of the many children who contracted AIDS in utero, and whose presence in the schools was also challenged by fearful parents and community groups in the mid-1980s.[77] Unconsciously, if not consciously, many Americans stigmatized the hemophiliac as they judged the culpability of the AIDS patient. In the late 1980s and early 1990s, few Americans understood this fact as well as people with hemophilia, including the children among them.

The deleterious impact of AIDS-related stigma on families with hemophilia became abundantly clear to many Americans after a highly publicized incident in 1987 in which the home of the Ray family was burned to the ground. The Ray household included three hemophilic boys (Ricky, Robert, Randy, aged ten, nine, and eight respectively) who were barred from attending their school in Arcadia, Florida, soon after they each tested positive for HIV. A court order in 1987 forced the school to readmit the Ray brothers in August but prompted a boycott of the school by many families. Their home was destroyed four days after the boys' court-ordered return to school. The Rays were not at home when the fire started, but the message was clear; they were not safe in their own community, and they soon left Arcadia.

The Ray story echoed that of Ryan White but was significantly more sinister, given that the stakes of symbolic violence had been raised. The Ray brothers, like White, became celebrated victims of the American public's intolerance of persons with AIDS. Cast nationally as innocent victims, these teenage boys who contracted AIDS through their hemophilia treatments were also victims of a system of medical management gone awry. Ricky received the most attention of the boys as the oldest and first to die. He succumbed to AIDS in 1992, but not before garnering national attention a year earlier by marrying, at the tender age of 14, his childhood sweetheart, Wenonah. Despite the impossibility of it, Ricky like so many people with hemophilia in the era asserted his desire to live a "normal" life.[78]

Above all, the burden of the AIDS stigma put in question the idea of social progress for Americans with hemophilia. After a decade of hope in which hemophilia could be seen as a malady whose management placed the patient within the spectrum of "normal" living, persons with hemophilia had grown accustomed to being open with others about their chronic illness. The stigmas associated with AIDS in the 1980s prompted many Americans with hemophilia to be tight-lipped about their HIV/AIDS status. Worse still, fears that many Americans would be unable to make meaningful distinctions between hemophilia and AIDS compelled people with hemophilia to keep their bleeder status under wraps as well. Or, as Andrew Flagg described his experience of acquiring AIDS from his hemophilia treatments, "The big impact of HIV, aside from the concern about getting sick, was the feeling that I needed to go underground again." It was a reaction that was commonly held but seldom mentioned at the time. Flagg first saw it publicized by a fellow sufferer in 1989. "There was an article in the *New York Times Magazine* by a hemophiliac who had essentially the same reaction [as I did]. He was starting to feel more comfortable about his hemophilia as a man and a person, then, suddenly because of his HIV, it wasn't something he wanted to tell anybody. He didn't know when or how he should bring it up."[79] That man in the *Times Magazine* was attorney and law teacher Peter Brandon Bayer. He was among only a handful of people with hemophilia who volunteered their stories for public scrutiny before the mid-1990s.

Most people with hemophilia not only shunned celebrity in these years; many rightfully feared it for what further burdens it might bring into their lives.[80] As early as 1985, leading AIDS activist Cindy Patton wrote of an anonymous man with hemophilia who had not only dubbed the "growing fear that hemophiliacs are dangerous to employ or to have in schools as 'hemophobia'" but also spoke to her "wryly of coming out of the 'clot closet.'" Patton saw it clearly: "Although 'innocent' of presumed sexual difference, the myths about hemophilia and taboo[s] about blood and bleeding make AIDS among hemophiliacs not quite 'clean' and best kept hidden."[81]

The assumption of "innocence" that frequently accompanied reportage and discussion of the transfusion-related AIDS epidemic was often cold comfort to people with hemophilia. What most Americans failed to get, as Peter Bayer stressed in 1989, was that the burden of AIDS only began with its devastating biological effects. "AIDS is more than a disease—it is a sociological event," he concluded after detailing for *Times* readers how his HIV-positive status had limited his "prospects for marriage, children and a normal sex life." Bayer had "become more philosophical" after two years of anger and bitterness about his fate but decided to publicize his story in the interest of public education. In one telling moment, Bayer related his discomfort at the comment of a well-meaning friend, who told him, "It's not fair because it's not your fault." Bayer's circumspect response appeared in the closing paragraphs of his essay: "HIV infection and AIDS are miserable conditions that nobody deserves. The issues of AIDS are not questions of culpability. The true concerns must be finding a cure, limiting the spread of the disease, comforting the afflicted and educating the ignorant and misinformed. . . . Indeed, an appropriate response to the AIDS crisis requires even more compassion and understanding for the afflicted." What Bayer understood better than many of his fellow Americans was that the label of innocence belonged to a judgmental society and culture that exempted certain people with AIDS from culpability while condemning others. Better, he suggested, to promote understanding of AIDS than to stigmatize anyone.[82]

The Trouble with Normal

Between 1982 and 1987, Americans with hemophilia had choices—albeit limited ones—about their condition and its treatment that might have limited the spread of AIDS to themselves or others. We have seen how most hemophilia treatment specialists in the United States encouraged their patients with moderate to severe forms of factor VIII and factor IX deficiency to continue using clotting factor concentrates. This was true even where physicians knew that AIDS was likely blood borne and that these products made from commercially pooled plasma were particularly vulnerable to contamination. Some physicians chose to advise their patients differently. And the patients, of course, had decisions to make as well. Most followed their doctor's orders; others disobeyed. Some avoided HIV infections by ignoring the consensus opinion among treatment specialists to keep using clotting factor concentrates. Others suffered immeasurably by disregarding their doctors' warning. In short, there was no "right" course of action for either physicians or their patients—none that was obviously safe given what was known and unknown at the time.

Historically meaningful goals such as "normalcy" mattered tremendously to patients and physicians as they reasoned—in uncertain times—about what they should do in the face of AIDS. The effects of untreated or undertreated hemophilia were widely believed to be of greater risk to the patient than the "unlikelihood" of contracting AIDS from a plasma product. Yet, as we have seen, this widely embraced calculation was based on incomplete evidence and assumptions that were grounded in the past history of "successful" hemophilia management. The AIDS crisis in the hemophilia community called on everyone—including patients, families, and physicians—to look to the recent past to determine the "best" course of action.

Among the most tragic events of the era are the choices made by those "disobedient" hemophilia patients who ignored medical advice that would have likely spared them and their families from HIV/AIDS. In the minority of cases where physicians chose alternative (albeit less convenient and potent) treatments like cryoprecipitate, these doctors met with strong resistance from both patients and professional colleagues who considered the use of concentrates as indispensable to the comprehensive care approach that had helped normalize the lives of people with hemophilia in the 1970s. Cleveland hematologist Oscar Ratnoff recalled an anecdote in which the president of the local hemophilia chapter accused him of "trying to change [his] lifestyle" by recommending cryoprecipitate instead of clotting factor. "Yes, I am," Ratnoff responded. That chapter president was not only a person with hemophilia but also a physician with a doctorate in immunology. Ratnoff claimed that the man's response was "representative of the general attitude" he found among patients and physicians committed to the NHF's consensus position.[83]

Understandably, most hemophilia patients and their families wanted to believe that AIDS or "fear of AIDS" would not impact the increasingly normal lifestyles to which they had become accustomed. Despite growing fears of contracting AIDS (or perhaps because of them), some of these patients and families actively resisted changes to their lifestyles where it impacted their sense of autonomy or "normalcy." Such individuals, like the physician-hemophiliac in Ratnoff's anecdote, tended to be people whose personal identity and lifestyle was heavily invested in the norms, practices, and ideals advanced throughout the nation's hemophilia community by the NHF, the hemophilia treatment centers (HTCs), and leading hemophilia advocates.

In short, many hemophilia patients and their families had become accustomed to a lifestyle that they wished to maintain in the face of AIDS.

To understand why an inflexible commitment to using clotting factor concentrates seemed rational to some very thoughtful people in the hemophilia community during the 1980s, it is critical to understand the culture that people with hemophilia, their families, physicians, and advocates inhabited and the way that clotting factor concentrates were portrayed vis-à-vis other treatment options. The culture surrounding hemophilia in Reagan-era America placed a premium on the forms of medical management that the hemophilia community had cultivated since the early 1950s. That culture fiercely contested the public's view of the hemophiliac as a fragile "invalid" who was incapable of either autonomy or normalcy. In fact, as the stories of Ryan White, Ricky Ray, and other hemophilia patients suggest, many people in the hemophilia community idealized and embraced "normalcy" all the more because of AIDS.

One of the lesser-publicized aspects of transfusion-related AIDS among hemophilia patients in the United States was the secondary epidemic of AIDS among the wives and girlfriends of HIV-infected hemophilic males that extended beyond the peak era of preventable transfusion-related HIV infections. There too, the attachment to normalcy and autonomy proved dangerous; and there, too, past history mattered. In his 1991 interview with onetime NHF education director and historian Susan Resnick, Ratnoff also recounted his concern about the wives of his HIV-positive hemophilia patients. In the 1980s, he often recommended to such couples that they practice "safe sex" with a condom, and often met resistance to such advice. He recalled: "Said one young wife with her husband's beaming approval, 'If I made him wear a condom, he wouldn't know I love him.'" When Ratnoff insisted that the couple use a condom, the husband became angry and switched to another doctor. The young wife contracted HIV and later died of the disease. From a public health perspective, this couple's attitude seemed irresponsible, yet when CDC immunologist Dale Lawrence began tracking the rate of HIV/AIDS infections among the wives of hemophilic men in the mid- to late 1980s, he learned that such experiences were not uncommon. By the time that Lawrence had completed his study, it was clear that the commitment to putatively "normal" sexual relations within hemophilia families had played a tragic role in creating a secondary epidemic. Like the majority of heterosexual Americans, the hemophilia community did not yet regard "safe sex" as "normal" sex between two loving, committed people. Ratnoff put a provocative spin on it, when emphasizing his disagreements with his "non-compliant" hemophilia patients: "They interpret 'normal' differently than I interpret it," he said. "What they want to be are normal risk-takers instead of normal people."[84]

The 1980s witnessed a rise in the social value of therapeutic order and control, as might be expected in a time when the general health of American society was becoming more important than the "right" of individuals to exercise complete control over their lives. The shift in the therapeutic terrain was embodied for Ratnoff and other doctors by the fact that even the most intimate behaviors of the hemophilia patient and his family required management in the interest of public health. Psychiatrist Robert Simon pointed out that "the sexually active hemophilia patient's most intimate interpersonal behavior has now become a vital aspect of medical compliance, in the form of safe sex."[85] Physicians treating hemophilia patients had a psychological, if not moral, incentive to be more confrontational with patients when they asserted a willingness to deviate from the doctor's orders. So whether doctors recommended that their patients stay on clotting factor concentrate or advised that patients use alternative treatments, the message that hemophilia patients and their families were getting was that they put their lives in jeopardy whenever they ignored their doctors.

Fortunately, a minority of people with moderate to severe hemophilia did escape HIV infection in the 1980s. Some did so by chance, if not dumb luck. Among these "lucky" hemophilia patients were those who were not receiving state-of-the-art care in the first place. The federal government had subsidized the costs of hemophilia care for patients under eighteen since the mid-1970s as well as for those adult patients who qualified for Medicare or Medicaid. That still left the majority of adult hemophilia patients at the mercy of the private insurance system to fund their health care. And many of these patients went uninsured or underinsured in the 1980s. Either they had reached the insurance company's annual or lifetime limits on medical treatment, or private insurers refused to cover their hemophilia altogether. Very few adult hemophilia patients—whether they were employed or not—could pay for concentrates or comprehensive care on their own. While it is unclear how many people were involved, this population of undertreated hemophilia patients experienced an unsettling paradox within the American health care system: their lack of access to concentrates, HTCs, and other sources of state-of-the-art hemophilia management likely spared some of them from HIV infection.

Other hemophilia patients avoided post-transfusion HIV by being selective about using clotting factor concentrates. This group was unusual, because it was often contingent on the patient following the advice of a hematologist or physician who went against the consensus in the hemophilia treatment community. These patients chose cryoprecipitate over concentrates, alternative therapies, and even no therapy at all. Tom Andrews described his own preference to go without concentrate: "The cautious among us developed a suspicious cast of mind that has been difficult to shed. A kind of wartime-rationing mentality set in, even after purified factor VIII concentrates became available: if at all possible, take the punishment and absorb the bleed." Later, in 1989, Andrews (on his physician's advice) resorted to infusions of desmopressin acetate (DDAVP), a synthetic clotting agent not derived from plasma. Because DDAVP stimulated what little active factor VIII was in Andrew's bloodstream, it increased his clotting ability up to 35% of normal. It was good for "bleeds of a non-life threatening nature" according to the card Andrews carried in his wallet. But best of all, it carried "no risk of infection." "Infusing it gave me a fever and chills," he later wrote, but it was "worth every shiver."[86]

Like many hemophilia patients, physicians too wanted to believe that AIDS would not compromise past gains, especially those clinical hematologists, like Los Angeles' Shelby Dietrich or New York City's Louis Aledort, who had each fought successfully in the 1970s to mainstream comprehensive care programs for hemophilia and keep them sustainable. As medical co-director at NHF, Aledort had a strategic plan for the 1980s that focused on extending comprehensive care and making it more affordable for all persons with bleeding disorders in the United States. Thus, at a time when President Reagan was slashing support to medical and social services, hemophilia specialists were utilizing their influence within the NHF to build on the dramatic successes of the 1970s. When these hemophilia treatment advocates suddenly found themselves dealing with AIDS beginning in 1982, there was a tendency among them to treat this emergent epidemic as a distraction from what they thought to be the more pressing issue of providing affordable, sustainable care to patients through comprehensive hemophilia clinics. It was a well-meaning and admirable outlook in some respects, but it inadvertently proved fatal for many hemophilia patients when doctors thought it prudent to minimize the growing evidence that AIDS was in the blood supply. Arguably, many of the hemophilia doctors who were most involved with the NHF in the early 1980s were least inclined to challenge the way things were being done. They resisted the idea that AIDS necessitated immediate and sweeping changes to the provision of hemophilia care. They too were focused on recently won norms and lifestyles.[87]

The result of such wishful thinking among leading hemophilia specialists and advocates in the United States was that most hemophilia patients and families were left in the dark about what was going on with AIDS, how AIDS related to their chosen lifestyle, and (most importantly) what might immediately be done to reduce their risks of contracting AIDS and other blood-borne diseases. Thus, even though hemophilia treatment specialists acted in what they believed were their hemophilia patients' best interests, they mostly failed them in the era of HIV-tainted blood products. For far too long, the message to patients and families was that it was "inappropriate" to respond to their fear of contracting AIDS by abandoning blood products. The NHF's own AIDS Task Force repeatedly urged "hemophiliacs . . . to maintain the use of clotting factor in their treatment of hemorrhagic episodes."[88] They told patients to trust their doctor's advice and treatment plan, and they emphasized to doctors that the risks of AIDS did not entail changes in treatment in most cases of hemophilia.

Plasma fractionation companies joined treatment specialists as advocates for this therapeutic approach. Such companies distributed newsletters and advertisements to their "consumers"—the health care professionals treating hemophiliacs—that detailed their dependency on one another as the recipe for success. For instance, in marketing its Profilate Antihemophilic Factor concentrate for factor VIII deficiency in 1981, the Alpha Therapeutic Corporation of Los Angeles characterized their product as "Part of a Great Team" that included the "hemophiliac," his "family," and "specialists" devoted to a "coordinated multidiscipline approach" to hemophilia care. The Profilate ad noted, "With such advances [clotting factor concentrates] . . . there is every reasonable hope that the hemophiliac can escape severely crippling deformity and subsequently live a life of relative normality" (fig. 7.1).[89]

As recognition grew that AIDS was in the blood supply, this dominant

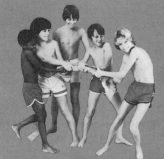
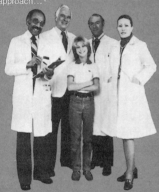
FIGURE 7.1. "Part of a Great Team" Clotting Factor Advertisement, Summer 1981.

message did not change dramatically. In December 1982, even as Alpha Therapeutic declared that it "ha[d] moved quickly to protect hemophilic patients by excluding plasma donors who may be potential carriers of AIDS," the company continued to advertise Profilate to health care professionals under the slogan "It Takes a Team" to maintain "the patient with hemophilia as an independent, self-supporting individual in his own community" (fig. 7.2). Alpha also made sure that physicians with hemophilia patients knew that "the National Hemophilia Foundation had recommended that existing treatment methods for hemophilic patients continue, since it is not yet clear what is causing AIDS" and that the company was working with the CDC "to help clarify whether the spread of AIDS is related to blood product use." Such companies did not deny that AIDS might be in the blood supply, but they argued that their actions were minimizing the threat, as they urged physicians to use their product to protect patients from their bleeding disorder.[90]

Nor did the message of the fractionation companies change once there was consensus that AIDS was caused by a blood-borne virus, for the simple reason that the blood industry, the FDA, and the medical profession had done far too little in the previous decade to address or prevent the spread of hepatitis in blood products. The fractionation companies, like hemophilia treatment specialists, knew from their experiences in the 1970s that most patients with severe to moderate hemophilia in the United States had already gotten one or another form of hepatitis from using pooled plasma products. New York hemophilia specialist Margaret Hilgartner described the clinical dilemma they faced on learning of AIDS in patients with severe hemophilia:

> Even though this might be the same disease that gays had, the discussion kept coming into the conversation: Was this going to be like hepatitis? Because if we had 72 percent [infected with hepatitis B], and some clinics had even higher percentages and were surviving, would these patients [with AIDS] then survive? Was it going to be as lethal? And if it wasn't going to be as lethal like it appeared to be in gays, did we really have to inform the patients to the same degree and worry about them?[91]

The consensus among hemophilia specialists was to treat AIDS among patients as they had treated hepatitis B infections—on a need-to-know basis.

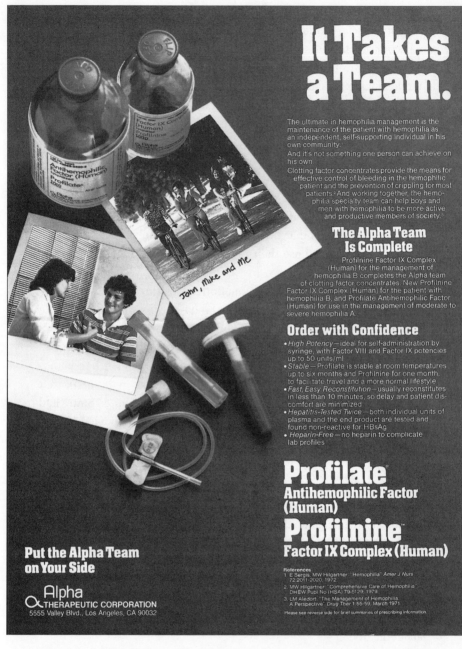

FIGURE 7.2. "It Takes a Team" Clotting Factor Advertisement, December 1982.

While some physicians were open with their patients that they had acquired hepatitis and that such infections could be lethal, physicians frequently emphasized the fact that hepatitis was not an immediate threat to the hemophiliac's life. Finally, professional consumers of blood products (including many hematologists) were also largely unaware in the early 1980s that there were experimental, yet promising technologies for killing blood-borne hepatitis viruses that the plasma industry had not aggressively embraced or publicized. The clotting factor concentrate's reputation of indispensability reinforced to physicians and patients alike that its benefits outweighed the known risks of contracting hepatitis as well as the uncertain but seemingly "small" risk of contracting AIDS.

Arguably, then, the hemophilia community's commitment to normalcy contributed to the tragedy of the hemophilia-AIDS catastrophe. The pursuit of a normal life put patients in greater danger because few people in the hemophilia treatment community were willing to recognize that AIDS constituted a crisis, one that made commitments to the usual norms of treatment incredibly dangerous. It was no longer obviously prudent, in other words, to treat clotting factor concentrates as the essential condition of effective comprehensive hemophilia care, as the "total care" approach of the late-1970s did. The fatal mistake was to assume that commercial clotting factor concentrates were solely responsible for the increased autonomy and normalcy that hemophilia patients experienced in the 1970s: that significant autonomy, and even normalcy, could not be delivered to patients without a comprehensive care system that treated commercial clotting factor concentrates as absolutely indispensable. And as the 1980s wore on, it became increasingly irresponsible for physicians to keep their patients in the dark about the realities of hepatitis, AIDS, and other transfusion-related infections.

"It Takes a Team": Healing, Culpability, and History

The hemophilia community endured an unexpected and incalculable loss from transfusion-related AIDS. After the problem was brought under control between 1987 and 1992, the hemophilia community sought to redress past mistakes. Hemophilia patients and families eventually realized they had been harmed by the industry that supplied their tainted plasma. Many patients felt betrayed by the NHF and the federal government, each of whom had failed to protect them. Some patients even lashed out at the physicians, nurses, and social workers who had urged them to use clotting factor concentrates during the 1980s. The de facto social contract that had long been promoted in the hemophilia community had been broken.

Peter Brandon Bayer eloquently captured this dynamic in the *New York Times Magazine*: "I did not 'contract' to receive this infection. I did not order it in exchange for money or other valuable consideration. I certainly did not want it. And it is a cruel and frustrating blow that the medication that allowed me at last to live a virtually normal life infected me with this virus."[92] Playing off the dual meaning of "contract," Bayer effectively evoked the issue that would consume the hemophilia community in the 1990s. Again the community would look back to its history, but this time to determine why the "contract" between patients and their advocates had fallen tragically short of being a "team" devoted to the best interests of people with hemophilia.

The collective experiences of the hemophilia community in the 1980s made it obvious that America's system for delivering effective medical care to hemophilia patients had not lived up to its promise and in many cases had killed those whom it was presumably designed to serve. This catastrophe was undoubtedly the product of human behaviors—a tragedy fashioned by a combination of mismanagement, denial, and even greed. Moreover, efforts to redress the high rates of HIV infection among persons with hemophilia led many parties to focus on uncertainties in the system and to ignore questions of culpability.

In the early 1990s, lawsuits and the emergence of two new hemophilia advocacy organizations—Hemophilia/HIV Peer Association and the Committee of Ten Thousand (COTT)—challenged the NHF for its dismal record of distributing effective information about AIDS and its inflexible defense of the extant systems of management. COTT leaders, for instance, believed that the NHF failed to work in the hemophilia patient's best interests by allying itself too closely with the commercial manufacturers of clotting factor concentrates and the doctors and treatment centers that profited from industry support.[93] These new hemophilia advocacy groups had much more in common with AIDS advocacy organizations of the era than did the NHF, and COTT was able to get a certain amount of recognition and justice for the victims of post-transfusion HIV. The leaders of COTT, which was largely composed of persons with hemophilia and HIV, also advocated important reforms in the oversight and management of the nation's blood supplies. That is to say, persons with hemophilia and HIV not only wanted recognition and justice for past mistakes but shared the concern of health professionals who wanted to prevent similar catastrophes in the future.[94]

The late 1990s witnessed the formal resolution of restitution efforts for most of the affected hemophilia patients and families. In 1997 a class action suit brought by COTT resulted in a negotiated settlement with the four major commercial companies that manufactured clotting factor concentrates. Each eligible victim, or surviving family, was awarded $100,000. Roughly 6,200 victims claimed a share of the settlement. The settlement was a bitter resolution for many of the surviving patients for they had little choice but to continue buying products from the same companies that had harmed them. In fact, for some patients, $100,000 was worth about year or two of concentrate, and certainly did not cover the lifelong treatment costs of HIV disease or post-transfusion hepatitis that were likely to kill them. Then, in 1998, the U.S. Congress passed the Ricky Ray Hemophilia Relief Act to provide additional monetary relief of another $100,000 per victim. To secure passage of the Ricky Ray legislation, Congress framed it as natural disaster relief—an "act of God"—rather than a tragedy facilitated by human choices and behavior. The class action and Ricky Ray "settlements" therefore admitted no guilt by industry or the government. In most respects, people with hemophilia were left on their own to sort out the social, economic, and political sources of neglect that led to their communal tragedy.

The breach of trust that occurred between hemophilia patients and their professional advocates in the 1980s and 1990s is still deeply felt today, which brings us to an important lesson of hemophilia of the AIDS era. As medical sociologist Charles Bosk pointed out in his classic 1981 study, *Forgive and Remember*, mechanisms for forgiving medical mistakes are as critical to physicians as remembrance and analysis of specific forms of failure.[95] Yet the medical profession's norms for dealing with mistakes are largely hidden and seldom detailed to patients or the public. Such norms risk leaving the false impression that physicians are prone to forgetting mistakes.

Not surprisingly, there has been some resistance within the hemophilia treatment community to dwelling on a system of medical management that, quite unintentionally, led to the premature deaths of so many. I opened this chapter by mentioning Louis Aledort's recent admonition to would-be historians of hemophilia: "Now is the time for healing, not finger-pointing." Aledort was chastising former CDC hematologist Bruce Evatt, whose account Aledort described as selective and self-serving.[96] It matters to history that Aledort and Evatt see these events differently, and even imperfectly. Both men were key actors in what happened in the 1980s. They and other participants should be encouraged to tell their versions of what happened both within and outside the hemophilia community. History is richer for it, particularly where lessons might be drawn from past events. But Aledort's rebuke of Evatt also begs a critical question: how should the history of such events be engaged so that it serves healing?

There is no simple solution to the question of history and healing in the recent history of hemophilia. Nor is it by any means clear what kinds of history would best promote healing while addressing the ironies of America's historical commitment to biomedical progress. But, as we advance the field of medicine, it does make sense for physicians, patients, historians, and others to engage in an honest dialogue about what happened to the hemophilia community during the AIDS era and to investigate its implications for our ongoing efforts to manage health and disease. For the sake of healing in particular, the spirit of that conversation needs to embrace both remembrance and forgiveness while giving full voice to the moral dimensions of the hemophilia patient's experience.[97]

Conclusion

The Governance of Clinical Progress
in a Global Age

In the early twentieth-first century, hemophilia stands alongside diabetes, asthma, cystic fibrosis, HIV disease, and a growing variety of other transformed pathologies to mark both the remarkable advances made by medicine in managing disease and the frustrating circumstances that those efforts have occasionally created. Nowhere has this history been more apparent than in developed countries like the United States, although similar stories can and have been told about chronic diseases elsewhere. This book has detailed much of the enterprise of hemophilia management as it evolved in American medicine and society over the past century. If we look back at these concerted efforts to manage hemophilia, what lessons does this history hold for the future governance of this enterprise in the United States and across the globe?

A Pathology of Progress, Revisited

The problem of governance as it relates to hemophilia begins with an appreciation of what disease management entails in its modern form. Historically, efforts to manage hemophilia have enjoyed some success—in a word, progress. But what does it mean to call hemophilia a "pathology of progress"? The opening of this book addressed this question by pointing to the narratives of technological progress and unfolding peril that have dominated the history of hemophilia since the advent of mass transfusions. Having detailed much of this history, the question can now be read in terms of the future governance of hemophilia and other chronic disease problems.

Hemophilia management can be defined as a technology-intensive commitment to alleviating the effects of a hereditary bleeding disorder. In fact, modern commitments to technological understanding of hemophilia not only predate medicine's characterizations of hemophilia as a bleeding disorder in the early twentieth century but also informed the earliest efforts to conceptualize hemophilia as a treatable malady. The ways that physicians have conceptualized hemophilia since the early nineteenth century have therefore been contingent upon the techniques that these same inquisitive physicians and scientists used to render the disease into something that other people could elucidate and transform. Print technologies, for instance, were instrumental in allowing Philadelphia physician John Otto to formulate the modern concept of hemophilia in 1803 and disseminate it to clinicians across the Atlantic Ocean. The paper tools of the genealogists allowed students of heredity to mark hemophilia as a disease with a distinctive sex-linked inheritance. Laboratory assays capable of measuring the delayed coagulation of hemophilic blood remade hemophilia into a distinctive bleeding disorder with a biochemical mechanism and clear rationale for its control. Today, genetic technologies have refined our understanding of hemophilia and its management to the level of genes, molecules, and DNA. The commitment to technology runs deep in medical efforts to control disease, to the point that any perceived progress we make in our efforts to manage hemophilia will always already be invested in some technological experience.

It is hardly surprising or accidental, then, that narratives of technological promise and peril pervade the recent history of hemophilia management or the histories of other chronic diseases. They do so because biomedical progress is a function of a technological way of being in the world. This is also why the question of governance is an appropriate one as we reflect on the past and move forward. Hemophilia's history—particularly its emergence and sustainability as a manageable disease—calls upon us to better understand what our commitments to biomedicine and its technological imperatives entail for present and future practice.

What then does this particular history, with all of its successes, failures, and ironies, tell us about the future of disease management for hemophilia and other chronic health problems? It is a worthy question as we enter a new century that seems increasingly invested in biotechnological ways of life. But addressing this question is made easier (and more consequential) if we see hemophilia as one among a rising number of transformed diseases that historian Charles Rosenberg has called "pathologies of clinical progress." This rubric captures several different aspects of "our present complaint": it speaks both to the "chronic-disease centered clinical environment" that ascended in medicine after greater control over infectious disease was achieved and to the powerful roles that laboratory and clinical science have played in creating "therapeutic modalities—such as insulin or dialysis—that have helped reconfigure the incidence and distribution of chronic illness." Indeed, such pathologies reflect a whole class of "medicine . . . developed and applied . . . then overprescribed." Rosenberg points to diabetes, chronic kidney disease, and "antibiotics—leading to selection for drug-resistant strains of pathogens" as prominent examples and concludes that the logic of such clinical progress speaks to "the need to integrate micro and macro levels of evolution in understanding the relationships among culture, environment, and diseases incidence."[1] Hemophilia can be added to the list of examples. But more importantly, Rosenberg's influential framing of the problem attunes us to the growth of altered disease that has not only become pervasive in the developed world but is threatening prospects for better health across the globe.

Collective commitments to biomedical science and technology have undoubtedly played a dominant role in the history of hemophilia since the 1930s, yet this book has also highlighted the prominent roles of gender, community, and other social factors in shaping how Americans treat hemophilia and the people affected by it. I therefore want to stress the necessity of interpreting "pathologies of clinical progress" in terms of the critical categories that shape people's experience of hemophilia and other chronic conditions.

Our understanding of the recent history of hemophilia would be impoverished if our efforts to narrate hemophilia's emergence as a manageable disease failed to account for the lived experience of hemophilia management and how it has changed over time. I have thus argued that understanding the unwanted as well as intended effects of the medical and social management of hemophilia requires sustained engagements with how this disease and its effects have been conceptualized by patients, families, and the lay public as well as by physicians, scientists, and other authorities. It matters not only that experts conceptualized hemophilia as a bleeding disorder that could be transmuted using increasingly potent transfusion technologies but also that they defined it as a disease that predominantly afflicts males. It also matters that patients and families have interpreted the efforts of doctors to "normalize" the hemophiliac's body and mind as consistent with their own aspirations for a healthy, more autonomous, and happy existence. The critical payoff to seeing the recent history of hemophilia through the lens of society and its evolving categories is that it puts us in a position to interpret critical events in ways that might otherwise leave important factors unexplained: like why the quest for "normal lives" was so important to postwar efforts to manage hemophilia, or how and why the AIDS catastrophe of the 1980s revealed this collective investment in normalization as a source both of strength and of eventual disappointment.

Autonomy without Normality: Hemophilia Activism in the 1990s

Hemophilia activism in the 1990s was both different and connected to the forms of advocacy that existed in the U.S. hemophilia community before AIDS, a fact that is worth considering in light of the continual need for good governance. We have already seen how transfusion-related AIDS radically changed how people within the nation's hemophilia community thought about their place in American medicine and society. For the most part, patients and their families had embraced medicine and its experts in the 1950s, 1960s, and 1970s; they had come to rely on technology-intensive interventions to achieve their aspirations for normalcy. Medical management therefore held special power for the hemophilia community; and, for better or worse, most patients, families, and physicians generally believed by 1980 that the "total care" model centered on the use of commercial clotting factor concentrates was a therapeutic arrangement that they could scarcely do without. The AIDS tragedy exposed the faults in the hemophilia community's prevailing assumption that "normal lives" were possible and, for many, destroyed it altogether. As such, many hemophilia activists in 1990s were driven not by the pursuit of normality but by a desire for social justice, more recognition of present risks and past harms, and a desire to see that hemophilia management in the future effectively served the goals of patient autonomy as well as improved health.

Hemophilia activists in the 1990s looked at the AIDS epidemic and the landscape that had grown up around people with hemophilia in the preceding decades and began to see just how risky an enterprise disease management actually was. In the United States, to be treated as a hemophiliac in 1980 was typically to depend on home care with occasional visits to a clinic or hospital for the comprehensive treatment that specialists could now provide.[2] Always vulnerable, hemophilia patients could nonetheless take solace from the fact that there was an expansive network of institutions, professionals, and lay advocates working to better their condition through disease management. The hemophilia treatment centers (HTCs), funded by the federal government, had already emerged as the backbone of this therapeutic landscape; many state-level governments were supporting HTCs as well.[3] But these HTCs could not have functioned effectively without the assistance of private and public laboratories, pharmaceutical and biotech firms, insurance companies, the federal agencies of the Department of Health and Human Services (FDA, CDC, NIH, Medicare, Medicaid, etc.), professional and trade associations, community blood banks, and an array of voluntary associations that included the American Red Cross and the National Hemophilia Foundation. It was this complex social network surrounding the treatment of hemophilia that became the focus of reform efforts by activists in the 1990s who wanted a great deal more than normalcy.

Thus, beginning in the late 1980s, many of the people most closely affected by the exigencies of this disease management system attempted to change it. In 1988, for instance, Dana Kuhn helped create the Man's Advocacy Network of the NHF (MANN) in order to pressure NHF membership to weaken the influence of the commercial plasma industry and those hemophilia specialists who were advocating strong ties to the industry. Kuhn's involvement with NHF followed his own tragic encounter with AIDS. As someone with mild hemophilia, Kuhn did not rely on clotting factor concentrates to facilitate normalcy. Yet, in 1983, at the age of forty-one, this seminary student, husband, and father of two children broke his foot playing basketball. His doctors gave him an infusion of factor VIII concentrate to play it safe. That one infusion infected him with HIV. By the time he learned of his infection in 1985, his wife was infected too. She died of AIDS a year later, leaving Kuhn with two young children to raise. Kuhn was understandably motivated to reform the NHF from the inside, but he met strong resistance. He left the NHF in 1993 after calling for an investigation of the organization's executive director, who later resigned.[4]

The hemophilia community took a little longer to confront AIDS than other sectors of the HIV-positive population.[5] As political scientist Patricia Siplon has noted, the "innocent victim" label was one critical impediment to the hemophilia community's involvement in AIDS activism. By the early 1990s, however, some men with hemophilia were embracing the similarities between them and gay men with AIDS rather than strive for the old "normalcy." These individuals formed new associations—the Committee of Ten Thousand (COTT) and the Hemophilia/HIV Peer Association (H/HIV Peer)—which openly challenged the competence of the NHF to advocate on behalf of persons with hemophilia. Leading persons with hemophilia in this alternative advocacy movement included COTT founders Jonathan Wadleigh and Tom Fahey, H/HIV Peer founder Michael Rosenberg, Greg Haas, Corey Dubin, and Dana Kuhn (now radicalized following his failed efforts to reform the NHF from within). With increased outside pressure, leading persons with hemophilia—such as Glenn Pierce and Val Bias—worked for reform within the NHF. But such reformers were not as disenchanted by the NHF's failures as those men who took their cues from recent AIDS activism.[6]

The COTT and H/HIV Peer Association were radical political organizations by comparison to the old forms of hemophilia management advocacy embodied at the NHF, and the radical character of these groups was widely evident where its members held the commercial plasma companies and the hemophilia doctors accountable for their actions during the 1980s. Infamously, the H/HIV Peer Association put out a "shame list" of doctors who had provided expert testimony in the courts for the plasma fractionators. Hematologist Louis Aledort was even labeled the "Mengele of the Hemophilia AIDS Holocaust" as activists lashed out.[7] The strategies of the new hemophilia groups mirrored the aggressive tactics of ACT-UP and other AIDS activists from the gay community. Like those earlier groups, they were successful on many levels.[8] The COTT and H/HIV Peer Association together pushed the federal government to review what happened to the hemophilia community, first in the form of 1994's Institute of Medicine hearing on

HIV and the blood supply and later in the passage of the Ricky Ray Hemophilia Relief Act of 1998. Simultaneously, they pressured the commercial plasma industry to deal with the implications of HIV-tainted concentrates. COTT, in particular, helped negotiate the 1997 settlement that gave many HIV-infected hemophilia families some modest financial relief.[9]

Another significant achievement of 1990s hemophilia activism was the appointment in 1995 of COTT president Corey Dubin to the Blood Products Advisory Committee of the FDA. Dubin became the first consumer advocate to have a voting role in the federal government's chief blood policy committee. When Dubin stepped down in 2000, COTT board member Terry Rice took his place.[10] This seat at the blood policy table was a concrete sign that the voices of persons with hemophilia had a prominent say in how the blood supply would be managed in the twenty-first century. Chief among the hemophilia community's concern was to prevent another AIDS-like tragedy from occurring, and Dubin and others were actively promoting greater vigilance against variant Creutzfeldt-Jakob disease (vCJD)— a potentially fatal form of transmissible spongiform encephalopathy—even as scientists and health authorities were trying to determine if its purported cause (a prion akin to the ones responsible for mad cow disease) is actually transmissible by blood and, if so, how to prevent its spread by transfusion of blood and plasma products.[11]

Since 1992, the prominent leadership roles that men with hemophilia have played in the broader advocacy movement signal what might be the most positive effect of the AIDS era: namely, that the American hemophilia community has now matured to the point that persons with hemophilia—not their parents, their physicians, or anyone else—are representing the experience, needs, and demands of the larger community. These activists have acquired scientific, medical, and political fluency that extends beyond their lived familiarity with hemophilia and its management. Thus, although the AIDS crisis decimated the hemophilia community, it also produced forms of activism that were a much needed antidote to the paternalism that had historically characterized the hemophilia advocacy movement in the United States. It also signaled the limits of normality. Normal was no longer a meaningful ideal for most people with hemophilia in the 1990s. For activists with hemophilia in particular, there was only a search for justice and a concerted commitment to achieving greater autonomy and health for the future.

The hemophilia activists who have made social justice and public health their focus since 1990 have proved themselves to be astute observers of history. As highlighted in this book, the recent past of hemophilia management well illustrates that the historic quest for normality—while flexible in its own ways—is too prone to complication and disappointment. Normal living is too elusive an ideal to serve disease management or the more critical goal of healing. Embracing extraordinary living and the autonomy it constitutes is better; it provides a more reliable passport to health.

There is No Normal, Only Vigilance

If normality is no longer an appealing goal for persons with hemophilia, the necessity to control this bleeding disorder and maximize health and autonomy remains as compelling as ever. As such, a hemophilia diagnosis for patient and family remains the first stage on a veritable odyssey. The Massie family effectively captured the reality of this modern passage (ca. 1958–75) in its appropriately titled memoir, *Journey*. Now, as then, managing hemophilia requires patients and their allies to negotiate a complex social and cultural system that renders hemophilia into a challenge that— despite its ever-present and risk-laden character—is considerably less burdensome than the disease would be in its "natural" state. Indeed, it is arguable that today's hemophilia family in the United States is more inclined than ever to think that this bleeding disorder—where adequately managed—should never be so burdensome as to entail a dramatic departure from theirs or society's expectations and norms for the healthy. The persistence of this belief is testimony to the past success of efforts to manage hemophilia as well as to the human spirit. Patients, families, or society should not aspire for less than improved health or autonomy. However, it is critically important given what is now known of past efforts to manage hemophilia and other diseases that we not overestimate our capacity for control. Our investments in technological fixes—even where they are successful—largely illustrate the need for greater circumspection and vigilance. Short of a complete cure (and arguably not even there), medical progress only gives rise to the need for more intensive management.

Thus, the enterprise of hemophilia management, along with its constitutive commitment to technological normalization, is undoubtedly alive and well in the twenty-first century. We now have synthetic clotting factor treatments that effectively stop hemophilic bleeding (without the risk of blood-borne infections) and even ongoing laboratory and clinical research that promises a "cure" in the form of techniques for replacing defective genes in patients with hemophilia. Yet, after the AIDS transfusion tragedy of the 1980s, normality as a marker of individual progress and existential meaning has lost much of its appeal. Consider, for instance, this made-for-television portrait of the hemophiliac's predicament that first aired on *Gideon's Crossing*, ABC's critically acclaimed medical drama, in February 2001. Derrick, a fictional hemophilia patient, asks Dr. Gideon if the new genetically engineered clotting factor he is about to receive will provide him with "a normal life"? The doctor responds: "There's no such thing as a normal life, Derrick. Everyone's life is different. Which means, I'm afraid, that you'll have to resign yourself to having a pretty extraordinary life."[12] Thus, even as normality wanes as an ideal for governing the aspirations and expectations of patients, extraordinary effort continues to be a hallmark of managing hemophilia.

Efforts to care for people with hemophilia should continue to change for the better. Yet, even as things change, what we are most likely to see in the twenty-first century are variations on themes that will be familiar to students of twentieth-century medicine and society. Today, the most fortunate children and adolescents with hemophilia in the United States rely not on plasma-derived clotting factor concentrates (which some have never had) but on concentrates synthesized in the laboratory using recombinant DNA technologies. Synthetic concentrates eliminate the risk of blood-borne pathogens like HIV and hepatitis C virus (HCV), but they have their own problems. They have been somewhat less potent than concentrates derived from human plasma (and thus require patients to infuse larger volumes of concentrate to control their bleeds). More troublesome, recombinant factor VIII and factor IX concentrates are an expensive commodity, prohibitively so for many hemophilia patients and their families. In fact, most hemophilia patients across the globe still rely on products derived from human plasma to manage their bleeding disorders, particularly beyond North America, Europe, Japan, and Australia. Even now there is not enough plasma-derived clotting factor to go around. It too remains an expensive as well as scarce commodity.

Cost remains the primary barrier to effective hemophilia care both in the United States and globally. Not only does human plasma continue to be a difficult resource to manage effectively, but its continued scarcity has also made the hemophilia patient's use of prophylactic infusions of concentrated clotting factor exceptional in most places. The inability of patients to practice such prophylaxis is itself a public health tragedy because hemophilia researchers from the late 1950s forward have demonstrated again and again that regular infusions of clotting factor (given independently of any symptoms) substantially reduce long-term disability as well as the incidence of bleeding and other symptoms.

Modern medicine and society have made remarkable progress in managing hemophilia since the 1950s, yet the persistent problem of cost means that things are not dramatically different today from what they were in the late 1960s when Dr. Kenneth Brinkhous told Robert Massie, "We've solved the scientific problem of concentrates, but we haven't solved the social problems." Society, he said, "is going to have to figure out a way to pay for this kind thing. The families simply can't do it by themselves."[13] The true test of progress in managing hemophilia has always hinged on giving patients access to state-of-the-art medicine. And while there has undoubtedly been progress in getting hemophilia patients the treatments they need in the United States, it has been a constant, humbling struggle, too.

Finally, the growing manageability of bleeding disorders has broadened hemophilia's significance within modern medicine and society beyond the patients and families that had traditionally been its principal victims. Those patients and families are still at the center of this drama, as they should be. Yet efforts to ease their disease-related burdens have required investments across society that, in both real and imagined ways, have connected the hemophilia patient's predicament to anyone who relies on safe and efficient blood services and modern health care systems for managing disease. Thus, modern medicine has transformed hemophilia into a problem that even the most self-interested societies cannot ignore. It is no longer merely a question of attending to the "special problems" of "categorical illness groups" or "fractional populations" like the hemophilia community (although this is still an enduring question).[14] After the tainted blood scandals of the 1980s and 1990s, compassion for the hemophilia patient's circumstance has been elevated into a necessary social duty and a requirement of responsible public health.

In fact, the problem of hemophilia has become so entwined with our systems of delivering safe and efficient blood services that to ignore this minority population is to risk violence to the whole population. To cite a concrete example of the danger here, public health authorities in the United Kingdom reported in May 2009 the first documented case of variant Creutzfeldt-Jakob disease in a person with hemophilia. Since the late 1990s, hemophilia activists have argued that this form of spongiform encephalopathy could be transmissible through transfusions of blood and plasma. The person in question was in his seventies and died of causes unrelated to vCJD, but traces of vCJD were found in his spleen at autopsy, and they very likely got there from his use of a tainted blood product. The evidence for blood-borne transmission of vCJD was compelling enough to cause the government to warn the public. As Chris James, chief executive of the U.K.'s Haemophilia Society noted, "It now looks like there is a real possibility of a link between receiving blood products and developing vCJD. What was a theoretical risk is now a suspected causal link." This news came the same week that the British government published its response to the well-publicized Archer inquiry that called in February 2009 for higher compensation of those hemophilia patients who received plasma products contaminated with HIV and HCV from the National Health Service in the 1970s and 1980s.[15]

What, then, does it mean for the future that our engagements with hemophilia in the past century have transformed this disease? No one, as far as I know, wants to go back to the days of bleeding, bruised, and crippled children. Yet there appears to be little choice at the current time but to sustain the project of hemophilia management and try to ensure that it effectively serves society as well as hemophilia patients and their families. It is even harder to say when, or if, a cure will be here. But if history provides any indication, we probably are further from a cure than media headlines, venture capitalists, and bullish scientists have been known to say. What we do have, at present, is a complex system for transforming hemophilia into a chronic, but manageable problem. This system has been around for decades now, and its lessons make it abundantly clear today that our past efforts intensify the requirement for vigilance rather than lessen it.

Globalization and Future Prospects

As suggested by the prevalence of hemophilia around the globe, the ways that experts have conceptualized and treated hemophilia over the course of the past century have had profound effects on aspects of the contemporary world that would—at first glance—seem far removed from a disease problem that most people would principally (and correctly) categorize as a personal and familial challenge. Although it is hardly obvious, past and present efforts to manage hemophilia have frequently impacted both the healthy and the sick. The fact that efforts to remedy hemophilia produce meanings and effects beyond patients and their families has not escaped the notice of journalists in the past two decades—particularly in light of the troubling issues raised by the management of bleeding disorders in the AIDS era. Two recent examples from the *New York Times* are suggestive of the social and political reach of the hemophilia problem and how management of the disease has frequently touched on issues of considerable importance to Americans as well as their neighbors, trading partners, and even enemies.

In May 2003, at a time when Americans were experiencing daily reports about SARS outbreaks in China, Walt Bogdanich and Eric Koli broke a story in the *Times* that highlighted the risks of globalization in a world where blood plasma is a multibillion-dollar commodity and "consumers" with bleeding disorders inhabit China and every other country on this planet. The journalists claimed that Cutter Biological, a division of the Bayer pharmaceutical company, sold millions of dollars of clotting concentrates to Asia and Latin America in the mid-1980s because the "product had proved unmarketable in the United States and Europe." Those clotting concentrates, which First World governments and consumers suspected of being tainted, did prove to be contaminated with the AIDS virus. Cutter/Bayer representatives have maintained, publicly at least, that the company did not knowingly sell tainted concentrates abroad. Bogdanich and Koli based their story on documents and interviews collected from American lawsuits filed on behalf of persons who had contracted HIV through similar blood products. The evidence demonstrated that Cutter Biological shipped its old, HIV-contaminated clotting concentrates for sale overseas in late February 1984 even though the company had already promised regulators in the United States and Europe that it would terminate all sales of the old product and begin selling "a new, safer product" that was heat-treated to reduce the risk of viral contamination. Allegedly, agents of Cutter Biological behaved illegally when they sought to clear their inventory of the old blood products. The most incendiary documents indicated that Cutter had continued to produce blood products using the old methods where they "had several fixed-price contracts and believed that the old product would be cheaper to produce." The results of these business decisions were disastrous, of course. In Taiwan alone, said Bogdanich and Koli, "more than 100 hemophiliacs got H.I.V. after using Cutter's old medicine." In emphasizing the extent of Cutter's malfeasance, Dr. Sidney Wolfe, director of the Public Citizen Health Research Group, told Bogdanich and Koli that the court documents they were scrutinizing were "the most incriminating internal pharmaceutical industry documents" he had seen in his three decades of monitoring the industry.[16]

The *Times* journalists sought to humanize as well as dramatize the documents detailing the industry's old but deadly business decision by interviewing surviving victims and participants in Taiwan and Hong Kong. By spring 1985, the commercial plasma industry was not disputing the connection between AIDS and unheated clotting factor concentrates, though it had frequently done so in the preceding year. Yet, of events in May 1985, Bogdanich and Koli wrote, "[when] the AIDS scare [had] reached hemophiliacs in Hong Kong, Cutter's distributor there placed an urgent call to Cutter headquarters" to ask for the new heat-treated product. "Sounding distraught, he told of an impending medical emergency. Hemophiliacs were frightened. Children were being infected with H.IV. Parents were hysterical. Couldn't the company send the new, safer product?" Cutter reportedly replied that "the new medicine was going to the United States and Europe," and that in Hong Kong and elsewhere only "a small amount was available for the 'most vocal patients.'"

This remarkable *Times* story was accompanied by a photograph of Lee Ching-Chang, the son of a Taiwanese farmer and "the only hemophiliac with H.I.V. willing to be photographed" because of the "despair, discrimination, job loss," and stigmas surrounding AIDS in China. Identified as an HIV carrier in 1986 and "too sick to work" by 2003, Mr. Lee said: "I am bitterly angry." As Bogdanich and Koli made clear for their readers, the vulnerability of these Chinese people with hemophilia was not just a function of their bleeding disorder. In the global economy of blood products, patients from poorer, less-developed nations (and continents) were subject to lesser treatment than their counterparts in the United States, the United Kingdom, or Germany. Quite simply, whether the executives at Cutter and other pharmaceutical companies articulated it or not, their actions in the

1980s and later demonstrated that they had valued the blood consumer in China less than an American or European one.[17]

Commercial plasma companies in the United States and Europe were clearly trying to recoup their investment in choosing how to distribute their different products. They did not want any plasma product to go to waste. In fact, hemophilia patients in China were not the only ones to feel that plasma fractionation companies were being valued more than their own lives. Americans, in all their diversity, have also been victims of such free market logic. It is well known, for instance, that in 1996 the Tokyo and Osaka District Courts awarded the Japanese victims of HIV-contaminated clotting factor concentrates the equivalent of $375,000 per individual, which was later amended upward to include a $1,500 a month stipend for each victim over his lifetime. Representatives of the Japanese government and five pharmaceutical companies made public apologies on March 14, 1996, before victims. Green Cross president Kawano Takehido bowed so deeply in one of these ceremonial apologies that his head reportedly touched the floor. It was a symbolic moment not only in Japan but in the United States as well. Many Americans with hemophilia were encouraged by this result and hoped that something similar would happen in the United States. When a class action settlement in the United States awarded only $100,000 to each victim or his family, many people in the American hemophilia community were angered by the fact that the lives of American hemophilia patients were not given as much value as the Japanese hemophilia patients. The companies involved were the same. The major difference was, as legal scholar Eric Feldman has shown, that hemophilia activism in Japan and the Japanese public was much more aggressive about holding the plasma industry responsible for its actions. The culture of accountability in Japan and the fact that many of these companies were American and European corporations trading in "foreign" blood gave Japanese hemophilia groups an advantage in generating public outrage over the tainted blood scandals of the 1980s.[18]

If the preceding 2003 hemophilia story by the *Times* is suggestive of social injustice in the age of globalization and AIDS, another *Times* story from October that year was even more indicative of the political dimensions of treatment inequities in hemophilia. In a story about the "struggle for Iraq," reporter Ian Fisher detailed the improving conditions of Iraqi "AIDS patients" following what the administration of President George W.

Bush was then calling the "liberation of Iraq." Upon the fall of Saddam Hussein's dictatorship, Muhanid Hassan was reportedly "astonished" to learn that "AIDS patients in most places outside of Iraq" were not quarantined. "'They don't separate them from others?' asked Mr. Hassan, [age] 42. 'Not in jail? Free?'" Fisher reported that Mr. Hassan was "a hemophiliac who earns a small living driving a taxi," and one of only seventy-two surviving HIV-positive "patients with blood disorders" in the new Iraq. Between 1985 and 1986, 244 Iraqis with blood disorders were infected with HIV by imported blood products. Then, in what Fisher calls a "cruel footnote in the history of Saddam Hussein's rule," people with bleeding disorders were rounded up, [and] their families taken hostage by the police if they fled." Mr. Hassan spent four years locked in a hospital though he never developed symptoms of AIDS. Another man, Khalid Ali Jabbar, avoided the incarceration of his five HIV-infected sons by moving them from house to house, only to lose them to AIDS anyway. In 1988 Mr. Hassan's mother said she had the opportunity to explain her distaste for the country's AIDS policy to Saddam Hussein. She recalled telling him, "It is like if you get food poisoning in a restaurant, instead of arresting the owners, you arrest the person who got sick." To this, Hussein supposedly replied, "I can't do anything for you. I am sorry. The problem is this war [with Iran]. I am very busy." According to Ian Fisher, it took Iraqi health officials more than six years to admit to the United Nations that it even had any AIDS cases in the country, and this neglect was "tied in part to a belief that AIDS is largely a Western illness of sex and drug abuse." Still other health officials admitted that "Mr. Hussein's vision of Iraq as a utopia under his leadership also made him hide the problem." Eventually, in 1991, Hussein did declare an "amnesty" for these AIDS victims.

Though Iraqi health officials welcomed the fact that they could now treat AIDS publicly after more than a decade of repression, they were also bracing for new HIV infections since the fall of Hussein's government. The sanctions that isolated Iraq from the rest of the world as well as the Draconian controls that characterized Hussein's handling of AIDS had kept HIV infections limited in the country. With the American and British occupation of Iraq came new opportunities for infection as well as a country with substantial needs beyond the health care.

Judging by the testimony of Fisher's informants, the situation for persons with bleeding disorders and AIDS may have actually worsened before it improved, particularly because the injustices of the Hussein regime were part of a broader culture of "intolerance" that seemed likely to persist in 2003. Thus, when asked what he planned to do in the new Iraq, twenty-nine-year-old Farid Khalis said, "I still can't tell anyone that I have H.I.V. In Iraq, people are ignorant. . . . Iraqi society will not tolerate us. They think this is only a sexual disease." When posed a similar question, Mr. Jabbar said that he wanted to leave Iraq and start life again with his wife and two remaining sons. He saw no end to the social stigma in Iraq. "For 16 years, my family, my neighbors, my brothers have all abandoned us," he said. Although no one in Mr. Jabbar's family had either hemophilia or AIDS in 2003, he could not bear to reconstruct his life in a country that had betrayed his five lost sons. In his mind, at least, the stigma of AIDS had effectively torn every bond of kinship his family knew. They were homeless and suffering despite having both a place to live and good health.[19]

These twenty-first-century stories confirm that hemophilia continues to play a role on the stage of world history. Another thing is also clear. People with hemophilia around the globe remain a vulnerable population despite the efforts by the World Federation of Hemophilia (WFH) and the World Health Organization to make modern hemophilia management available globally. In fact, in 2004, as Brian O'Mahony looked back on the forty-year history of the WFH, he characterized ongoing efforts to "introduce, improve, and maintain haemophilia care worldwide," as a "back to the future" enterprise.[20] Presumably, O'Mahony was serious about replicating past successes; but given the troubles that have accompanied much of that past success, his "back to the future" trope is a questionable characterization of ongoing efforts to advance the health prospects of the global hemophilia population. Avoiding past mistakes is critical, of course, to any effort to replicate past successes. And, in all fairness to O'Mahony, the WFH has proved committed to learning from the past in its recent efforts to promote hemophilia management around the world.

Still, if our local, national, and international governance of the problem of hemophilia is to build upon past lessons, we must come to grips with the undesired as well as intended effects of our past progress. That includes arranging our social and political priorities in ways that make individual autonomy as well as health increasingly central to the mission of governance while also maximizing the greater health of minority as well as majority populations.

The Irony of the "Wild-Type" Cure

Our capacity to make sense of biomedical progress in the management of hemophilia has been constantly challenged in the past century by the unforeseen, undesirable, and occasionally ironic entailments of our efforts to improve our health. But it can rightfully be argued that the high infection rates of HIV and hepatitis viruses among people with hemophilia might have been lessened or prevented with more foresight and vigilance. What if blood bankers and the plasma industry had put the health and safety of their consumers first by treating hepatitis B virus as an imminent threat? What if the federal government had effectively ensured the quality of blood and plasma supplies? What if physicians and public health authorities had been more proactive with their patients about the potential risks of transfusion-related infections?

Such questions all presuppose that better management is the principal remedy to any form of medical progress in the fight against hemophilia or any other disease. Certainly, efforts to manage disease and promote health more responsibly should be applauded. This would reduce the unforeseen troubles and unmitigated tragedies that our past investments in medical progress have occasionally produced. But while researching *The Bleeding Disease*, I grew increasingly concerned about those investments in progress that can be categorized as biomedical (i.e., heavily invested in a resolutely biotechnological way of experiencing the world). Commitments to progress—and particularly those invested in biotechnology—will almost always have unintended effects. Preventable disasters, however, have been an all-too-common part of the enterprise of hemophilia management. Avoiding such outcomes while managing our expectations of biomedicine's promise therefore becomes critical as we move forward.

When I was first introduced to hemophilia research in 1993, early gene transfer research promised the ultimate solution to hemophilic bleeding: a genetic cure that would replace the defective clotting factor gene found in the bodies of patients.[21] Optimism for experimental gene therapy became more muted in 1998 after the death of Jesse Gelsinger and a few other patients who had undergone experimental gene transfer for their genetic ailments.[22] None of these patients had hemophilia, but their deaths undoubtedly impacted the culture surrounding research for genetic cures of hemophilia in the early twenty-first century. Still, even before 1998, hemophilia researchers working on gene transfer seemed to me more cautious and circumspect than other boosters of gene therapy—largely because of the tumultuous events surrounding transfusion-related AIDS and hepatitis. These hemophilia researchers have remained cautiously optimistic about gene therapy as the field matured in the past decade. As of 2010, studies of gene transfer for hemophilia remain a promising biotechnological solution to controlling bleeding disorders, but few people are saying (as many researchers and venture capitalists said in the mid 1990s) that a working gene cure for hemophilia is five to ten years away.[23] History does not hold the key to when a veritable cure or solution to hemophilia will arrive. That time may never come, or it may be right around the corner. But history does hold some lessons, and, above all, it suggests that—short of some remarkable advance—we are most likely to see in the coming years improved technologies, practices, and systems for managing hemophilia and other genetic diseases across the lifetime of a patient.

For the latter reason, I conclude this book with a little-appreciated fact in the recent history of hemophilia that speaks forcefully to what the future holds—namely, the fact that recently a small number of people with hemophilia have had their clotting factor deficiency *cured* by means of liver transplantation. It may surprise readers to learn that liver transplantation can cure hemophilia. It certainly surprised me when I heard about it in the 1990s. In fact, when circulating an early draft of this book to a handful of experts in 2007, one of my readers (an M.D. with a Ph.D. in history) warned me against saying that transplantation could cure hemophilia. As a professor of medicine working at an American university with a thriving transplant center, he told me that he had never heard of it. Cut it, he suggested. Technically, my expert adviser was correct. Liver transplantation is not being used as treatment for hemophilia per se. Since the late 1990s, however, a growing number of adult hemophilia patients have received liver transplantations to treat the advanced liver disease they had acquired from one or more transfusions of HCV-infected plasma. The amazing thing about these aggressive, last-ditch efforts to manage hepatitis C in hemophilia patients is that the new livers correct the patient's primary bleeding disorder.

The first successful liver transplants in human patients with hemophilia A occurred between 1985 and 1987, the result of teamwork by highly skilled hematologists and transplant surgeons working at the University of

Pittsburgh and Northwestern University.[24] This surgical breakthrough built upon studies in the late 1960s and early 1970s using hemophilic dogs that suggested that the liver played an essential in the synthesis of clotting factor VIII and that liver transplant could effectively correct the defect found in hemophilic dogs (with the factor VIII deficiency). Dr. Kenneth Brinkhous, who was thoroughly familiar with these studies, told me in the mid-1990s that transplantation experiments were nothing short of a demonstration that gene transfer represents the ultimate cure for hemophilia. He then described liver transplantation for hemophilia as a form of what he fondly called "wild-type" gene therapy. Surgeons, he opined, had effectively replaced the defective genes in the patient's liver by giving the patient a healthy organ (whose cells included fully functional factor VIII genes capable of manufacturing clotting proteins in the patient's bloodstream). Brinkhous was then claiming that work conducted in his laboratories and among his colleagues had already pointed the way toward cure. And the research on gene transfer techniques that became all the rage in the 1990s was—at least in his way of thinking—an outgrowth of those earlier physiological and transplantation experiments on his hemophilic dogs.[25] Brinkhous's interpretation of the past and future of hemophilia research has only become more compelling to me since that discussion. More recently, as I have combed the Internet and medical literature for news of hemophilia advances (including gene transfer experimentation as well as innovative liver transplants), it does seem valid to borrow O'Mahony's trope and assert that today's cutting-edge hemophilia research is a kind of "back to the future" enterprise.

As I write in 2010, there are still a significant number of Americans with hemophilia who are alive today despite being infected with HIV and HCV in the 1980s (if not earlier). With advances in AIDS treatment, HIV infection itself became a chronic, manageable disease by the late 1990s. So it is not at all clear today that HIV disease is more likely to kill an HIV-positive hemophilia patient today than his primary bleeding disorder. However, those hemophilia patients who acquired hepatitis C via their treatments have not been so fortunate. In the past decade, HCV infections have emerged as the biggest threat to life among those (HIV+ and HIV−) hemophilia patients who survived the tumultuous eighties.

Today, liver transplantation is becoming better known as a remedy for hemophilia patients even though physicians are recommending it only to those patients who would otherwise die of the end-stage liver disease (associated with HCV). This unheralded and largely unwanted development might very well be the ultimate irony in the history of hemophilia management. Certainly, it is a "cure" that no sane person would choose.

The well-publicized transplant of Robert Massie Jr. is a case in point. In July 2009 Bob, at fifty-three years old, underwent a rare form of liver replacement for his end-stage hepatitis C infection (a domino transplant for HCV). Like many other people with hemophilia and advanced HCV, the transplant has cured him of his clotting factor deficiency. Bob maintains an active blog on his Web page (bobmassie.org) that details the roller-coaster experience that is liver transplantation coupled with the complex management of his life-threatening HCV infections. And while Bob no longer has to worry about a fatal bleed due to his inherited deficiency of factor VIII, he and a few other patients in his situation are still engaged in a constant and extraordinary effort to manage their health. That struggle, as foretold in his parents' 1975 memoir *Journey*, continues his personal odyssey through American medicine and society. Among Bob Massie's recent posts to his blog: "I know that people have been wondering what has happened in the transplant saga, and that many of you have been hoping or assuming that no news is good news. Unfortunately this is has not been entirely true. . . . Nonetheless, I think I now can describe the developments in the proper context, without giving too bright or too dark a picture." He thus proceeded to describe an accumulation of fluid in his belly following the surgery (e.g., ascites). He might have also described the complicated array of drugs he takes to prevent his immune system from rejecting his new organ, or the continued treatments of his hepatitis C infection that could damage his new liver as it had the old one. Thus, Bob Massie's blog entries in 2009 and 2010 provide compelling testimony that side effects and complications of medical management now govern his life.[26]

If the past of hemophilia management is a reliable measure of the future, this unwanted cure of hemophilia by liver transplantation may very well prove to be the rule rather than exception in the ongoing biomedical effort to manage genetic disease. I hope not. But looking at the track record, can one bet against it with any confidence? Certainly, the recent history of hemophilia suggests that ironic outcomes are an intrinsic danger to biomedical efforts to manage disease; they seem no less integral to the enterprise than extraordinary effort and vigilance. Thus, insofar as the majority of people remain resolute about medical progress in this biotechnological age of ours, it makes sense to wonder whether we should continue to tolerate the ironic effects of disease management—or aggressively root them out.

In any case, the AIDS crisis is not the only irony borne out of hemophilia's transformation into a manageable disease. There have been many incongruities along the way. Some of these ironies emerge from the effects of technology. Some reflect cultural and social preferences for interpreting the disease and its treatment in gendered terms. Some undoubtedly arise from views about the contested rights and responsibilities of people with disease or disability. And frequently these ironies have reflected widely shared aspirations to "normalize" the experiences of people with chronic diseases like hemophilia. The history of hemophilia management is replete with troubling ironies. But, more importantly, these ironic effects of medical progress can be instructive as well. In other words, the fact that disease management is not a story of steady progress is not cause for overwhelming negativity or cynicism. It merely signals the need to grapple with the powers and limitations of our aspirations to heal and improve ourselves.

NOTES

Preface

1. See Wolfgang Saxon, "K. M. Brinkhous, 92; Helped Develop Hemophilia Treatment," *New York Times*, Dec. 25, 2000, p. B7; William W. McLendon, "Kenneth M. Brinkhous, M.D.: Obituary," *Journal of the American Medical Association* 285 (2001): 1093; Joe W. Grisham and J. Charles Jennette, "Kenneth Merle Brinkhous, M.D., 1908–2000: In Memoriam," *American Journal of Pathology* 159 (July 2001): 3–4; and Gilbert White II and Harold R. Roberts, "Kenneth M. Brinkhous: Investigator, Teacher, Administrator, and Gene Therapist," *Molecular Therapy* 3 (April 2001): 421–22.

2. Bruno Latour and Steve Woolgar, *Laboratory Life: The Construction of Scientific Facts* (repr., Princeton: Princeton University Press, 1986).

3. Bruno Latour, "Give Me a Laboratory and I Will Raise the World," in Karin Knorr-Cetina and Michael Mulkay, eds., *Science Observed* (Beverly Hills, CA: Sage Publications, 1983), pp. 141–70.

4. The core of my 1997 master's thesis in history was published as Stephen Pemberton, "Canine Technologies, Model Patients: The Historical Production of Hemophiliac Dogs in American Biomedicine," in Susan Schrepfer and Philip Scranton, eds., *Industrializing Organisms: Introducing Evolutionary History* (New York: Routledge, 2004), pp. 191–213.

Introduction

1. See Chris Feudtner, *Bittersweet: Diabetes, Insulin, and the Transformation of Illness* (Chapel Hill: University of North Carolina Press, 2003).

2. See Gerald Grob, *The Deadly Truth: A History of Disease in America* (Cambridge, MA: Harvard University Press, 2005), and Charles Rosenberg, *Our Present Complaint: American Medicine, Then and Now* (Baltimore: Johns Hopkins University Press, 2007).

3. Susan Resnick, *Blood Saga: Hemophilia, AIDS, and the Survival of a Community* (Berkeley: University of California Press, 1999).

4. See, e.g., George Getze, "Normal Lives Possible: New Shots Protect Hemophilia Victims," *Los Angeles Times*, May 13, 1964, p. B1.

5. These statistics are representative of the national picture, though they come from one Cleveland Hospital. Paul K. Jones and Oscar D. Ratnoff, "The Changing Prognosis of Classic Hemophilia (Factor VIII 'Deficiency')," *Annals of Internal Medicine* 114 (1991): 641–48.

6. Ronald Bayer, "Blood and AIDS in America: The Making of a Catastrophe," in Eric Feldman and Ronald Bayer, eds., *Blood Feuds: AIDS, Blood, and the Politics of Medical Disaster* (New York: Oxford University Press, 1999), pp. 33–35.

7. Resnick, *Blood Saga*, p. ix; Bayer, "Blood and AIDS in America"; and Douglas Starr, *Blood: An Epic History of Medicine and Commerce* (New York: Alfred A. Knopf, 1998).

8. Lauren B. Leveton, Harold C. Sox Jr., and Michael A. Stoto, eds., *HIV and the Blood Supply: An Analysis of Crisis Decisionmaking* (Washington, DC: National Academy Press, 1995).

9. See Edward Tenner, "Medicine: Conquest of the Catastrophic," and "Medicine: The Revenge of the Chronic," in *Why Things Bite Back: Technology and the Revenge of Unintended Consequences* (New York: Vintage Books, 1997), pp. 33–89, quote on p. 56.

10. Charles B. Kerr, "The Fortunes of Haemophiliacs in the Nineteenth Century," *Medical History* 7 (1963): 359–70, quote on p. 359.

11. The discursive and temporal dislocations characteristic of the AIDS epidemic are given expert expression in Paula Treichler's *How to Have Theory in an Epidemic: Cultural Chronicles of AIDS* (Durham, NC: Duke University Press, 1999); John Nguyet Erni, *Unstable Frontiers: Technomedicine and the Cultural Politics of "Curing" AIDS* (Minneapolis: University of Minnesota Press, 1994), pp. 69–88; William Haver, *The Body of This Death: Historicity and Sociality in the Time of AIDS* (Stanford, CA: Stanford University Press, 1996); and Alexander García Düttmann, *At Odds with AIDS: Thinking and Talking about a Virus* (Stanford, CA: Stanford University Press, 1996).

12. Donna Boone, preface to Donna Boone, ed., *Comprehensive Management of Hemophilia* (Philadelphia: F. A. Davis, 1973), p. ix.

13. See, e.g., Sander Gilman, *Disease and Representation: Images of Illness from Madness to AIDS* (Ithaca: Cornell University Press, 1988), and John Williams-Searle, "Cold Charity: Manhood, Brotherhood, and the Transformation of Disability, 1870–1900," in Paul K. Longmore and Lauri Umanski, eds., *The New Disability History: American Perspectives* (New York: New York University Press, 2001), pp. 157–86.

14. See Michael Kimmel, *Manhood in America: A Cultural History* (New York: Free Press, 1996).

15. Anxieties about gender in the hemophilia community also surfaced in the

late 1980s when feminists within the fold of the bleeding disorders community challenged the National Hemophilia Foundation's dominant focus on male patients. See Resnick, *Blood Saga*, and Treichler, *How to Have Theory in an Epidemic*, pp. 42–98, 244–45.

16. See Nayan Shah, *Contagious Divides: Epidemics and Race in San Francisco's Chinatown* (Berkeley: University of California Press, 2001), especially pp. 251–55. More generally, see William Connolly, *Politics and Ambiguity* (Madison: University of Wisconsin Press, 1987), pp. 3–16; Nikolas Rose, *The Power of Freedom: Reframing Political Thought* (New York: Cambridge University Press, 1999); and Barbara Cruikshank, *The Will to Empower: Democratic Citizens and Other Subjects* (Ithaca: Cornell University Press, 1999).

17. See Rayna Rapp and Faye Ginsberg, "Enabling Disability: Rewriting Kinship, Reimagining Citizenship," *Public Culture* 13 (2001): 533–56.

18. See Richard Titmuss, *The Gift Relationship: From Human Blood to Social Policy*, rev. ed. (New York: New Press, 1997); Starr, *Blood*; and Feldman and Bayer, *Blood Feuds*.

19. See Georges Canguilhem, *The Normal and the Pathological* (New York: Zone Books, 1991), and François Ewald, "Norms Discipline, and the Law," *Representations* 30 (Spring 1990): 146–54.

20. See Shah, *Contagious Divides*, and Douglas Baynton, "Disability and the Justification of Inequality in American History," in Longmore and Umanski, *The New Disability History*, pp. 33–57. More generally, see Erving Goffman, *Stigma: Notes on the Management of Spoiled Identity* (New York: Simon and Schuster, 1963).

21. The most prominent examples are Robert K. Massie, *Nicholas and Alexandra* (New York: Dell Publishing, 1967); Robert Massie and Suzanne Massie, *Journey* (New York: Alfred A. Knopf, 1975); Resnick, *Blood Saga*; and Starr; *Blood*.

22. See Charles Rosenberg and Janet Golden, eds., *Framing Disease: Studies in Cultural History* (New Brunswick, NJ: Rutgers University Press, 1992); Jacalyn Duffin, *Lovers and Livers: Disease Concepts in History* (Toronto: University of Toronto Press, 2005).

23. See Robert Hudson, *Disease and Its Control: The Shaping of Modern Thought* (Westport, CT: Greenwood Press, 1983); William Arney and Bernard Bergen, *Medicine and the Management of Living: Taming the Last Great Beast* (Chicago: University of Chicago Press, 1984); David Weatherall, *Science and the Quiet Art* (New York: W. W. Norton, 1995); and Sherwin Nuland, *Wisdom of the Body* (New York: Alfred Knopf, 1997).

24. Goffman, *Stigma*.

Chapter 1: The Emergence of the Hemophilia Concept

1. "Tracing Parentage by Eugenic Tests," *New York Times*, September 23, 1921, p. A8.

2. G. Isley Ingram, "The History of Haemophilia," *Journal of Clinical Pathology* 29 (June 1976): 469–79.

3. On the relationship between natural history and the practical focus of most historians, see Daniel Lord Smail, *On Deep History and the Brain* (Berkeley: University of California Press, 2008). On genetic knowledge's characterization as a form of writing, see Lily Kay, *Who Wrote the Book of Life? A History of the Genetic Code* (Stanford, CA: Stanford University Press, 2000).

4. See William Bulloch and Paul Fildes, "Haemophilia," in Karl Pearson, ed., *Treasury of Human Inheritance*, vol. 1 (London: Cambridge University Press, 1912), pp. 169–354; occasionally referenced as *Eugenics Laboratory Memoirs XII, Francis Galton Laboratory for National Eugenics, University of London* (London: Dulau, 1911), parts V and VI, sec. XIVa. See also Edward B. Krumbhaar, "John Conrad Otto and the Recognition of Hemophilia," *Bulletin of the Johns Hopkins Hospital* 46 (1930): 123–40; and Fred Rosner's essays, "Hemophilia in the Talmud and Rabbinic Writings," *Annals of Internal Medicine* 70 (April 1969): 833–37, and "Hemophilia in Rabbinic Texts," *Journal of the History of Medicine and Allied Sciences* 49 (1994): 240–50.

5. George Canguilhem, *The Normal and the Pathological* (New York: Zone Books, 1991), pp. 140–41, 199.

6. Susan Resnick, *Blood Saga: Hemophilia, AIDS, and the Survival of a Community* (Berkeley: University of California Press, 1999), pp. 8–9.

7. John C. Otto, "An Account of an Hemorrhagic Disposition Existing in Certain Families," [New York] *Medical Repository* 6 (1803): 1–4; "Account of Singular Cases of Hemorrhage [Letter of Dr. E. H. Smith to Dr. Benjamin Rush, April 9, 1794; Letter of Dr. John Coats to John B. Bordley, May 27, 1803; and Letter of Charles W. Binny to Dr. John Coats, June 1, 1803]," *Philadelphia Medical Museum* 1 (1805): 284–88; John Hay, "Account of a Remarkable Hemorrhagic Disposition Existing in Many Individuals of the Same Family," *New England Journal of Medicine and Surgery* 2 (1813): 221–25; William Buel and Samuel Buel, "An Account of a Family Predisposition to Hemorrhage," *Transactions Physico-Medical Society of New York* 1 (1817): 304; Reynell Coates, "Observations on Hereditary Hemorrhage," *North American Medical and Surgical Journal* 6 (July 1828): 37–53. Critical scholarship on these discoveries includes Victor McKusick, "The Earliest Record of Hemophilia in America [Obituary of Isaac Zoll]," *Blood* 19 (1962): 243–44; Victor McKusick, "Hemophilia in Early New England: A Follow-

Up of Four Kindreds in Which Hemophilia Occurred in the Pre-Revolutionary Period," *Journal of the History of Medicine and Allied Sciences* 17 (1962): 342–65; and Victor McKusick and Samuel Rapaport, "History of Classical Hemophilia in a New England Family," *Archives of Internal Medicine* 110 (August 1962): 144–49.

8. Otto, "An Account of an Hemorrhagic Disposition Existing in Certain Families," 1.

9. Ibid., 3.

10. On the fallacy of "precursors" in the history of science, see George Canguilhem, "The History of the History of Science," in François Delaporte, ed., *A Vital Rationalist: Selected Writings of George Canguilhem* (Cambridge, MA: MIT Press, 1994), pp. 49–51.

11. The best historical treatment of Otto remains Krumbhaar's "John Conrad Otto and the Recognition of Hemophilia." Much of what is written about Otto relies on Isaac Parrish, "Biographical Memoir of John C. Otto," *Transactions of the College of the Physicians of Philadelphia* 1 (1845): 303–18.

12. See Bulloch and Fildes, "Haemophilia," pp. 172–73, on points of dissemination.

13. Lisa Rosner, "Thistle on the Delaware: Edinburgh Medical Education and Philadelphia Practice, 1800–1825," *Social History of Medicine* 5 (1992): 19–40.

14. Otto, "An Account of an Hemorrhagic Disposition Existing in Certain Families," 1.

15. Ibid., 1–2.

16. John Redman Coxe, "Singular Cases of Hemorrhagy," *Philadelphia Medical Museum* 1 (1805): 286–90.

17. Otto, "An Account of an Hemorrhagic Disposition Existing in Certain Families," 2–3.

18. Ibid., 3–4.

19. John Hay, an American physician, is widely credited in the Anglophone literature with the first accurate description of the sex-linked inheritance in hemophilia in 1813. Hay worried about the transmission of hemophilia because his son had married the daughter of a hemophiliac. He traced hemophilia in his daughter-in-law's family into the early eighteenth century, finding the now-familiar inheritance pattern. Hay's article did not have the influence of Otto's publication, despite having great familiarity with the disease because of his extended family. The value of Hay's contribution was frequently overlooked in Europe until the 1870s. For this reason, Christian Friedrich Nasse (1820) and other German investigators are more properly credited with disseminating the notion that transmission of hemophilia followed a relatively predictable sex-linked pattern. See Oscar Ratnoff, "Why Do People Bleed?" in Maxwell Wintrobe, ed.,

Blood, Pure and Eloquent (New York: McGraw-Hill, 1980), p. 626; Alan Rushton, *Genetics and Medicine in the United States, 1800–1922* (Baltimore: Johns Hopkins University Press, 1994), pp. 4–8; and Peter S. Harper, *A Short History of Medical Genetics* (New York: Oxford University Press, 2008), pp. 20–25.

20. John Wickham Legg, *Treatise on Haemophilia, Sometimes Called the Hereditary Haemorrhagic Diathesis* (London: H. K. Lewis, 1872), pp. 28, 39.

21. Anonymous, "Bemerkungen uber eine besondere Neigung zu Blutungen in gewissen Familien," in *Sammlung auserlesener Abhandlungen zum Gebrauche praktischer Aerzte* 22, no. 2 (Leipzig, 1805): 275. The journal's "editor," Christian Erhard Kapp, may have been the author. See Bulloch and Fildes, "Haemophilia," pp. 170, 198.

22. The quote is from the 1793 German case report that has since been attributed to Georg Wilhem Chistoph Consbruch (1764–1837) of Bielefeld, from the reprint and translation of Consbruch's original text communicated in Krumbhaar, "John Conrad Otto and the Recognition of Hemophilia," pp. 126–27. See also Bulloch and Fildes, "Haemophilia," p. 171.

23. See Thomas H. Broman, *The Transformation of German Academic Medicine, 1750–1820* (New York: Cambridge University Press, 1996), and George Weisz, "Specialization in the German-Speaking World," in *Divide and Conquer: A Comparative History of Medical Specialization* (New York: Oxford University Press, 2006), pp. 44–62.

24. See Johanna Bleker, "To Benefit the Poor and Advance Medical Science: Hospitals and Hospital Care in Germany, 1820–1870," in Manfred Berg and Geoffrey Cocks, eds., *Medicine and Modernity: Public Health and Medical Care in Nineteenth- and Twentieth-Century Germany* (Cambridge: Cambridge University Press, 1997), p. 24.

25. Christian Friedrich Nasse's seminal work on hemophilia is "Von einer erblichen Neigung zu tödtlichen Blutungen," *Archiv für medizinische Erfahrung im Gebiete der praktischen Medizin und Staatsarzneikunde, hrsg. Von Horn, Nasse und Henke* (Berlin, May–June 1820), p. 385.

26. Bulloch and Fildes, "Haemophilia," pp. 172, 199.

27. English-language literature on Schönlein, with references to the German scholarship, includes Erwin Ackerknecht, "Johann Lucas Schoenlein, 1793–1864," *Journal of the History of Medicine and the Allied Sciences* 19 (1964): 131–38; Johanna Bleker, "Between Romantic and Scientific Medicine: Johann Lukas Schoenlein and the Natural History School," *Clio Medica* 18 (1983): 191–201; Timothy Lenoir, "Review of Johanna Bleker, Die naturhistorische Schule 1825–1845: Ein Beitrag zur Geshichte der klinschen Medizin in Deutscheland," *Isis* 73 (1982): 459; Timothy Lenoir, "Laboratories, Medicine, and Public Life in Ger-

many, 1830–1849: Ideological Roots of the Institutional Revolution," in Andrew Cunningham and Perry Williams, eds., *The Laboratory Revolution in Medicine* (Cambridge: Cambridge University Press, 1992), pp. 14–71; Johannes Hierholzer, Christel Hierholzer, and Klaus Hierholzer, "Johann Lukas Schönlein and His Contribution to Nephrology and Medicine," *American Journal of Nephrology* 14 (1994): 467–72; and Thomas Schlich, "Review of Johanna Bleker, Eva Brinkschulte, and Pascal Grosse, eds., *Kranke und Krankheiten im Juliusspital zu Würzburg, 1819–1829: Zur frühen Geschichte des Allgemeinen Krankenhauses in Deutschland," Bulletin of the History of Medicine* 71 (1997): 346–47.

28. Ackerknecht, "Johann Lucas Schoenlein," 131–38, quote on p. 136.

29. Friedrich Hopff, *Über die Haemophilie oder die erbliche Anlage zu tödtlichen Blutungen* (Würzberg: C. W. Becker, 1828).

30. For a detailed interpretation of this word history, see Kenneth Brinkhous, "A Short History of Hemophilia, with Some Comments on the Word 'Hemophilia,'" in K. M. Brinkhous and H. C. Hemker, eds., *Handbook of Hemophilia* (Amsterdam: Excepta Medica, 1975), pp. 3–7.

31. Ludwig Grandidier, *Die Haemophilie oder die Bluterkrankheit, nach eigenen und fremden Beobachtungen monographisch bearbeitet* (Leipzig: Otto Wigand, 1855). The second edition appeared in 1877.

32. Hermann Immermann provides the most comprehensive review of the nineteenth-century German literature on hemophilia that is presently available in English translation. See H. Immermann, "Haemophilia," trans. A. Brayton Ball, in H. von Ziemssen and Albert H. Buck, eds., *Cyclopaedia of the Practice of Medicine* (New York: William Wood, 1878), 17:3–104, especially pp. 3–5, 9–10.

33. Ibid., p. 84.

34. On the unreliability of Grandidier's statistics, see Legg, *Treatise on Haemophilia*, pp. 30–32, and, especially, Bulloch and Fildes, "Haemophilia," p. 172.

35. See Johanna Bleker, Eva Brinkschulte, and Pascal Grosse, eds., *Kranke und Krankheiten im Juliusspital zu Würzburg, 1819–1829: Zur frühen Geschichte des Allgemeinen Krankenhauses in Deutschland* (Husum, Germany: Matthiesen, 1995), and Schlich, "Review of *Kranke und Krankheiten im Juliusspital zu Würzburg, 1819–1829.*"

36. Legg, *Treatise on Haemophilia*, p. 2, n. 2.

37. Charlotte Zeepvat aptly uses the phrase "open secret" in *Prince Leopold: The Untold Story of Queen Victoria's Youngest Son* (Phoenix Mill, Gloucestershire: Sutton Publishing, 1998), p. 175. Physicians, geneticists, and medical historians have long taken an interest in royal hemophilia. Haldane's seminal essay "Blood Royal" is among the earliest contributions to this literature; it appeared in various forms between 1939 and 1940. See J. B. S. Haldane, "Blood Royal: A

Study of Haemophilia in the Royal Families," *Modern Quarterly: London Leftist Quarterly* 2 (April 1938): 129–39; "Blood Royal: The Dramatic Story of How Hemophilia Has Affected the Recent History of the World," *Living Age* 356 (March 1939): 26–31; and *Adventures of a Biologist* (New York: Harper & Brothers, 1940).

Key sources that highlight the British royal family include Hugo Iltis, "Haemophilia: The Royal Disease and the British Royal Family," *Journal of Heredity* 39 (April 1948): 113–16; Victor A. McKusick, "The Royal Hemophilia," *Scientific American* 213 (1965): 88–95; Frederick Cartwright, *Disease and History* (New York: Thomas Crowell, 1972), pp. 167–96; G. I. C. Ingram, "The History of Haemophilia," *Journal of Clinical Pathology* 29 (1976): 469–79; W. T. W. Potts, "Royal Hemophilia," *Journal of Biological Education* 30 (Autumn 1996): 207–17; D. M. Potts and W. T. W. Potts, *Queen Victoria's Gene: Haemophilia and the Royal Family* (Phoenix Mill, Gloucestershire: Sutton Publishing, 1995); and Alan Rushton, *Royal Maladies: Inherited Diseases in the Ruling Houses of Europe* (Victoria, BC: Trafford Publishing, 2008), pp. 1–32.

38. "The Haemorrhagic Diathesis," *British Medical Journal* 1 (April 5, 1884): 686.

39. William Osler, "Haemophilia," in William Pepper and Louis Starr, eds., *A System of Practical Medicine*, vol. 3 (Philadelphia: Lea Brothers, 1885), p. 934.

40. Zeepvat, *Prince Leopold*, p. 14.

41. Ibid., pp. 13–16.

42. Ibid., pp. 14, 20–21, and Legg, *Treatise on Haemophilia*, pp. 99–100.

43. Theo Aronson, *Grandmama of Europe*, (Indianapolis: Bobbs-Merrill, 1973), pp. 170–72.

44. Legg, *Treatise on Haemophilia*, pp. 32–33.

45. Ibid., pp. 126–27.

46. Ibid.

47. Ibid., pp. 32–35.

48. See Haldane, "Blood Royal," *Modern Quarterly*; "Blood Royal," *Living Age*; and *Adventures of a Biologist*.

49. Haldane, "Blood Royal," *Living Age*, p. 31.

50. Legg, *Treatise on Haemophilia*, pp. 39–40.

51. Immermann, "Haemophilia," p. 31.

52. Bulloch and Fildes found only three papers concerning hemophilia in people of African descent, including W. V. M. Koch, "Haemophilia Occurring in Malaria," *British Medical Journal* 1 (June 7, 1890): 1301–2. Julian Herman Lewis found six other reports when writing "Hemophilia," in *The Biology of the Negro* (Chicago: University of Chicago Press, 1942), pp. 250–51. These were Hadlock,

"Hemorrhagic Diathesis, 'Clinic' of Cincinnati," *Transactions of the Academy of Medicine* 7 (1874): 241; Walter Steiner, "Haemophilia in the Negro," *Johns Hopkins Medical Bulletin* 11 (1900): 44–47; Louis Buck, "Haemophilia in the Negro," *Medical Record* 58 (1900): 149; D. J. Pachman, "Hemophilia in Negroes," *Journal of Pediatrics* 10 (1937): 809; Noble Crandall, "Hemophilia in the Negro," *American Journal of the Medical Sciences* 192, no. 6 (December 1936): 745–51; Eugene P. Campbell, "Hemophilia in the Negro: Report of a Case," *Medical Annals of the District of Columbia* 8 (1939): 294–95, 316. Other known cases include J. Rosenbloom, "A Warning against the Use of Arsphenamin in the Treatment of Syphilis in a Hemophiliac," *Journal of Laboratory and Clinical Medicine* 9 (1923): 57; J. H. Taylor, "A Case of Haemophilia in a Negro," *Journal of the South Carolina Medical Association* 19 (1923): 665; J. Muir, "Heredity in Hemophilia in South Africa," *Journal of the Medical Association of South Africa* 2 (1928): 599; I. N. Kuglemass, "The Diagnosis and Management of Hemophilia in Childhood," *New York State Journal of Medicine* 32 (1932): 660; E. L. Rypins, "Roentgen Ray as Aid in Diagnosis of Hemophilia," *American Journal of Roentgenology* 31 (1934): 597; C. E. Prip Buus, "Articular Changes in Hemophilia," *Acta Radiol.* 16 (1935): 503; Carroll LaFleur Birch, *Hemophilia: Genetic and Clinical Aspects* (Urbana: University of Illinois Press, 1937); and Robert Nesbitt and Julius Richmond, "Hemophilia in the Negro," *Journal of Pediatrics* 34 (1949): 315–21.

53. Nesbitt and Richmond, "Hemophilia in the Negro," pp. 315–21, quotes on pp. 319–20.

54. John Hay can also be credited with demonstrating in 1813 that sex characteristics might be used as a principle for deciding what constituted a legitimate hemophilia diagnosis; yet as detailed in notes 7 and 19 above, Nasse's study (ca. 1820) was far more influential.

55. See Brinkhous, "A Short History of Hemophilia, with Some Comments on the Word 'Hemophilia,'" especially pp. 4–7.

56. Legg, *Treatise on Haemophilia*, p. 31.

57. John Eric Erichsen, "Haemorrhagic Diathesis," in *The Science and Art of Surgery* (Philadelphia: Henry Leas's Son, 1881), pp. 912–13. See also Thomas D. Dunn, "Haemophilia," *American Journal of the Medical Sciences* 85 (January 1883): 68–83, especially p. 73.

58. John Wickham Legg, "Haemophilia," in Thomas Clifford Allbutt, ed., *A System of Medicine*, vol. 9 (London: MacMillan, 1898), pp. 548–55, quote on p. 553.

59. Bulloch and Fildes, "Haemophilia," quotes on pp. 169, 174–76.

60. *Monumental* is the adjective repeatedly used in the history of hemophilia literature to describe the work of Bulloch and Fildes. See Ingram, "The History

of Haemophilia"; Brinkhous, "A Short History of Hemophilia, with Some Comments on the Word 'Hemophilia'"; Resnick, *Blood Saga*; and E. M. Tansey and D. A. Christie, eds., *Haemophilia: Recent History of Clinical Management, Welcome Witnesses to Twentieth Century Medicine*, vol. 4 (London: Wellcome Trust, 1999).

61. Bulloch and Fildes, "Haemophilia," pp. 177–81, especially p. 179.

62. See Daniel Kevles, *In the Name of Eugenics: Genetics and the Uses of Human Heredity* (Cambridge, MA: Harvard University Press, 1995), pp. 41–49, and Georges Canguilhem, "On the History of the Life Sciences since Darwin," in *Ideology and Rationality in the History of the Life Sciences* (Cambridge, MA: MIT Press, 1988), pp. 103–23.

63. Legg, "Haemophilia," pp. 127–28.

64. Immermann, "Haemophilia," quotes on pp. 26, 89–91.

65. See Kevles, *In the Name of Eugenics*, p. 48, and Charles Davenport, *Heredity in Relation to Eugenics* (New York: Henry Holt, 1911).

66. J. B. S. Haldane, "The Origin of Hereditary Disease by Mutation: The Possibilities of Negative Eugenics," in *Heredity and Politics* (New York: Norton, 1938), pp. 73–111, quote on p. 88.

67. See Grandidier, *Die Haemophilie*, and Birch, *Hemophilia*.

68. Amram Scheinfeld, *You and Heredity*, (New York: Frederick Stokes, 1939), pp. 130–32, 162, 189, 329, 377.

69. Ibid., p. 377.

70. See Haldane, "Blood Royal," *Living Age*, quote on p. 30; and F. A. E. Crew, "Haldane as a Geneticist," in K. R. Dronamragju, ed., *Haldane and Modern Biology* (Baltimore: Johns Hopkins University Press, 1968), p. 16.

71. Scheinfeld, *You and Heredity*, p. 406. See also p. 353.

72. Ibid., p. 405.

73. Ibid., p. 406.

74. Ibid. See, e.g., pp. 335–54, 377, 381–84, 405–6.

Chapter 2: The Scientist, the Bleeder, and the Laboratory

1. Robert Gywn Macfarlane, "Almroth Edward Wright," in Gywn Macfarlane, *Alexander Fleming: The Man and the Myth* (New York: Oxford University Press, 1985), pp. 47–56. See also Michael Dunnill, *The Plato of Praed Street: The Life and Times of Almroth Wright* (London: Royal Society of Medicine Press, 2000), especially pp. 32–35; Michael Worboys, "Almroth Wright at Netley: Modern Medicine and the Military in Britain, 1892–1902," in Roger Cooter, Mark Harrison, and Steve Sturdy, eds., *Medicine and Modern Warfare* (Amsterdam: Editions Rodopi, 1999), pp. 77–97; and Wai Chen, "The Laboratory as Business: Sir

Almroth Wright's Vaccine Programme and the Construction of Penicillin," in Andrew Cunningham and Perry Williams, eds., *The Laboratory Revolution in Medicine* (New York: Cambridge University Press, 1992), pp. 245–92.

2. Almroth E. Wright, "On the Method of Determining the Condition of Blood Coagulability for Clinical and Experimental Purposes, and on the Effect of the Administration of Calcium Salts in Haemophilia and Actual or Threatened Hemorrhage [Preliminary Communication]," *British Medical Journal* 2 (July 29, 1893): 223–25. Wright followed his preliminary report with "On the Methods of Increasing and Diminishing the Coagulability of the Blood with Especial Reference to Their Therapeutic Employment," *British Medical Journal* 2 (1894): 57–61.

3. Wright utilized thin-walled capillary tubes to measure clotting times of whole blood (drawn from a finger prick). His method was influential but not entirely novel. German hematologists utilized whole blood clotting times in the 1880s following the work of Vierordt (1878) and Hasebroek (1882), but these methods were not used to say anything about hemophilic blood. In the early 1900s, at least one influential investigator, Hermann Sahli, contested Wright's claim that a prolonged whole blood clotting time was a defining mark of hemophilic blood. By 1910, however, there was near universal agreement on the matter. See, e.g., Oscar Ratnoff, "Why Do People Bleed?" in Maxwell Wintrobe, ed., *Blood, Pure and Eloquent* (New York: McGraw-Hill, 1980), pp. 601–57, and Charles Owen, *A History of Blood Coagulation* (Rochester, MN: Mayo Foundation for Medical Education and Research, 2001), pp. 191–98.

4. By 1913 there were at least thirty-two published methods for taking the whole blood clotting time. After 1914 in the United States, the clotting time was usually done by the method of Lee and White or by that of Howell. See Roger Irving Lee and Paul Dudley White, "A Clinical Study of the Coagulation Time of the Blood," *American Journal of Medical Sciences* 145 (1913): 495–503, and William Henry Howell, "Condition of the Blood in Hemophilia, Thrombosis, and Purpura," *Archives of Internal Medicine* 13 (1914): 76–95.

5. James Wardrop, *On the Curative Effects of the Abstraction of Blood* (Philadelphia: Waldie, 1837), pp. 9–10. The British edition appeared as *On Blood Letting* earlier in London in 1834.

6. See John Wickham Legg, *Treatise on Haemophilia, Sometimes Called the Hereditary Haemorrhagic Diathesis* (London: H. K. Lewis, 1872), especially pp. 28, 33, 83, 92, 99–100, and Hermann Immermann, "Haemophilia," trans. A. Brayton Ball, in H. von Ziemssen and Albert H. Buck, eds., *Cyclopaedia of the Practice of Medicine* (New York: William Wood, 1878), 17:3–104, especially pp. 14, 30–31, 50–63.

7. See Immermann, "Haemophilia," pp. 10, 44–45, 55, 62–64, 66–70.

8. Immermann, "Haemophilia," quote on p. 75, and William Osler, "Haemophilia," in William Pepper and Louis Starr, eds., *A System of Practical Medicine*, vol. 3, *Diseases of the Respiratory, Circulatory, and Haemopoetic Systems* (Philadelphia: Lea Brothers, 1885), pp. 931–39, quote on p. 937.

9. A dramatic overview is available in Douglas Starr, *Blood: An Epic History of Medicine and Commerce* (New York: Alfred Knopf, 1998), pp. 3–16. See also Bernard J. Ficarra, "The Evolution of Blood Transfusion," *Annals of Medical History*, 3rd ser., 4 (1942): 305–6, and Diamond, "A History of Blood Transfusion," in Wintrobe, *Blood Pure and Eloquent*, pp. 659–88.

10. On Blundell's work, see Kim Pelis, "Transfusion, with Teeth," in James Bradburne, ed., *Blood: Art, Power, Politics, and Pathology* (New York: Prestel, 2002), pp. 175–91, and Susan Lederer, *Flesh and Blood: Organ Transplantation and Blood Transfusion in Twentieth-Century America* (New York: Oxford University Press, 2008), pp. 34–36.

11. Kim Pelis, "Blood Standards and Failed Fluids: Clinic, Lab, and Transfusion Solutions in London, 1868–1916," *History of Science* 39 (2001): 185–213.

12. Samuel Lane, "Hemorrhagic Diathesis: Successful Transfusion of Blood," *Lancet* 35, no. 896 (October 31,1840): 185–88.

13. Account and all quotes from ibid.

14. William Osler, "Haemophilia," in *Principles and Practice of Medicine*, 4th ed. (New York: Appleton, 1901).

15. William Henry Howell, "The Condition of the Blood in Hemophilia, Thrombosis, and Purpura," *Archives of Internal Medicine* 13 (January 1914): 76–95, quote on p. 89.

16. Frank Boulton, "Thomas Addis; Scottish Pioneer in Haemophilia," *Journal of the Royal College of Physicians of Edinburgh* 33, no. 2 (2003): 135–42, and Derek Doyle, "Thomas Addis of Edinburgh and the Coagulation Cascade: 'for the greatest benefit done to practical medicine,'" *British Journal of Haematology* 132, no. 3 (February 2006): 268–76.

17. Ernest W. Hey Groves, "A Clinical Lecture on the Surgical Aspects of Haemophilia," *British Medical Journal* 1 (March 16, 1907): 611–14. See also William Bulloch and Paul Fildes, "Haemophilia," in Karl Pearson, ed., *Treasury of Human Inheritance*, vol. 1 (London: Cambridge University Press, 1912), pedigree 500.

18. Thomas Addis, "The Coagulation of the Blood in Man," *Quarterly Journal of Experimental Physiology* 1 (1908): 304–44, and "The Ineffectiveness of Calcium Salts and of Citric Acid as Used to Modify the Coagulation Time of the Blood for Therapeutic Purposes," *British Medical Journal* 1 (August 24, 1909): 997, 1151–52, 1269–70.

19. Paul Morawitz's clotting theory first appeared as "Die Chemie der Blutger-innung," *Ergebnisse der Physiologie* 4 (1905): 307–423; translated as *The Chemistry of Blood Coagulation*, trans. Robert C. Hartmann and Paul F. Guenther (Springfield, IL: Charles C. Thomas Publishers, 1958).

20. Boulton, "Thomas Addis; Scottish Pioneer in Haemophilia," p. 136. Morawitz had studied these patients, and his studies are documented in pedigree 389 of Bulloch and Fildes, "Haemophilia."

21. See Thomas Addis, "The Ineffectiveness of Calcium Salts and of Citric Acid," and T. Addis, "Hereditary Haemophilia: Deficiency in the Coagulability of the Blood the Only Immediate Cause of the Condition," *Quarterly Journal of Medicine* 4 (1910): 14–32. The completed study appeared as Thomas Addis, "The Pathogenesis of Haemophilia," *Journal of Pathology and Bacteriology* 15 (1911): 427–52.

22. See Boulton, "Thomas Addis; Scottish Pioneer in Haemophilia," and Doyle, "Thomas Addis of Edinburgh and the Coagulation Cascade."

23. See Susan Resnick, *Blood Saga: Hemophilia, AIDS, and the Survival of a Community* (Berkeley: University of California Press, 1999), pp. 20–25.

24. William Henry Howell, "Condition of the Blood in Hemophilia, Thrombosis, and Purpura," *Archives of Internal Medicine* 13 (1914): 76–95, quote on p. 89. On general theories of blood coagulation, see Owen, *A History of Blood Coagulation*, and Ratnoff, "Why Do People Bleed?"

25. Howell likened antithrombin to a native form of hirudin (the soluble protein that leeches excrete to keep blood liquid as they draw it from their host). He believed antithrombin prevented thrombin from acting on fibrinogen (thereby delaying clot formation). Today, there are four types of antithrombin that play a role in hemostasis and thrombosis. It seems an open historical question as to what type of "antithrombin" Howell and other early twentieth-century investigators actually isolated. See W. H. Howell, *A Text-Book of Physiology for Medical Students and Physicians*, 4th ed. (Philadelphia: W. B. Saunders, 1911), p. 453, and W. H. Seegers, J. F. Johnson, and C. Fell, "An Antithrombin Reaction to Prothrombin Activation," *American Journal of Physiology* 176 (January 1954): 97–103.

26. Howell, "Conditions of the Blood in Hemophilia," p. 92.

27. See Louis B. Jaques, "The Howell Theory of Blood Coagulation: A Record of the Pernicious Effects of a False Theory," *Canadian Bulletin of Medical History* 5 (1988): 143–65, and Madison Bentley, "A Psychologist's Reflections upon Howell's 'Physiology,'" *American Journal of Psychology* 60 (July 1947): 420–32.

28. George R. Minot and Roger I. Lee, "The Blood Platelets in Hemophilia," *Archives of Internal Medicine* 17 (1916): 474–95, quote on p. 495. The period is recounted in Roger Irving Lee, *The Happy Life of a Doctor* (Boston: Little, Brown,

1956), p. 35, and Francis M. Rackemann, *The Inquisitive Physician: The Life and Times of George Richards Minot* (Cambridge, MA: Harvard University Press, 1956), pp. 182–84.

29. Roger Lee and Paul White, "A Clinical Study of the Coagulation Time of Blood," *American Journal of Medical Science* 145 (1913): 495–503.

30. On the wave of transfusion experimentation in the early twentieth century, see Lederer, *Flesh and Blood*, pp. 32–66.

31. Minot and Lee, "The Blood Platelets in Hemophilia," quotes on p. 485.

32. Ibid., p. 475.

33. See James A. Marcum, "The Origin of the Dispute over the Discovery of Heparin," *Journal of the History of Medicine and Allied Sciences* 55 (2000): 37–55.

34. W. H. Howell and E. B. Cekada, "The Cause of the Delayed Clotting in Hemophilic Blood," *American Journal of Physiology* 78 (November 1926): 500–511, quote on p. 511.

35. Howell's mature views on hemophilia vis-à-vis his theory of clotting were published in 1935 and 1939. Here, Howell laid to rest Addis's notion that hemophilia was due to a qualitative defect in prothrombin, but (after 1937) he also began to question the viability of the platelet hypothesis. Ongoing research at Harvard's Thorndike Laboratory had effectively suggested the actual delay in clotting was likely due to an unknown "globulin" (clotting factor) in the plasma. See W. H. Howell, "Theories of Blood Coagulation," *Physiological Reviews* 15 (July 1935): 435–70, and W. H. Howell, "Hemophilia: The Wesley M. Carpenter Lecture," *Bulletin of the New York Academy of Medicine* 15 (January 15, 1939): 3–26.

36. See Joel Howell, *Technology in the Hospital* (Baltimore: Johns Hopkins University Press, 1997), and Keith Wailoo, *Drawing Blood: Technology and Disease Identity in Twentieth-Century America* (Baltimore: Johns Hopkins University Press, 1997).

37. William Castle, "The Conquest of Pernicious Anemia," in Wintrobe, *Blood, Pure and Eloquent*, pp. 283–18. See also Wailoo, *Drawing Blood*, pp. 99–133.

38. Paul Émile-Weil published a study in 1905 declaring that he had transfused small amounts of human and bovine blood serum into hemophilia patients, correcting the whole blood clotting time in several of them. This may very well be the first reported transfusion experiment after Lane's 1840 transfusion. This was not a whole blood transfusion, and the only way a transfusion of serum would have corrected delayed coagulation in a hemophilia patient is if that patient had hemophilia B, not classical hemophilia. Factor VIII is absent in serum,

whereas factor IX is present. See Paul Émile-Weil, "L'hemophilie. Patholgénie et sérothérapie," *Presse Médicale* 2 (1905): 673–76, and Ratnoff, "Why Do People Bleed?" pp. 630, 32.

39. Thomas Addis, "The Effect of Intravenous Injections of Fresh Human Serum and of Phosphated Blood on the Coagulation Time of the Blood in Hereditary Haemophilia," *Proceedings of the Society for Experimental Biology and Medicine* 14 (1916): 19–23.

40. Lederer, *Flesh and Blood*, pp. 32–66.

41. See Addis, "The Effect of Intravenous Injections of Fresh Human Serum," and Boulton, "Thomas Addis; Scottish Pioneer in Haemophilia."

42. See Kim Pelis, "Taking Credit: The Canadian Army Medical Corps and the British Conversion to Blood Transfusion in WWI," *Journal of the History of Medicine* 56 (2001): 238–77, especially pp. 243–44; Lederer, *Flesh and Blood*, pp. 32–67; and Peter English, *Shock, Physiological Surgery, and George Washington Crile: Medical Innovation in the Progressive Era* (Westport, CT: Greenwood Press, 1980).

43. In 1914–15 there were three simultaneous studies that proposed using sodium citrate in this way. Lewisohn's was the only one written in English, and it gained the most recognition in the coming years. See Pelis, "Taking Credit," pp. 243–44.

44. See Reuben Ottenberg, "The Effect of Sodium Citrate on Blood Coagulation in Hemophilia," *Proceedings of the Society for Experimental Biology and Medicine* 13 (1916): 104–6. On Ottenberg's contribution, see Lederer, *Flesh and Blood*, pp. xii, 146. See also Addis, "The Effect of Intravenous Injections of Fresh Human Serum." There is no explicit evidence in Minot and Lee's hemophilia transfusion of 1916 that an anticoagulant was used. That experiment was published after Ottenberg's as well. See again Minot and Lee, "The Blood Platelets in Hemophilia."

45. Boulton, "Thomas Addis; Scottish Pioneer in Haemophilia," quote on p. 139. See also Addis, "The Effect of Intravenous Injections of Fresh Human Serum." The best published account of William White's health history is found in E. W. H. Groves, "A Clinical Lecture upon the Surgical Aspects of Haemophilia with Special Reference to Two Cases of Volkmann's Contracture Resulting from This Disease," *British Medical Journal* 1 (March 16, 1907): 611–14.

46. See Addis, "The Effect of Intravenous Injections of Fresh Human Serum," and Boulton, "Thomas Addis; Scottish Pioneer in Haemophilia." Addis employed sodium phosphate as his anticoagulant ("one part of 5 per cent . . . to three parts of blood"), rather than a weak sodium citrate solution that was the standard after Lewisohn and Ottenberg.

47. See Lederer, *Flesh and Blood*, pp. 143–64, and Louis K. Diamond, "The Story of Our Blood Groups," in Wintrobe, *Blood, Pure and Eloquent*, pp. 691–717.

48. As Kim Pelis has explained, the view that blood transfusion took off after Landsteiner's discovery is a persistent myth in the history of medicine. See "Taking Credit," p. 239. See also Lederer, *Flesh and Blood*.

49. Douglas B. Kendrick, *Blood Program in World War II* (Washington, DC: Office of the Surgeon General, Department of the Army, 1964), pp. 1–27, quote p. 4.

50. See Roger I. Lee, "A Simple and Rapid Method for the Selection of Suitable Donors for Transfusion by the Determination of Blood Groups," *British Medical Journal* 2 (November 24, 1917): 684–85; Kendrick, "Historical Note"; and Pelis, "Taking Credit."

51. Starr, *Blood*, p. 53.

52. Transfusion history narratives were greatly affected by Keynes's version of events. See ibid., p. 55, and especially Pelis, "Taking Credit."

53. The story is effectively told in Douglas Starr, "Prelude to a Blood Bath," in *Blood*, pp. 72–87, but should be read in light of Pelis, "Taking Credit."

54. Lee, *The Happy Life of a Doctor*, quotes on pp. 29–30, 35.

55. Kenneth M. Brinkhous, "Harry P. Smith (1895–1972): Pathologist, Teacher, Investigator, and Administrator," *American Journal of Clinical Pathology* 63 (1975): 605–8.

56. See George W. Corner, *George Hoyt Whipple and His Friends: The Life-Story of a Nobel Prize Pathologist* (Philadelphia: J. B. Lippincott, 1963).

57. See Maxwell M. Wintrobe, *Hematology, the Blossoming of a Science: A Story of Inspiration and Effort* (Philadelphia: Lea & Febiger, 1985).

58. See E. D. Warner, K. M. Brinkhous, and H. P. Smith, "The Titration of Prothrombin in Certain Plasmas," *Archives of Pathology* 18 (1934): 587.

59. Michael Bliss, *The Discovery of Insulin* (Chicago: University of Chicago Press, 1982), and Wailoo, *Drawing Blood*, pp. 99–133.

60. See K. M. Brinkhous, H. P. Smith, and E. D. Warner, "Plasma Protein Level in Normal Infancy and in Hemorrhagic Disease of the Newborn," *American Journal of Medical Sciences* 193 (1937): 475–80, and Ratnoff, "Why Do People Bleed?" pp. 617–18.

61. Armand J. Quick, Margaret Stanley-Brown, and Frederick W. Bancroft, "A Study of the Coagulation Defect in Hemophilia and in Jaundice," *American Journal of Medical Science* 190 (1935): 501–11. See Edith Ebel, *The Quick Tests: The Life and Work of Dr. Armand J. Quick* (Blacksburg, VA: Pocahontas Press, 1995), and Ratnoff, "Why Do People Bleed?" p. 612.

62. E. D. Warner, K. M. Brinkhous, and H. P. Smith, "A Quantitative Study

of Blood Clotting: Prothrombin Fluctuations under Experimental Conditions," *American Journal of Physiology* 114 (1936): 667–75.

63. Jaques, "The Howell Theory of Blood Coagulation," p. 150.

64. Ratnoff, "Why Do People Bleed?" p. 612. For a lucid and independent account of the controversy over the one-stage and two-stage prothrombin essays, see Robert Gwyn Macfarlane, "Russell's Viper Venom, 1934–1936," *British Journal of Haematology* 13 (1967): 437–51, especially pp. 443–44.

65. See Robert D. Langdell, John B. Graham, and Kenneth M. Brinkhous, "Prothrombin Utilization during Clotting: Comparison of Results with the Two-Stage and One-Stage Methods," *Proceedings of the Society of Experimental Biology and Medicine* 74 (1950): 424–27, and Kenneth M. Brinkhous, Robert D. Langdell, and John B. Graham, "The Problem of Prothrombin Determinations in Serum," in Joseph E. Flynn, ed., *Blood Clotting and Its Allied Disorders: Transactions of the Third Josiah Macy, Jr. Conference* (New York: Josiah Macy, Jr. Foundation, 1950), pp. 208–11.

66. Corner, *George Hoyt Whipple and His Friends*, p. 98.

67. Kenneth M. Brinkhous, interview by Susan Resnick, November 29, 1991. Courtesy of Susan Resnick.

68. My narrative is based on Brinkhous's recollections of the 1990s, as they were related to Susan Resnick in her 1991 interview and to me on two different occasions, in 1994 and 1995. Quote from K. M. Brinkhous, "Understanding Factor VIII," Karl Landsteiner Award Lecture, annual meeting of the American Association of Blood Banks, San Diego, November 17, 1994.

69. Brinkhous detailed the experience in "Hemophilia: Pathophysiologic Studies and the Evolution of Transfusion Therapy," *American Journal of Clinical Pathology* 41 (April 1964): 342–51.

70. This history is told in greater depth in Stephen Pemberton, "Canine Technologies, Model Patients: The Historical Production of Hemophiliac Dogs in American Biomedicine," in Susan Schrepfer and Philip Scranton, eds., *Industrializing Organisms: Introducing Evolutionary History* (New York: Routledge, 2004), pp. 191–213.

71. Kenneth Brinkhous, "A Study of the Clotting Defect in Hemophilia: The Delayed Formation of Thrombin," *American Journal of the Medical Sciences* 198 (October 1939): 509–16, quote on p. 515, and Roy Kracke, *Diseases of the Blood* (Philadelphia: J. B. Lippincott, 1941).

72. Ratnoff, "Why Do People Bleed?" p. 629.

73. Arthur J. Patek Jr. and Richard P. Stetson, "Hemophilia. I. The Abnormal Coagulation of the Blood and Its Relation to the Blood Platelets," *Journal of Clinical Investigation* 15 (1936): 531–42. Only the theory of Addis seemed to

satisfy Patek's belief that the defect in hemophilia was due to a qualitative change in plasma prothrombin. See p. 540.

74. The phrasing is Francis Rackemann's in *The Inquisitive Physician*, p. 184.

75. Arthur J. Patek Jr. and F. H. L. Taylor, "Hemophilia. II. Some Properties of a Substance Obtained from Normal Human Plasma Effective in Accelerating the Coagulation of Hemophilic Blood," *Journal of Clinical Investigation* 16 (1937): 113–24, quote on p. 123.

76. Ratnoff, "Why Do People Bleed?" p. 629.

77. Brinkhous, "A Study of the Clotting Defect in Hemophilia: The Delayed Formation of Thrombin," pp. 509–16, and "Clotting Defect in Hemophilia: Deficiency in a Plasma Factor Required for Platelet Utilization," *Proceedings of the Society for Experimental Biology and Medicine* 66 (1947): 117–20. Brinkhous and colleagues began describing classic hemophilia as a deficiency of "antihemophilic factor" (AHF) in a series of publications between 1950 and 1952 to reflect the postwar consensus that classic hemophilia was likely a deficiency of a plasma factor. In the same era, prominent research groups at Harvard and Oxford independently concluded in the same era that the deficient plasma factor was a globulin (i.e., a serum protein distinct from albumin). Jessica Lewis, Laskey Taylor, and others at Harvard first coined the term *antihemophilic globulin* (AHG) in 1946 in the second issue of *Blood*. See J. H. Lewis, H. J. Tagnon, C. S. Davidson, G. R. Minot, and F. H. L. Taylor, "The Relation of Certain Fractions of the Plasma Globulins to the Coagulation Defect in Hemophilia," *Blood* 1 (1946): 166–72.

78. Rackemann, *The Inquisitive Physician*, pp. 183–84.

79. The patients were Russell White, Edward Woogmaster, James Smith, and Victor Marotta. See Patek and Stetson, "Hemophilia. I," p. 542.

80. Frances Burns, *Boston Globe*, September 24, 1954, as quoted in Rackemann, *The Inquisitive Physician*, pp. 183–84.

81. Ratnoff, "Why Do People Bleed?" p. 602.

82. See Starr, *Blood*, pp. 88–46.

83. Jessica H. Lewis, "Experiments of Nature," *Journal of the American Medical Association* 179 (March 31, 1962): 1011–12.

Chapter 3: Vital Factors in the Making of a Masculine World

1. Helen Furnas, "I've Got the Lonesomest Disease!" *Saturday Evening Post* 226 (November 21, 1953): 24–25, 110, 114, 117, 119.

2. Robert L. Rosenthal, O. Herman Dreskin, and Nathan Rosenthal, "A New Hemophilia-Like Disease Caused by Deficiency of a Third Plasma Thromboplastin Factor," *Proceedings of the Society of Biological and Experimental Medicine*

82 (1953): 171–74; R. L. Rosenthal, "Hemophilia and Hemophilia-Like Diseases Caused by Deficiencies in Plasma Thromboplastin Factors," *American Journal of Medicine* 17 (July 1954): 57–68; R. L. Rosenthal, O. H. Dreskin, and N. Rosenthal, "Plasma Thromboplastin Antecedent (PTA) Deficiency: Clinical, Coagulation, Therapeutic and Hereditary Aspects of a New Hemophilia-Like Disease," *Blood* 10 (February 1955): 120–31; and R. L. Rosenthal, "The Present Status of Plasma Thromboplastin Antecedent (PTA) Deficiency," in K. M. Brinkhous, ed., *Hemophilia and Hemophiliod Diseases: International Symposium* (Chapel Hill: University of North Carolina Press, 1957), pp. 116–23.

3. See William Bulloch and Paul Fildes, "Haemophilia," in Karl Pearson, ed., *Treasury of Human Inheritance*, vol. 1 (London: Cambridge University Press, 1912), pp. 169–354; occasionally referenced as *Eugenics Laboratory Memoirs XII, Francis Galton Laboratory for National Eugenics, University of London* (London: Dulau, 1911), parts V and VI, sec. XIVa.

4. The medical literature was mixed on the question of whether hemophilic males could be "transmitters" before the rise of Mendelianism. Mendel's laws demonstrated clearly that males could transmit hemophilia through their daughters to their grandsons, effectively "skipping" a generation. As detailed in chapter 1, Nasse's law (1820) affirmed that the daughters of affected males transmit the disease and allowed for this possibility. In 1877, however, Hermann Lossen of Heidelberg, Germany, denied that affected males transmit the hemophilia on the basis of extensive work with the Mampel family. The Mampels not only had a long history of hemophilic bleeding but had been studied since the 1820s. The belief that affected males are not transmitters of hemophilia was occasionally called the law of Lossen where the Mampel family studies were held to be paradigmatic in the late nineteenth and early twentieth centuries. Bulloch and Files supported the law of Lossen on methodological grounds in 1911, saying that "it cannot be said that a generation is 'skipped' unless that generation includes unaffected males." See, e.g., Bulloch and Fildes, "Haemophilia," pp. 185, 267–71; Reginald Ruggles Gates, *Heredity in Man* (London: Constable, 1929), p. 205; and C. B. Kerr, "The Fortunes of Haemophiliacs in the Nineteenth Century," *Medical History* 7 (1963): 359–70.

5. In 1930, C. A. Mills reported transmission of hemophilia through the male as a novel find, therefore suggesting that Mendelianism took a while to penetrate into American hematology. See C. A. Mills, "The Transmission of Hemophilia," *Journal of the American Medical Association* 94 (May 17, 1930): 1571–72, and C. A. Mills, "Hemophilia," *Journal of Laboratory and Clinical Medicine* 17 (June 1932): 932.

6. Paul Clough, "Hemophilia," in *Diseases of the Blood* (New York: Harper and Brothers, 1929), p. 236.

7. The diagnostic criteria can be found in H. Joules and R. G. Macfarlane, "Pseudo-Haemophilia in a Woman," *Lancet* 1 (March 26, 1938): 715–18.

8. Carroll LaFleur Birch, *Hemophilia: Clinical and Genetic Aspects* (Urbana: University of Illinois Press, 1937), p. 40.

9. Carroll LaFleur Birch, "Hemophilia," *Proceedings of the Society for Experimental Biology and Medicine* 28 (April 1931): 752–53.

10. R. G. Macfarlane, "Russell's Viper Venom, 1934–64," *British Journal of Haematology* 13 (1967): 437–51, quote on p. 439.

11. "Successfully Treats Two for Hemophilia: Chicago Woman Doctor Arrests Inherent Bleeding by Use of Ovarian Extract," *New York Times*, March 15, 1931, p. A15.

12. Birch's first publication on hemophilia was "Hemophilia," in *Proceedings of the Society for Experimental Biology and Medicine* (April 1931). Press coverage quoted from "Successfully Treats Two for Hemophilia." See also "Ovaries for Bleeders," *Time* 18 (July 13, 1931): 45. On the inception of Birch's thinking, see Carroll Birch, "Hemophilia," *Journal of the American Medical Association* 99 (November 5, 1932): 1566–72, quote on p. 1566.

13. Carroll Birch, "Hemophilia and the Female Sex Hormone," *Journal of the American Medical Association* 97 (July 31, 1931): 244.

14. Birch, "Hemophilia," quote on p. 1571.

15. See Robert Brown and Fuller Albright, "Estrin Therapy in a Case of Hemophilia," *New England Journal of Medicine* 209 (September 28, 1933): 630–32; Jacob Brem and Jerome Leopold, "Ovarian Therapy: Relationship of the Female Sex Hormone to Hemophilia," *Journal of the American Medical Association* 102 (January 20, 1934): 200–202; and Richard Stetson, Claude Forkner, William Chew, and Murray Rich, "Negative Effect of Prolonged Administration of Ovarian Substances in Hemophilia," *Journal of the American Medical Association* 102 (April 7, 1934): 1122–26.

16. Birch, *Hemophilia*, p. 38. Not until the 1960s, following the work by Mary Lyon and others on the processes of X chromosome inactivation, was it found that the functional X chromosome protects the female carrier of hemophilia (X^HX) from the expression of bleeding symptoms that might otherwise be occasioned by the female carrier's abnormal X^H chromosome.

17. Ibid., pp. 40–42, 44, 62–65. Birch was able to test blood samples of a few of these suspected female bleeders using the standard coagulation time test but nothing more sophisticated.

18. Bulloch and Fildes, "Haemophilia," p. 174.

19. On the idiosyncratic terminology employed by Birch, see H. Grüneberg, "Review of *Haemophilia: Clinical and Genetic Aspects*," *Eugenics Review* 29 (1938): 277–78.

20. See Paul M. Aggeler and Salvatore P. Lucia, *Hemorrhagic Disorders: A Guide to Diagnosis and Treatment* (Chicago: University of Chicago Press, 1949), p. 31.

21. Clough, "Hemophilia," p. 236.

22. See Birch, *Hemophilia*, p. 40. See also, for comparison, Mildred Warde, "Haemophilia in the Female," *British Medical Journal* 2 (October 6, 1923): 599–600; Madge Thurlow Macklin, "Heredity in Hemophilia," *American Journal of the Medical Sciences* 175 (February 1928): 218–24, especially p. 222; and Gates, *Heredity in Man*, pp. 207–8.

23. See Kenneth M. Brinkhous and John B. Graham, "Occurrence of Hemophilia in Females," *Journal of Laboratory and Clinical Medicine* 34 (1949): 1587–88, K. M. Brinkhous and J. B. Graham, "Hemophilia in the Female Dog," *Science* 111 (June 30, 1950): 723–24, and K. M. Brinkhous, J. B. Graham, G. D. Penick, and R. D. Langdell, "Studies on Canine Hemophilia," in Joseph Flynn, ed., *Blood Clotting and Allied Problems: Transactions of the Fourth Conference, January 22–23, 1951* (New York: Josiah Macy, Jr. Foundation, 1951), pp. 51–118. The history of this canine hemophilia colony is detailed in Stephen Pemberton, "Canine Technologies, Model Patients: The Historical Production of Hemophiliac Dogs in American Biomedicine," in Susan Schrepfer and Philip Scranton, eds., *Industrializing Organisms: Introducing Evolutionary History* (New York: Routledge, 2004), pp. 191–213.

24. M. C. Isreales, H. Lempert, and E. Gilbertson, "Haemophilia in the Female," *Lancet* 1 (1951): 1375, and C. Merskey, "The Occurrence of Haemophilia in the Human Female," *Quarterly Journal of Medicine* 20 (1951): 299. There was also a debate as to whether female "conductors" or "carriers" manifested detectable symptoms of a bleeding disorder. See C. Merskey and R.G. Macfarlane, "The Female Carrier of Haemophilia," *Lancet* 1 (1951): 487, and A. Margolius and O. Ratnoff, "A Laboratory Study of the Carrier State in Classic Hemophilia," *Journal of Clinical Investigation* 35 (1956): 1316–23.

25. See Rosenthal, Dreskin, and Rosenthal, "New Hemophilia-Like Disease Caused by Deficiency of a Third Plasma Thromboplastin Factor." A short, but fuller account of its discovery is found in Oscar Ratnoff, "Why Do People Bleed?" in Maxwell M. Wintrobe, ed., *Blood, Pure and Eloquent* (New York: McGraw Hill, 1980), pp. 623–24.

26. See Rosenthal, "The Present Status of Plasma Thromboplastin Antecedent (PTA) Deficiency."

27. For reviews, see Uri Seligsohn, "Factor XI in Haemostasis and Thrombosis: Past, Present and Future," *Thrombosis and Haemostasis* 98 (2007): 84–89, and K. Gomez and P. Bolton-Maggs, "Factor XI Deficiency," 14 (2008): 1183–89.

28. See Susan Resnick, *Blood Saga: Hemophilia, AIDS, and the Survival of a Community* (Berkeley: University of California Press, 1998), pp. 20–25, and Ratnoff, "Why Do People Bleed?" p. 611.

29. On the thromboplastin generation test, see R. Biggs and A. Stuart Douglas, "The Thromboplastin Generation Test," *Journal of Clinical Pathology* 6 (1953): 23–29, and R. Biggs, A. S. Douglas, and R. G. Macfarlane, "Formation of Thromboplastin in Human Blood," *Journal of Physiology* 119 (1953): 89–101. On history, see R. Biggs, "Thirty Years of Haemophilia Treatment at Oxford," *British Journal of Haematology* 13 (1967): 452–63, and E. M. Tansey and D. A. Christie, eds., *Haemophilia: Recent History of Clinical Management*, vol. 4, *Wellcome Witnesses to Twentieth Century Medicine* (London: Wellcome Trust, 1999), especially pp. 3–8.

On the original partial thromboplastin time test (PTT), see Robert D. Langdell, Robert H. Wagner, and Kenneth M. Brinkhous, "Effect of Antihemophilic Factor on One-Stage Clotting Tests," *Journal of Laboratory and Clinical Medicine* 41 (1953): 637–47, and Kenneth M. Brinkhous, Robert D. Langdell, George D. Penick, John B. Graham, and Robert H. Wagner, "Newer Approaches to the Study of Hemophilia and Hemophiliod States," *Journal of the American Medical Association* 154 (1954): 481–86.

30. On the advantages of the PTT, see Ratnoff, "Why Do People Bleed?" p. 622, and Kenneth M. Brinkhous and Frederick A. Dombrose, "Partial Thromboplastin Time," in David Seligson, ed., *CRC Handbook Series in Clinical Laboratory Science, Section I: Hematology*, vol. 3 (Boca Raton, FL: CRC Press, 1980), pp. 221–46, especially pp. 221 and 230.

31. A. J. Patek and R. P. Stetson, "Hemophilia. I. The Abnormal Coagulation of the Blood and Its Relation to the Blood Platelets," *Journal of Clinical Investigation* 15 (1936): 531–42, and A. J. Patek and F. H. L. Taylor, "Hemophilia. II. Some Properties of a Substance Obtained from Normal Human Plasma Effective in Accelerating the Coagulation of Hemophilic Blood," *Journal of Clinical Investigation* 16 (1937): 113–24. See E. L. Lozner and F. H. L. Taylor, "Coagulation Defect in Hemophilia: Studies of Clot-Promoting Activity Associate with Plasma Euglobin in Hemophilia," *Journal of Clinical Investigation* 18 (1939): 821–25; George Minot and F. H. L. Taylor, "Hemophilia: The Clinical Use of Antihemophilic Globulin," *Annals of Internal Medicine* 26 (1947): 341–52; and K. M. Brinkhous, "Clotting Defect in Hemophilia: Deficiency in a Plasma Factor Re-

quired for Platelet Utilization," *Proceedings of the Society for Experimental Biology and Medicine* 66 (1947): 117–20.

32. During the war, at least seven pharmaceutical companies held contracts to produce albumin and/or other plasma fractions for military use. These included Armour Laboratories, Cutter Laboratories, Eli Lily Laboratories, E.R. Squibb, Lederle Laboratories, Upjohn Co., and Sharp and Dohne. See Douglas M. Surgenor, *Edwin J. Cohn and the Development of Protein Chemistry* (Cambridge, MA: Harvard University Press, 2001), especially pp. 129–30, 140.

33. See the seminal article by Edwin J. Cohn et al., "Preparation and Properties of Serum and Plasma Proteins: IV. A System for the Separation into Fractions of the Protein and Lipoprotein Components of Biological Tissues and Fluids," *Journal of the American Chemical Society* 68 (March 1946): 459–75; and Surgenor, *Edwin J. Cohn and the Development of Protein Chemistry*, especially pp. 227, 238–41.

34. Edwin J. Cohn, "Blood Proteins and Their Therapeutic Value" *Science* 101 (January 19, 1945): 51–56; "The Separation of Blood into Fractions of Therapeutic Value," *Annals of Internal Medicine* 26 (1947): 341–352; and "The History of Plasma Fractionation," in E. C. Andrus et al., eds., *Advances in Military Medicine* (Boston: Little, Brown, 1948), pp. 364–443.

35. On the public campaign for plasma fractionation, see "Man of Blood," *Newsweek* 25 (May 14, 1945): 106; John F. Fulton, "Penicillin, Plasma Fractionation, and the Physician," *Atlantic Monthly* 176 (September 1945): 107–13; "Blood Fractionation Process Patented," *Science News Letter* 48 (December 15, 1945): 377; Charles A. Janeway, "Blood and Blood Derivatives—A New Public Health Field," *American Journal of Public Health* 36 (January 1946): 1–14, quote on p. 1; and Douglas M. Surgenor, "Blood," *Scientific American* 190 (February 1954): 54–62.

36. As historian Angela Creager has effectively argued, plasma fractionation reflected the circumstances of American science and society in the 1940s while accelerating, if not initiating, modern medicine's growing dependence on biotechnology. Her reading of Cohn's work (including his patent efforts) is critical for understanding university-industry collaboration in the mid-twentieth century as well as interpreting blood's rising status as a commodity in the era. See Angela N. H. Creager, "Biotechnology and Blood: Edwin Cohn's Plasma Fractionation Project, 1940–1953," in Arnold Thackray, ed., *Private Science: Biotechnology and the Rise of the Molecular Sciences* (Philadelphia: University of Pennsylvania Press, 1998), pp. 39–64, especially 53–54, and Angela N. H. Creager, "Producing

Molecular Therapeutics from Human Blood: Edwin Cohn's Wartime Experience," in Soraya de Chadarevian and Harmke Kamminga, eds., *Molecularizing Biology and Medicine: New Practices and Alliances, 1910s-1970s* (Amsterdam: Harwood Academic Publishers, 1998), pp. 107–37, especially pp. 126–29.

37. On plasma fractionation and hemophilia, see G. R. Minot, C. S. Davidson, J. H. Lewis, H. J. Tagnon, and F. H. L. Taylor, "Coagulation Defect in Hemophilia: Effect in Hemophilia, of Parentaeral Administration, of Fraction in Plasma Globulins Rich in Fibrinogen," *Journal of Clinical Investigation* 24 (1945): 704–7; and Cohn, "The History of Plasma Fractionation," pp. 432–33.

38. Owren first presented his preliminary results to colleagues at the Norwegian Academy of Science in 1944. The full announcement came in Paul A. Owren, "Parahaemophilia: Haemorrhagic Diathesis Due to Absence of Previously Unknown Clotting Factor," *Lancet* 252 (April 5, 1947): 446–48. Later in 1947, Owren defended and published this research for his Ph.D. See Paul A. Owren, "Coagulation of Blood: Investigations on New Clotting Factor," *Acta Med Scand* (suppl.) 194 (1947): 1–327. Biographical details are available in Kenneth M. Brinkhous and Helge Stormorken, "Obituary: Paul A. Owren, M.D. 1905–1990," *Thrombosis and Haemostasis* 64 (1990): 341–42. A comprehensive account of the factor V discovery can be found in Helge Stormorken, "The Discovery of Factor V: A Tricky Clotting Factor," *Journal of Thrombosis and Haemostasis* 1 (2003): 206–21. There was some initial skepticism about Owren's findings, and Armand Quick disputed them aggressively. See Armand J. Quick, "Components of Prothrombin Complex," *American Journal of Physiology* 151 (November 1947): 63–70; Ratnoff, "Why Do People Bleed?" pp. 610–14.

39. Pavlovsky believed the results pointed to the existence of an anticoagulant factor in the plasma that inhibited the capacity of the patient's blood to clot. See Alfredo Pavlovsky, "Contribution to the Pathogenesis of Hemophilia," *Blood* 2 (1947): 185–91. See also M. R. Castex, A. Pavlovsky, and C. Simonetti, "Contributión al estudio de la fisopatogenia de la hemofilia," *Medicina, Buenos Aires* 5 (1944): 16, and Pavlovsky's own account of his work, entitled "Antecedents," submitted to Maxwell Myer Wintrobe for publication in *Hematology: The Blossoming of a Science*. See box 82, "Biographies for *Hematology: The Blossoming of a Science*, O–Q," folder 10: "Pavlovsky, Alfredo," Maxwell Myer Wintrobe Papers, Accn. #954, Manuscripts Division, J. Willard Marriott Library, University of Utah.

40. The pivotal studies on the discovery of factor IX deficiency were (in order of their appearance): Paul M. Aggeler, Sidney G. White, M. B. Glendenning, et al., "Plasma Thromboplastin Component (P.T.C.) Deficiency: A New Disease Resembling Hemophilia," *Proceedings of the Society of Experimental Biology and*

Medicine 79 (1952): 692–94; Irving Schulman and C. H. Smith, "Hemorrhagic Disease in an Infant Due to Deficiency of a Previously Undescribed Clotting Factor," *Blood* 7 (1952): 794–807; and R. Biggs, A. Stuart Douglas, R. G. Macfarlane, R. G. Dacie, J. V. Pitney, W. R. Merskey, and J. R. O'Brien, "Christmas Disease: A Condition Previously Mistaken for Haemophilia," *British Medical Journal* 2 (1952): 1378–82.

41. Sidney G. White, Paul M. Aggeler, and Mary Beth Glendenning, "Plasma Thromboplastin Component (PTC): A Hitherto Unrecognized Blood Coagulation Factor: Case Report of PTC Deficiency," *Blood* 8 (February 1953): 101–24; Sidney G. White, Paul M. Aggeler, and Byron E. Emery, "Plasma Thromboplastin Component (PTC): Potency of Plasma Fractions," *Proceedings of the Society for Experimental Biology and Medicine* 83 (1953): 69–71; and Paul M. Aggeler, Theodore H. Spaet, and Byron E. Emery, "Purification of Plasma Factor B (Plasma Thromboplastin Component) and Its Identification as a Beta2 Globulin," *Science* 119 (June 4, 1954): 106–7.

42. Schulman and Smith, "Hemorrhagic Disease in an Infant Due to Deficiency of a Previously Undescribed Clotting Factor."

43. Biggs et al., "Christmas Disease: A Condition Previously Mistaken for Haemophilia," quotes on p. 1382.

44. On the evolving relation between disease identity and treatment in this era, see Keith Wailoo, *Drawing Blood: Technology and Disease Identity in Twentieth-Century America* (Baltimore: Johns Hopkins University Press, 1997); Jeremy Greene, *Prescribing by Numbers: Drugs and the Definition of Disease* (Baltimore: Johns Hopkins University Press, 2007); and Nicholas Rasmussen, *On Speed: The Many Lives of Amphetamine* (New York: New York University Press, 2008).

45. Paul Giangrande, "Six Characters in Search of an Author: The History of the Nomenclature of Coagulation Factors," *British Journal of Haematology* 121 (2003): 703–12, especially pp. 704–5. See also Alastair Robb-Smith, *Life and Achievements of Professor Robert Gwyn Macfarlane FRS: Pioneer in the Care of Haemophiliacs* (London: Royal Society of Medicine, 1993); Rosemary Biggs, Christine Lee, Charles Rizza, and Tilly Tansey, "Witnessing Medical History: An Interview with Dr. Rosemary Biggs," *Haemophilia* 4 (1998): 769–77; and Tansey and Christie, *Haemophilia: Recent History of Clinical Management.*

46. See, for instance, the call for parents of hemophiliacs to have their boys tested for Christmas disease in the *Bulletin of the Midwest Chapter of the Hemophilia Foundation, Inc.* (Chicago) 2, no. 8 (August 1954), David Street, editor, in folder "National Hemophilia Foundation Correspondence, 1954," Kenneth M. Brinkhous Papers, Francis Owen Blood Research Laboratory, University of North Carolina at Chapel Hill.

47. See the editorial, "Blood Coagulation and the Clinical Pathologist," *Journal of Clinical Pathology* 6 (February 1953): 1–2.

48. See, e.g., the recommendations in hematologist Benjamin Alexander's "Medical Progress: Coagulation, Hemorrhage and Thrombosis," *New England Journal of Medicine* 252 (1955): 432–42, 484–94, 526–35.

49. Theodore H. Spaet, "Recent Progress in the Study of Hemophilia," *Stanford Medical Bulletin* 13 (February 1955): 24–47, especially pp. 32, 34–35.

50. Paul M. Aggeler, Sidney G. White, and Theodore H. Spaet, "Deutero-hemophilia: Plasma Thromboplastin Factor B Deficiency, Plasma Thromboplastin Component (PTC) Deficiency, Christmas Disease, Hemophilia B," *Blood* 9 (1954): 246–53.

51. William Dameshek, "Introduction to 'Symposium: What Is Hemophilia?'" *Blood* 9 (March 1954): 244–45, quote on p. 244.

52. See R. Biggs and R. G. Macfarlane, *Human Blood Coagulation and Its Disorders* (Springfield, IL: Charles C. Thomas, 1953; 2nd ed., 1957). Nearly four hundred articles on blood coagulation appeared in the 1949–50 academic year (1st ed., p. 3), and more than six hundred appeared in the 1953–54 academic year (2nd ed., p. 3). Citations on blood clotting and related subjects from the *Index Medicus* for 1945–55 corroborate this claim.

53. Dameshek, "Introduction," p. 244.

54. Traditionally, Aggeler's group might be credited along with two other research groups with the simultaneous discovery of factor IX deficiency, also known variously as hemophilia B and Christmas disease. See P. M. Aggeler, S. G. White, M. B. Glendenning, et al., "Plasma Thromboplastin Component (P.T.C.) Deficiency: A New Disease Resembling Hemophilia," *Proceedings of the Society of Experimental Biology and Medicine* 79 (1952): 692–94; I. Schulman and C. H. Smith, "Hemorrhagic Disease in an Infant Due to Deficiency of a Previously Undescribed Clotting Factor," *Blood* 7 (1952): 794–807; and R. Biggs, A. S. Douglas, R. G. Macfarlane, et al., "Christmas Disease: A Condition Previously Mistaken for Haemophilia," *British Medical Journal* 2 (1952): 1378–82.

55. Dameshek, "Introduction," p. 244.

56. Ibid.

57. Armand Quick, *The Hemorrhagic Diseases and the Physiology of Hemostasis* (Springfield, IL: Charles C. Thomas, 1942), pp. 209–10.

58. See, for instance, Clough, "Hemophilia," pp. 236–43, and Nathan Rosenthal, "Hemorrhagic Diatheses," in Hal Downey, ed., *Handbook of Hematology* (New York: Paul B. Hoeber, 1938), 1:501–51.

59. See, e.g., the three Symposium contributions, Mario Stefanini, "Hemophilia: Specific Entity or Syndrome?"; Leandro Tocantins, "Hemophilic Syndromes

and Hemophilia"; and Fritz Koller, "Is Hemophilia a Nosologic Entity?" *Blood* 9 (March 1954): 73–80, 281–85, 286–90.

60. Quote from Spaet, "Recent Progress," p. 24.

61. Dameshek, "Introduction," p. 245.

62. See T. Koller and W. R. Merz, eds., *Thrombose und Embolie, Referate der I. Thrombosis and Embolism, Proceedings* (Basel: B. Schwabe, 1955).

63. Description and quotations from Wright's speech are excerpted from a undated, typed manuscript in Kenneth Brinkhous, "History of International Committee on the Nomenclature of the Blood Clotting Factors, 1954–59," in folder "History of International Society of Thrombosis and Haemostasis," Brinkhous Papers.

64. See Koller and Merz, *Thrombose und Embolie*. The committee itself was composed of some of the world's most distinguished clotters. Between 1954 and 1959, its U.S. members were Benjamin Alexander, Kenneth Brinkhous, Leandro Tocantins, Armand Quick, and Walter Seegers.

65. The history of the nomenclature committee is recounted in serial form in *Thrombosis et Diathesis Haemorrhagica, Supplementum* vols. 2–6 (1958–61). See also Giangrande, "Six Characters in Search of an Author."

66. "The Nomenclature of Blood Clotting Factors" *Journal of the American Medical Association* 180 (June 2, 1962): 733–35.

67. See box 78, folder 8: "Koller, Fritz," Wintrobe Papers.

68. See F. Duckert, P. Flückiger, M. Matter, and F. Koller, "Clotting Factor X: Physiologic and Physico-Chemical Properties," *Proceedings of the Society of Experimental Biology and Medicine* 90 (October 1955): 17–22; and C. Hougie, E. M. Barrow, and J. B. Graham, "Stuart Clotting Defect. I. Segregation of an Hereditary Hemorrhagic State from the Heterogeneous Group Heretofore Called 'Stable Factor' (SPCA, Proconvertin, Factor VII) Deficiency," *Journal of Clinical Investigation* 36 (March 1957): 485–96.

69. All quotes and analysis in the preceding discussion pertain to Furnas, "I've Got the Lonesomest Disease!"

70. As an example of this confusion, see the response by Kenneth Brinkhous to a query by Robert Lee Henry and the Hemophilia Foundation, Inc., requesting clarification of an abstract that Brinkhous and his colleagues had presented at a recent AMA meeting, entitled "Newer Approaches to the Study of Hemophilia and Hemophilia-Like States." K. M. Brinkhous to Robert Lee Henry, June 4, 1953, in folder "National Hemophilia Foundation Correspondence, 1953," Brinkhous Papers.

71. *The Hemophilia Foundation, Inc. Newsletter*, July 1954, p. 2, Brinkhous Papers.

72. Furnas, "I've Got the Lonesomest Disease!" pp. 25, 119. See also "His Parents Refused to Let This Boy Die," *McCall's Magazine*, May 1951, pp. 46–47, 80–94, and Pearl P. Puckett, "Calling All Bleeders," *American Mercury* 79 (August 1954): 73–74.

73. Spaet, "Recent Progress," p. 24.

74. See Aggeler, Spaet, and Emery, "Purification of Plasma Factor B," and Aggeler, White, and Spaet, "Deuterohemophilia: Plasma Thromboplastin Factor B Deficiency."

75. Kenneth Brinkhous, folder "National Hemophilia Foundation Correspondence, 1954," Brinkhous Papers, and Resnick, *Blood Saga*, p. 36.

76. Furnas, "I've Got the Lonesomest Disease!" p. 119.

77. R. G. Macfarlane, "An Enzyme Cascade in the Blood Clotting Mechanism, and Its Function as a Biochemical Amplifier," *Nature* 202 (1964): 498–99, and Earl W. Davie and Oscar D. Ratnoff, "Waterfall Sequence for Intrinsic Blood Clotting," *Science* 145 (1964): 1310–11. Accounts of this work are available in Robb-Smith, *Life and Achievements of Professor Robert Gwyn Macfarlane*; Ratnoff, "Why Do People Bleed?"; Charles A Owen Jr., *A History of Blood Coagulation* (Rochester, MN: Mayo Foundation for Medical Education and Research, 2001); and Cecil Hougie, *Thrombosis and Bleeding: An Era of Discovery* (Victoria, BC: Trafford Publishing, 2004).

Chapter 4: Normality within Limits

1. "A Time to Be Alive," *Medic*, vol. 3 (Narberth, PA: Alpha Video Distributors, 2006). James E. Moser, creator; Ted Post, director; Frank LaTourette, producer; Worthington Miner, executive producer; and Art and Jo Napolean, teleplay. Other than Richard Boone as Dr. Konrad Styner and Edmund Penny as Intern Carl, medical personnel in the episode were played by real doctors and nurses: A. J. Connick Doran, M.D.; Lynn Ward Wiseman, M.D.; Shirley Haile, R.N.; and Marei K. Marshall, R.N. On the history of *Medic*, see Joseph Turow, "No Compromise with Truth," in *Playing Doctor: Television, Storytelling, and Medical Power* (New York: Oxford University Press, 1989), pp. 25–45, and Turow, "Medic," in Horace Newcomb, ed., *The Encyclopedia of Television*, 2nd ed. (Chicago: Fitzroy Dearborn, 2004), pp. 1467–68.

2. Peter Jones, "Forty Years of Progress in Global Hemophilia Care," and David Page, "Remembering Frank Schnabel," *Hemophilia World* 10, no. 1 (March 2003): 1–9, 10–11, quote on p. 10. Essays reprinted in Canadian Hemophilia Society, *50 Years to Remember: A Souvenir Booklet* (Montreal: Canadian Hemophilia Society, 2003).

3. On Schnabel, see Douglas Starr, *Blood: An Epic History of Medicine and Commerce* (New York: Alfred Knopf, 1998), pp. 242–45, 281.

4. See, e.g., Donald Bateman, "The Good Bleed Guide: A Patient's Story," *Social History of Medicine* 7 (Spring 1994): 126.

5. See Helen Furnas, "I've Got the Lonesomest Disease!" *Saturday Evening Post* 226 (November 21, 1953): 24–25, 110, 114, 117, 119, and Susan Resnick, *Blood Saga: Hemophilia, AIDS, and the Survival of a Community* (Berkeley: University of California Press, 1999), pp. 20–36.

6. See Starr, *Blood*.

7. See Alton Blakeslee's argument for a "new kind of citizenship" in *Blood's Magic for All* (New York: Public Affairs Committee, November 1948), also known as Public Affairs Pamphlet No. 145. See also Starr, *Blood*, and Sarah Chinn, "'Liberty's Life Stream': Blood, Race, and Citizenship in World War II," in *Technology and the Logic of American Racism* (New York: Continuum Press, 2000), pp. 93–140.

8. "Blood of Friends Sends Boy Home," *New York Times*, January 27, 1949, p. A25.

9. "Boy's Life Hangs on Blood Gifts," *New York Times*, April 18, 1950, p. A19. See also "Hemophilia Victim Gets Gifts of Blood," *New York Times*, April 19, 1950, p. A26.

10. Charles Carmen, interview by Susan Resnick, Independence, Ohio, September 12, 1990. Courtesy of Susan Resnick.

11. See Resnick, *Blood Saga*. On the history and character of voluntary health organizations in this era, see David Sills, *The Volunteers: Means and Ends in a National Organization* (Glencoe, IL: Free Press, 1957), and Richard Carter, *The Gentle Legions: National Voluntary Health Organizations in America* (New Brunswick, NJ: Transaction, 1992).

12. Pearl P. Puckett, "Calling All Bleeders," *American Mercury* 79 (August 1954): 73–74.

13. Ibid.

14. Susan Resnick, "The History of the National Hemophilia Foundation: A Half Century Overview," *Hemaware* 3 (October 1988): 12–19. For more details, see Nathan Smith, *A History of the National Hemophilia Foundation, 1948–1984* (New York: National Hemophilia Foundation, 1984), and Resnick, *Blood Saga*.

15. Resnick, *Blood Saga*, p. 34.

16. Letter from Robert Lee Henry to Kenneth Brinkhous, January 12, 1951, with accompanying pamphlet, entitled *A Message of Special Interest to Hospitals and Doctors from the National Hemophilia Foundation, Inc.*, in folder "National Hemophilia Foundation Correspondence, 1950–52," Kenneth M. Brinkhous

Papers, Francis Owen Blood Research Laboratory, University of North Carolina at Chapel Hill. Quotes are from the pamphlet. See also Jodie Landes Corngold, "Robert Lee Henry, The Founder of the National Hemophilia Foundation," *Hemaware* 3 (October 1988): 9.

17. Furnas, "I've Got the Lonesomest Disease!" p. 24.

18. Mary Gooley's testimony in Resnick, *Blood Saga*, p. 35.

19. "His Parents Refused to Let This Boy Die," *McCall's Magazine*, May 1951, pp. 46–47, 80–94, quote on p. 86.

20. Resnick, "The History of the National Hemophilia Foundation," p. 13, and *Blood Saga*, pp. 33–36.

21. Resnick, *Blood Saga*, p. 35, and "His Parents Refused to Let this Boy Die," pp. 46–47, 80, 82, 86, 88, 90, 94.

22. See, e.g., "Hemophilia Clinic Designated," *New York Times*, April 16, 1957, p. A37.

23. Resnick, *Blood Saga*, pp. 2, 35.

24. Susan Lindee, *Moments of Truth in Genetic Medicine* (Baltimore: Johns Hopkins University Press, 2006), p. 159.

25. Elaine Tyler May, *Homeward Bound: American Families in the Cold War Era* (New York: Basic Books, 1990), p. 26.

26. Joseph Veroff, Richard Kulka, and Elizabeth Douvan, *The Inner American: A Self-Portrait from 1957 to 1976* (New York: Basic Books, 1981), p. 194.

27. Resnick, *Blood Saga*, p. 35.

28. "Certificate of Incorporation of the Hemophilia Foundation, Inc.," in Smith, *A History of the National Hemophilia Foundation, 1948–1984*, appendix B.

29. Letter from Robert Lee Henry to Kenneth Brinkhous, December 2, 1953, in folder "National Hemophilia Foundation Correspondence, 1953," and Dr. Peter Vogel, "Minutes of the Meeting of the Medical Advisory Council of the Hemophilia Foundation, May 2, 1954," in folder "National Hemophilia Foundation Correspondence, 1954," Brinkhous Papers.

30. Chapter information based on author's review of folders "National Hemophilia Foundation Correspondence," for the years 1953 to 1960, Brinkhous Papers.

31. Smith, *A History of the National Hemophilia Foundation, 1948–1984*, p. 5, and Resnick, *Blood Saga*, p. 35.

32. Undated report by Robert Lee Henry, "The Hemophilia Foundation, Inc. Annual Report to Sufferers [concerning 1951]," in folder "National Hemophilia Foundation Correspondence, 1950–52," Brinkhous Papers.

33. "His Parents Refused to Let This Boy Die," p. 82.

34. These events are drawn from six letters, found in folders "National He-

mophilia Foundation Correspondence," for years 1955 and 1956, Brinkhous Papers: Letter from Mrs. C., King's Mountain, North Carolina, to the Hemophilia Foundation, June 25, 1955; Letter from Margaret Hexter to Mrs. C., July 20, 1955; Memorandum from Rebecca Randolph, Social Service Department, N.C. Memorial Hospital to Kenneth Brinkhous, August 12, 1955; Letter from Margaret Hexter to M. P. Rudolph, M.D., Chief, Crippled Children's Section, State Board of Health, Raleigh, North Carolina, October 24, 1956; Letter from Margaret Hexter to Kenneth Brinkhous, October 24, 1956; Letter from Kenneth Brinkhous to Margaret Hexter, November 23, 1956; and Letter from Margaret Hexter to Kenneth Brinkhous, November 29, 1956. The family name of the patients is omitted to protect their privacy.

35. Smith, *A History of the National Hemophilia Foundation, 1948–1984*, p. 6.

36. "Special Meeting of Board of Trustees of the Hemophilia Foundation, Convened at 2:00 P.M., Saturday, September 29, 1956, at the Morrison Hotel, Chicago, Illinois," in folder "National Hemophilia Foundation Correspondence, 1956," Brinkhous Papers.

Henry's count of "under 2,000 members" is a reference to the number of individual patients that the NHF registered in 1956, which was actually 2,128 patients (inclusive of the 37 female bleeders who were registered). The NHF also gathered information on citizenship and location. Only 1,448 patients were affiliated with U.S.-based chapters; 19 were affiliated with the Montreal chapter, and 624 were unaffiliated. "National Hemophilia Foundation Analysis of Registered Hemophiliacs, Jan. 1, 1957," in folder "National Hemophilia Foundation Correspondence, 1957," Brinkhous Papers.

37. The conference proceedings are published as Kenneth M. Brinkhous, ed., *Hemophilia and Hemophiliod Diseases: International Symposium* (Chapel Hill: University of North Carolina Press, 1957).

38. See David Oshinsky, *Polio: An American Story* (New York: Oxford University Press, 2006).

39. The minutes list these women only by last name. The official foundation communications often referred to women just by their last name or by their husband's name. They were Margaret B. Hexter (Mrs. George J. Hexter), Gertrude M. Bernstein (Mrs. Mark Bernstein), Mrs. Segal (probably Mrs. Norton Segal), and Mrs. Dorothy W. White. "Special Meeting of Board of Trustees of the Hemophilia Foundation," September 29, 1956, in folder "National Hemophilia Foundation Correspondence, 1956," Brinkhous Papers.

40. Letter from Armand Quick to Kenneth Brinkhous, March 12, 1957, in folder "National Hemophilia Foundation Correspondence, 1957," Brinkhous Papers.

41. Anthony Britten, "A Little Freedom for the Hemophiliac," *New England Journal of Medicine* 283 (November 5, 1970): 1051.

42. Quotes from Martin C. Rosenthal, "Minutes of the Subcommittee of the Medical Advisory Council," December 9, 1957. See also Letter from Martin Rosenthal to Kenneth Brinkhous, October 28, 1957; Letter from Brinkhous to Rosenthal, November 12, 1957; Letter from Brinkhous to Cutter Laboratories, December 13, 1957; and "Memorandum on Concentration of Antihemophilic Factor," from Samuel Moss, Executive Secretary of NIH Hematology Study Section to Chief, NIH Division of Research Grants; all in folder "National Hemophilia Foundation Correspondence, 1957," Brinkhous Papers.

43. Robert Littell, "Bearer Is a Hemophiliac," *Reader's Digest* 74 (April 1959): 214–20, quotes on pp. 214–15. The original article appeared in nonabridged form in the Canadian periodical *Liberty*, February 1959. The *Reader's Digest* version was edited to appeal to an American audience.

44. On the critical relation of credibility to stigma, see Erving Goffman, *Stigma: Notes on the Management of Spoiled Identity* (New York: Simon and Schuster, 1963), pp. 2–19.

45. Ralph Zimmerman, *Mingled Blood*, (New York: National Hemophilia Foundation, 1956), six-page pamphlet, found at National Library of Medicine, Bethesda, MD, and in folder "National Hemophilia Foundation Correspondence, 1956," Brinkhous Papers.

46. Paul K. Jones and Oscar Ratnoff, "The Changing Prognosis for Classic Hemophilia," *Annals of Internal Medicine* 114 (1991): 646.

47. "A Time to Be Alive."

48. Turow, "No Compromise with Truth," p. 26. Dow Chemical initially ran full-page ads in many newspapers and magazines. See, e.g., *TV Guide*, September 11, 1954, p. 12. The reviews are "The Man behind the 'Medic,'" *Look*, 18 (November 30, 1954): 100; "Doctor!" *Newsweek* 46 (November 20, 1955): 94; and "Strong Medicine," *TV Guide*, October 9, 1954, p. 21.

49. NBC aired the show as a rerun on June 20, 1955, after its premiere on January 31. See "On Television," *New York Times*, January 31, 1955, p. A29, and "TV Programs This Week," *New York Times*, June 19, 1955, p. X13.

50. *Bulletin of the Midwest Chapter of the Hemophilia Foundation, Inc.* (Chicago) 3, no. 2 (February 1955), in folder "National Hemophilia Foundation Correspondence, 1955," Brinkhous Papers.

51. Letter from Margaret B. Hexter, Foundation Secretary, to Dr. K. M. Brinkhous, December 28, 1955, and letter of response, December 31, 1955, in folder "National Hemophilia Foundation Correspondence, 1955," Brinkhous Papers.

52. "Television Discovers New Brand of Hemophilia on Mystery Show (Cour-

tesy of Midwest Chapter Bulletin)," in *Bulletin of the New York Chapter of the Hemophilia Foundation, Inc.* 2, no. 14 (April 1954): p. 3, in folder "National Hemophilia Foundation Correspondence, 1956," Brinkhous Papers. The review is anonymous, but I have assigned the reviewer a female gender as a stylistic choice.

53. *Hemophilia Foundation, Inc. Newsletter*, July 1954, p. 1, in folder "National Hemophilia Foundation Correspondence, 1955," Brinkhous Papers.

54. Charles Carmen, interview by Susan Resnick.

55. Salvatore Lucia, "Hemophilia," in Howard F. Conn, ed., *Current Therapy, 1950* (Philadelphia: W. B. Saunders, 1950), p. 164 (emphasis added). This view, which was concisely stated by San Francisco hematologist Salvatore Lucia in the 1950, 1951, and 1952 editions of *Conn's Current Therapy*, meant that hemophilic children should be denied strenuous exercise and participation in sports.

56. Charlotte L. Endres, "The Hard Life of Edward Smith," *Today's Health* 36 (1958): 26–27; "Two's Company: David and Chris Daly," *Saturday Evening Post* 232 (January 23, 1960): 39–39; and Suzanne Massie in Robert Massie and Suzanne Massie, *Journey*, (New York: Alfred A. Knopf, 1975), pp. 28–29.

57. Maurice Leonard, "Hemophilia," in Howard F. Conn, ed., *Current Therapy, 1953* (Philadelphia: W. B. Saunders, 1953), p. 218.

58. Leonard, "Hemophilia," p. 152.

59. Anthony F. De Palma, "Management of Hemophilic Arthopathy," in Brinkhous, *Hemophilia and Hemophiliod Diseases*, p. 234.

60. All quotes from Dorothy White, *Home Care of the Hemophilic Child* (New York: National Hemophilia Foundation, 1958), 14 pages, quote on p. 1. The National Hemophilia Foundation published and circulated White's pamphlet in 1959 and 1960. Copy available at the National Library of Medicine, Bethesda, MD.

61. Letter from Kenneth Brinkhous to Martin Rosenthal, August 18, 1958, commenting on Dorothy White, "Home Care of the Hemophilic Child," a typescript manuscript, in folder "National Hemophilia Foundation Correspondence, 1958," Brinkhous Papers.

62. White, *Home Care of the Hemophilic Child*, p. 1.

63. Ibid., p. 2.

64. Ibid., p. 14.

65. Mrs. Robert Lauder, "Letter-to-Editor, Hemophilia," *Saturday Evening Post* 236 (June 8, 1963): 22, writing in response to Robert Massie, "They Live on Borrowed Blood," *Saturday Evening Post* 236 (May 4, 1963): 32–34.

66. White, *Home Care of the Hemophilic Child*, p. 2.

67. Philip Wylie, *Generation of Vipers*, 2nd ed. (New York: Rinehart, 1955). On Wylie and "momism" in America, see Michael Kimmel, *Manhood in America: A Cultural History* (New York: Free Press, 1996).

68. Anonymous, "Hemophilia—A Lifetime Hazard," *New England Journal of Medicine* 273 (December 30, 1965): 1493–94.

69. Resnick, "Interview with Marvin Gilbert," January 4, 1991, New York City. Courtesy of Susan Resnick.

70. Littell, "Bearer Is a Hemophiliac," p. 215.

71. See "Donors Aid Blood," *New York Times*, January 17, 1955, p. A23, "Transfusions Failing: Duke Hospital Says Hemophilia Patient Has Turn for Worse," *New York Times*, January 24, 1955, p. A15; "Transfusions in Vain: Hemophiliac Dies after Getting Record 400 Pints of Blood," *New York Times*, January 25, 1955, p. A27; "Record," *Time* 65 (February 7, 1955): 48.

72. Hemophilia continues to be extraordinarily costly. In 2001, for example, Duke Hospital spent five million dollars to treat one patient with acquired hemophilia. More the 95% of the cost was for blood products. See Ron Winslow, "Intensive Care: One Patient, 34 Days in the Hospital, a Bill For $5.2 Million, He Had Internal Bleeding; Doctors at Duke Spared No Effort to Control It," *Wall Street Journal*, August 2, 2001, p. 1.

73. A sampling from the *New York Times*, from 1949–55 suggests the ubiquity of the subject: "Blood of Friends Sends Boy Home," January 27, 1949, Books Section, p. 25; "Three Ailing Brothers Get Shop as Gift," March 5, 1950, p. A11; "Boy's Life Hangs on Blood Gifts," April 18, 1950, p. A19; "Child 'Bleeder' Improves: Florida Boy Flown Here May Soon Be Going Home," March 26, 1952, p. A25; "Thirty Yachtsmen to Donate Blood," September 11, 1952, p. A29; "Forty Sailors to Donate Blood for Children Who Need Stockpile to Combat Hemophilia," October 9, 1952, p. A35; "168 Transfusions Futile," January. 11, 1955, p. A27; Gertrude Samuels, "The Red Cross—People Helping People," March 6, 1955, Sunday Magazine, p. 13. Such stories continued with amazing frequency through the 1960s. See, e.g., "Man with 586 Blood Brothers," *Ebony* 22 (February 1967): 56–62.

74. "Daily Gift of Life: Student Blood Donors Keep Hemophiliac in School," *Life* 40 (April 30, 1956): 141–42.

75. Littell, "Bearer Is a Hemophiliac."

76. Page, "Remembering Frank Schnabel," pp. 10–11.

Chapter 5: The Hemophiliac's Passport to Freedom

1. See Kenneth M. Brinkhous, Edward Shanbrom, Harold R. Roberts, William P. Webster, Lajos Fekete, and Robert H. Wagner, "A New High-Potency Glycine Precipitated Anti-Hemophilic (AHF) Concentrate: Treatment of Classical Hemophilia and Hemophilia with Inhibitors," *Journal of the American Medical Association* 205 (August 26, 1968): 613–17.

2. Richard D. James, "Hope for 'Bleeders,'" *Wall Street Journal*, March 26, 1968, p. 1. See also "Clotting Concentrate Is Approved for Sale to the Hemophiliac," *New York Times*, March 26, 1968, p. A37. For media coverage of studies involving the Hyland concentrates, see, e.g., Jane E. Brody, "Hemophilia Gains Shown in Three Tests," *New York Times*, January 26, 1966, p. A14; Jane E. Brody, "New Hope for the Hemophiliac," *New York Times*, January 30, 1966, p. E10; George Getze, "Normal Lives Possible: New Shots Protect Hemophilia Victims," *Los Angeles Times*, May 13, 1966, p. B1; "Blood Shots Will Help Hemophiliacs," *Washington Post*, May 13, 1966, p. A25; and Patricia Deutsch and Ron Deutsch, "One Man's Fight against Hemophilia," *Today's Health* 45 (August 1967): 40–42, which was reprinted in condensed from as "Dr. Thelin's Fight against Hemophilia," *Reader's Digest* 91 (August 1967): 90–94.

3. James, "Hope for 'Bleeders.'"

4. Quote from "Passport to Freedom for the Hemophiliac," a four-page mail advertisement printed in February 1970 for the high-potency (human) AHF concentrate manufactured by Courtland Scientific Products, a Division of Abbott Laboratories, based in North Chicago, Illinois. The product was made to the same specifications as the 1968 Hyland AHF concentrate, although the manufacturer was different. Advertisement in folder "Antihemophilia Products," Kenneth M. Brinkhous Papers, Francis Owen Blood Research Laboratory, University of North Carolina at Chapel Hill.

5. Susan Resnick, *Blood Saga: Hemophilia, AIDS, and the Survival of a Community* (Berkeley: University of California Press, 1999), p. 56.

6. Robert Massie, "They Live on Borrowed Blood," *Saturday Evening Post* 236 (May 4, 1963): 32–34.

7. Fund-raising pamphlet entitled *Hemophilia Is a National Health Problem*, distributed by the Intermountain Chapter of the National Hemophilia Foundation, Salt Lake City, Utah. The pamphlet was accompanied by letter from L. Howard Marcus, campaign chairman of the Intermountain Chapter of the National Hemophilia Foundation dated February 28, 1962. Source found in box 49, "Professional Organization, N–P," folder 4 "National Hemophilia Foundation—Intermountain Chapter," Maxwell Myer Wintrobe Papers, Accn. #954, Manuscript Division, J. Willard Marriott Library, University of Utah, Salt Lake City.

8. David Binder, "Blood Shortage Worsening Here," *New York Times*, March 26, 1962, pp. A1 and A26.

9. "Meeting the Blood Problem: Editorial," *New York Times*, April 3, 1962, p. A38.

10. Binder, "Blood Shortage Worsening Here," p. 26.

11. Ibid., p. 1. See also Lawrence Galton, "6,000,000 Pints of Blood Is Not Enough," *New York Times*, March. 29, 1964, p. SM38. Data on blood donation and supply in the 1950s and the early 1960s are faulty and notoriously difficult to interpret, as shown by Richard Titmuss, *The Gift Relationship: From Human Blood to Social Policy*, rev. ed. (New York: New Press, 1997), especially pp. 97–122.

12. Douglas Starr, *Blood: An Epic History of Medicine and Commerce* (New York: Alfred Knopf, 1998), pp. 188–89.

13. Binder, "Blood Shortage Worsening Here."

14. Bernard Segal, "Blood for Hemophiliacs: To the Editor," *New York Times*, April 14, 1962, p. A24.

15. *Blood Banks and Antitrust Laws. Hearings before the Subcommittee on Antitrust and Monopoly of the Committee of the Judiciary, U.S. Senate, 88th Cong., second session, pursuant to S. res. 262, on S. 2560 on August 18, 19, and 20, 1965* (Washington, DC: U.S. Government Printing Office, 1964), quote on pp. 2–3. See also Titmuss, *The Gift Relationship*, pp. 101–3, and Starr, *Blood*, pp. 196–97, 201–6.

16. Congress would revisit these issues repeatedly in the coming years. See *Proposed Antitrust Exemption for Certain Blood Banks. Hearings before the Subcommittee on Antitrust and Monopoly of the Committee of the Judiciary, U.S. Senate, 90th Cong., first session, pursuant to S. res. 26, on S. 1945 on August 1, 1967* (Washington, DC: U.S. Government Printing Office, 1964) and *Blood Assurance Act of 1979. Hearing before the Subcommittee on Health and Scientific Research of the Committee on Labor and Human Resources, U.S. Senate, 96th Cong., second session, on S. 1610 to provide for a National Blood Exchange Program and for Other Purposes, May 21, 1980* (Washington, DC: U.S. Government Printing Office, 1980).

17. Binder, "Blood Shortage Worsening Here."

18. Massie, "They Live on Borrowed Blood," p. 34.

19. Ibid., p. 33.

20. See *Blood Banks and Antitrust Laws*, pp. 157–212.

21. See Alfred Katz, "On Being a Citizen: The Social Participation of Hemophiliacs," in *Hemophilia: A Study in Hope and Reality* (Springfield, IL: Charles C. Thomas, 1970), pp. 97–104.

22. Segal, "Blood for Hemophiliacs: To the Editor."

23. See William Chafe, "The Paradox of Change: American Society in the Postwar Years," in *The Unfinished Journey: America since World War II*, 3rd ed. (New York: Oxford University Press, 1995), pp. 111–45; Warren Susman and Edward Griffin, "Did Success Spoil the United States? Dual Representations in Post-

war America," in Lary May, ed., *Recasting America: Culture and Politics in the Age of Cold War* (Chicago: University of Chicago Press, 1989), pp. 19–37; and Gary A. Donaldson, *Abundance and Anxiety: America, 1945–1960* (Westport, CT: Praeger, 1997).

24. Massie, "They Live on Borrowed Blood."

25. Harvey J. Klein and David J. Anstee, *Mollison's Blood Transfusion in Clinical Medicine*, 11th ed. (Malden, MA: Blackwell Publishing, 2005), pp. 777–78.

26. Starr, *Blood*, pp. 207–8.

27. See Howard Rusk, "The Blood Center—II: No Mere 'Drugstore,' Agency Plans Major Research Effort to Save Lives," *New York Times*, March 7, 1965, p. A61.

28. See Robert K. Cutter, "The Drug Manufacturers' Dilemma," *Hospital Management* 91 (February 1961): 46–47.

29. Starr, *Blood*, p. 208.

30. See Getze, "Normal Lives Possible."

31. Starr, *Blood*, p. 207.

32. Judith Graham Pool, Edward J. Hershgold, and Albert B. Pappenhagen, "High Potency Antihaemophilic Factor Concentrates Prepared from Cryoglobulin Precipitate," *Nature* 203 (July 18, 1964): 312. See Kenneth M. Brinkhous, "Judith Graham Pool," in Barbara Sicherman and Carol Hurd Green, eds., *Notable American Women, the Modern Period: A Biographical Dictionary* (Cambridge, MA: Harvard University Press, 1980), pp. 553–54.

33. Judith Graham Pool and Angela E. Shannon, "Production of High-Potency Concentrates of Antihemophilic Globulin in a Closed-Bag System: Assay in Vitro and in Vivo," *New England Journal of Medicine* 273 (December 30, 1965): 1443–47, quote on p. 1443.

34. See Judith G. Pool and Jean Robinson, "Observations on Plasma Banking and Transfusion Procedures for Haemophilic Patients Using Quantitative Assay for Antihaemophilic Globulin," *British Journal of Haematology* 5 (1959): 24–30.

35. Kenneth M. Brinkhous, "Plasma Antihemophilic Factor, Biological and Clinical Aspects," *Sang* 25 (1954):738–41, and Resnick, *Blood Saga*, pp. 40–41.

36. Maxwell M. Wintrobe, *Hematology, the Blossoming of a Science* (Philadelphia: Lea & Febiger, 1985), pp. 425–26.

37. "Clot Substance Isolated," *Science News Letter* 87 (April 24, 1965): 259.

38. Resnick, *Blood Saga*, p. 42.

39. Ibid., p. 44.

40. "Help for Hemophiliacs," *Time* 92 (August 16, 1968): 66–67. See also "Strategy for the Future," in Kenneth M. Brinkhous, "Changing Prospects for Children with Hemophilia," *Children* 17 (November–December 1970): 222–25.

41. See Kenneth M. Brinkhous, "A Short History of Hemophilia, with Some Comments on the Word 'Hemophilia,'" in K. M. Brinkhous and H. C. Hemker, eds., *Handbook of Hemophilia* (Amsterdam: Excepta Medica, 1975), pp. 3–20, and Kenneth M. Brinkhous, "Pathophysiologic Studies and the Evolution of Transfusion Therapy," *American Journal of Clinical Pathology* 41 (April 1964): 342–51.

42. James, "Hope for 'Bleeders.'" Key clinical studies leading to the marketing of the glycine-precipitated AHF concentrate included William P. Webster, Harold R. Roberts, G. Murray Thelin, Robert H. Wagner, and Kenneth M. Brinkhous, "Clinical Use of a New Glycine-Precipitated Antihemophilic Faction," *American Journal of the Medical Sciences* 250 (December 1965): 643–51; Charles F. Abilgaard et al., "Treatment of Hemophilia with Glycine-Precipitated Factor VIII," *New England Journal of Medicine* 275 (September 1966): 471–75; and Edward Shanbrom and G. Murray Thelin, "Long-Term Prophylaxis of Severe Hemophilia: Clinical and Laboratory Evaluation of a New Potent Concentrate," *Abstracts of Papers Presented at the 11th Congress of the International Society of Hematology, Sydney, Australia* (1966), p. 249, which appeared in revised form as Edward Shanbrom and G. Murray Thelin, "Experimental Prophylaxis of Severe Hemophilia with a Factor VIII Concentrate," *Journal of the American Medical Association* 208 (June 9, 1969): 1853–56.

43. Baxter had first promised to market a factor VIII concentrate as a "biological" in 1966, under a license from the National Institutes of Health. The NIH granted that license in March 1968. The FDA later assumed regulatory control of biologicals in 1972. See, e.g., "Baxter Labs Unit Says It Will Market a New Antihemophilic Product," *Wall Street Journal*, May 16, 1966, p. 12. On the trading irregularities, see "Baxter Labs' New Drug," *Wall Street Journal*, March 26, 1968, p. 25.

44. James, "Hope for 'Bleeders'"; Victor Hillery, "Abreast of the Market," *Wall Street Journal*, March 27, 1968, p. 33.

45. See, e.g., "Cutter Labs Says It Has Approval to Sell Product for Treating Hemophilia," *Wall Street Journal*, April 4, 1969, p. 3.

46. "Passport to Freedom for the Hemophiliac."

47. Quote from a four-page Hyland advertising pamphlet, entitled *Hemophil, Antihemophilic Factor (Human), Method Four: For Modern Management of Hemophilia A*, which was published by Hyland Division Travenol Laboratories, Inc., Costa Mesa. California in 1969–70. Advertisement in folder "Antihemophilia Products," Brinkhous Papers.

48. "Wall Street Journal Article on Hemophilia," *National Hemophilia Foun-*

dation Chapter Bulletin, March 26, 1968, box 49: "Professional Organization, N–P," folder 3: "National Hemophilia Foundation—Executive Bulletin," Wintrobe Papers.

49. Martin C. Rosenthal, "Method Four—AHF Concentrate," *Medical Bulletin of the National Hemophilia Foundation*, March 1968, box 49: "Professional Organization, N–P," folder 3: "National Hemophilia Foundation—Executive Bulletin," Wintrobe Papers.

50. Martin C. Rosenthal, "Method Four—AHF Concentrate," *Medical Bulletin of the National Hemophilia Foundation* (March 28, 1968), box 49, folder 3, Wintrobe Papers.

51. Ibid.

52. See "Cutter Labs Says It Has Approval to Sell Product for Treating Hemophilia."

53. Shelby Dietrich, interview with Susan Resnick, October 25, 1990, Pasadena, California. Courtesy of Susan Resnick. It is unclear from the interview what film about Rasputin Dietrich recalls here. She merely refers to it as the Rasputin film that predated *Nicholas and Alexandra* (1971). If Dietrich's memory is correct, she may have seen the 1932 film, *Rasputin and the Empress*, starring John and Ethel Barrymore.

54. Quotes from Getze, "Normal Lives Possible," and "Blood Shots Will Help Hemophiliacs." See also Shelby L. Dietrich, *Hemophilia: A Total Approach to Treatment and Rehabilitation* (Los Angeles: Orthopaedic Hospital, 1968).

55. Getze, "Normal Lives Possible."

56. Paul K. Jones and Oscar Ratnoff, "Changing Prognosis of Classical Hemophilia (Factor VIII 'Deficiency')," *Annals of Internal Medicine* 114 (1991): 644.

57. Alfred H. Katz, "Some Psychosocial Problems in Hemophilia," *Social Casework* 40 (1959): 321–26, quotes on pp. 321, 323.

58. Ibid., p. 322.

59. Ibid., pp. 321, 324.

60. Anthony F. De Palma, "Management of Hemophilic Arthopathy," in Kenneth Brinkhous, ed., *Hemophilia and Hemophiliod Diseases: International Symposium* (Chapel Hill: University of North Carolina Press, 1957), 234.

61. Katz, "Some Psychosocial Problems in Hemophilia," p. 324.

62. Alfred Katz and Jacqueline MacAfee Husek, *Social and Vocational Adaption of the Hemophiliac Adult*, (Los Angeles: UCLA School of Public Health, 1965), quote on p. 1. This report was later revised and published as Katz, *Hemophilia: A Study in Hope and Reality* (see note 21). See also Alfred H. Katz, "Social Adaptation in Chronic Illness: A Study of Hemophilia," *American Journal of*

Public Health 53 (October 1963): 1666–75, and Florence B. Goldy and Alfred H. Katz, "Social Adaptation in Hemophilia," *Children* 10 (September–October 1963): 189–93.

63. Paraphrased from Katz, *Social and Vocational Adaption of the Hemophiliac Adult*, pp. 8–20, and Katz, *Hemophilia: A Study in Hope and Reality*, pp. 16–24.

64. Katz, *Social and Vocational Adaption of the Hemophiliac Adult*, p. 74, and Katz, *Hemophilia: A Study in Hope and Reality*, p. 106.

65. Katz, *Social and Vocational Adaption of the Hemophiliac Adult*, p. 81. In the longer quotation, the ellipsis appears in Katz's text.

66. "The Daredevil Gesture," *Marcus Welby, M.D*, season 1 (Universal City Studies/Shout Factory LLC, 2010), disc 7, episode 2. The American Broadcasting Company originally aired the episode on March 17, 1970. David Victor, creator and executive producer; Jerome Ross, writer; Steven Spielberg, director; Robert Young, Dr. Marcus Welby; James Brolin, Dr. Steven Kiley; Frank Webb, Larry Bellows; Marsha Hunt, Mrs. Bellows.

67. See *The Irony of Growth and Progress: Annual Report, 1970–71* (New York: National Hemophilia Foundation, 1971), 15 pp., quotes on p. 4 and 8, in folder "National Hemophilia Foundation, 1972," Brinkhous Papers.

Chapter 6: Autonomy and Other Imperatives of the Health Consumer

1. The television spot, entitled "Eric-60," received an "Award of Excellence" from the American Institute of Graphic Arts and was cited as one the fifty best commercials and advertisements produced in the United States in 1969. The context of advertisements is outlined in "Coordinated National Campaign Underway: Agency Slogans Tie Materials Together," *National Hemophilia Foundation News Letter* 6 (January 1970): 1–3, in folder "NHF Correspondence, 1970," Kenneth M. Brinkhous Papers, Francis Owen Blood Research Laboratory, University of North Carolina at Chapel Hill. The text of the commercial appears in *Hemophilia Act of 1973: Hearing before the Subcommittee on Health of the Committee on Labor and Public Welfare, United States Senate, Ninety-third Congress, First Session, on S. 1326 to Amend the Public Health Service Act to Provide for Programs for the Diagnosis and Treatment of Hemophilia, November 15, 1973* (Washington: U.S. Government Printing Office, 1974), pp. 31–36, quotes on pp. 31–32, 36.

2. Nathan Smith, "Economic Implications" in David Green, ed., *Hemophilia: A Manual of Outpatient Management* (Springfield, IL: Charles Thomas, 1973), pp. 70–76, quote on p. 75.

3. See Barron Lerner, *The Breast Cancer Wars: Hope, Fear, and the Pursuit of*

a Cure in Twentieth-Century America (New York: Oxford University Press, 2001); Keith Wailoo, *Dying in the City of the Blues: Sickle Cell Anemia and the Politics of Race and Health* (Chapel Hill: University of North Carolina Press, 2001); Alonzo Plough, *Borrowed Time: Artificial Organs and the Politics of Extending Lives* (Philadelphia: Temple University Press, 1986); and Steven Peitzman, *Dropsy, Dialysis, and Transplant: A Short History of Failing Kidneys* (Baltimore: Johns Hopkins University Press, 2007).

4. Paul Starr, *The Social Transformation of American Medicine* (New York: Basic Books, 1982), pp. 379–419.

5. Richard Nixon used the phrase "massive crisis" in a July 1969 press conference. See the *New York Times*, July 11, 1969. This source figures prominently in Starr, *The Social Transformation of American Medicine*, and Susan Resnick, *Blood Saga: Hemophilia, AIDS, and the Survival of a Community* (Berkeley: University of California Press, 1998).

6. Starr, *The Social Transformation of American Medicine*, p. 382.

7. See Robert Massie and Suzanne Massie, *Journey* (New York: Alfred Knopf, 1975).

8. Resnick, *Blood Saga*, p. 56.

9. Wailoo, *Dying in the City of the Blues*, p. 166. See also Keith Wailoo, *How Cancer Crossed the Color Line* (New York: Oxford University Press, 2011).

10. The politics of these categorical illness communities are described in relation to cystic fibrosis and sickle cell disease in Keith Wailoo and Stephen Pemberton, *The Troubled Dream of Genetic Medicine: Ethnicity and Innovation in Tay-Sachs, Cystic Fibrosis and Sickle Cell Disease* (Baltimore: Johns Hopkins University Press, 2006).

11. Resnick, *Blood Saga*, pp. 60–62, quotes on p. 62.

12. Lee S. Goldsmith, "Brief of the National Hemophilia Foundation as *Amicus Curiae*," submitted in the Supreme Court of Illinois Case of *Cunningham v. MacNeal Memorial Hospital*, November 1970, in folder "NHF Medical Advisory Council, 1970," Brinkhous Papers. See also Douglas Starr, *Blood: A History of Medicine and Commerce* (New York: Alfred Knopf, 1998), pp. 207–30.

13. See, e.g., "In Cold Blood," *Newsweek* 69 (May 1, 1967): 82; "Reversing the Plasma Rules," *Science News* 93 (April 20, 1968): 373; "Crackdown on Plasma," *Time* 92 (July 19, 1968): 54; "Closing Down the Pool," *Newsweek* 72 (July 22, 1968): 55; Harold Schmeck, "The Perils of Blood Transfusions," *New York Times*, November 3, 1968, p. E11; Walter Rugaber, "Prison Drug and Plasma Projects Leave Fatal Trail," *New York Times*, July 29, 1969, p. A1; "Why There Is Peril from Some Blood Donors/New Epidemic in U.S. Venereal Disease," *New York Times*, July 19, 1970, p. E6; "Plasma Problems: Protecting the Donors," *Science News* 98

(August 8, 1970): 113; "Policing the Plasma Plants," *Time* 96 (August 17, 1970): 43; "Sweating Blood," *Time* 96 (October 19, 1970): 57.

14. Douglas Surgenor, "NHLI Study of Blood Banking in the United States," September 1971, folder "NHF Medical Advisory Council, 1971," Brinkhous Files. See also Starr, *Blood*, p. 207.

15. Surgenor, "NHLI Study of Blood Banking in the United States," p, 2. The relevant RFP was NHLI no. 71-24.

16. See, e.g., James M. Stengle, "The Hemophiliac's Demand on Blood Resources: The Magnitude of the Problem," *Annals of the New York Academy of Science* 240 (1975): 155. Stengle chaired the NHLI's Blood Resources Advisory Committee in the early 1970s.

17. Surgenor, "NHLI Study of Blood Banking in the United States," p. 3.

18. Representations of the hemophilia patients as "chronic blood users" and "burdens to blood supply" were pervasive in the late 1960s and early 1970s. See, e.g., Dudley Dalton, "Hope Is Offered to Hemophiliacs at Long Island Medical Center," *New York Times* March 14, 1971, p. BQ101, and "Two Hemophiliac Boys Face Crisis: Blood Component Supply Ebbs," *Los Angeles Times*, January 3, 1972), p. A12.

19. National Heart Lung Institute, National Blood Resource Program, *NHLI's Blood Resource Studies*, vol. 1, *Supply and Use of the Nation's Blood Resources*, DHEW Publication No. 73-417, vol. 2. *Federal and State Regulation of the Nation's Blood Resource*, DHEW Publication No. 73-417, and vol. 3, *Pilot Study of Hemophilia Treatment in the United States*, DHEW Publication No. 73-419 (Washington, DC: U.S. Department of Health, Education, and Welfare, 1972).

20. Surgenor, "NHLI Study of Blood Banking in the United States," pp. 4–5.

21. Most regions of the United States where specialized treatments were traditionally unavailable had lower concentrations of hemophilia patients than census counts for the general male population indicate they should. See NHLI, *Pilot Study*, pp. 56, 106.

22. NHLI, *Pilot Study*, pp. 83–94.

23. The 25,500 population estimate in the NHLI, *Pilot Study* (pp. 44–46) was revised downward in 1976 to 13,287 severe and moderate hemophilia patients. See "Halving Hemophilia," *Medical World News*, July 25, 1977, p. 11.

24. NHLI, *Pilot Study*, pp. 135–38, 160–62.

25. Ibid., pp. 50–53.

26. Drs. Harvey Alter and Jay Hoofnagle, interviews by Stephen Pemberton, National Institutes of Health, Bethesda, MD, July 29–30, 1998.

27. On the failures of health care reform in the 1970s, see Colin Gordon, *Dead*

on *Arrival: The Politics of Health Care in Twentieth-Century America* (Princeton: Princeton University Press, 2007), pp. 243–51.

28. Resnick, *Blood Saga*, p. 65.

29. NHLI, *Pilot Study*, p. 183.

30. Ibid., p. 234.

31. Programs were not only appearing in the United States in the early 1970s, but in other countries as well. These countries included England, Canada, Australia, Germany, and France. See Jan van Eys, "Home Transfusion for Hemophilia," in Margaret Hilgartner, ed., *Hemophilia in Children* (Littleton, MA: Publishing Sciences Group, 1976), pp. 185–200.

32. NHLI, *Pilot Study*, p. 234.

33. Jack Lazerson, "The Prophylactic Approach to Hemophilia A," *Hospital Practice* 6 (February 1971): 107. See also Jack Lazerson, "Hemophilia Home Transfusion Program," *Journal of Pediatrics* 81 (1972): 330.

34. Anthony F. A. Britten, "A Little Freedom for the Hemophiliac," *New England Journal of Medicine* 283 (November 5, 1970): 1051–52.

35. Ibid., 1052.

36. S. Frederick Rabiner and Margaret C. Telfer, "Home Transfusion for Patients with Hemophilia A," *New England Journal of Medicine* 283 (November 5, 1970): 1011–15.

37. Ibid.

38. Ibid.

39. Charles Abilgaard, interview by Susan Resnick, October 23, 1990, Sacramento, CA, pp. 4–5. Courtesy of Susan Resnick.

40. The story of Jim Garner, covered by *Life* magazine in 1956, suggests that home transfusion care had multiple origins. The story includes a photo of Jim's wife, Mrs. Evelyn Garner, giving him a home infusion of plasma. The photo caption calls Mrs. Garner a "trained lab technician." See "Daily Gift of Life: Student Blood Donors Keep Hemophiliac in School," *Life* 40 (April 30, 1956): 141–42.

41. Resnick, *Blood Saga*, p. 36.

42. Halden presented "The Fort Worth Story," to the Annual Meeting for the National Hemophilia Foundation," on Friday, October 10, 1969 at the Drake Hotel, Chicago. He also gave two papers in 1970: E. Richard Halden Jr. "Principles of Therapy in the Hemophilic with Emphasis on the Physiological Concentrate for Home Transfusion," paper presented at the seventeenth State Tri-Regional Home Transfusion Seminar, Fort Worth, Texas, August 22, 1970; and E. Richard Halden Jr. "Discussion as Panel Member on 'An Introduction to Home Transfusion Therapy,'" paper presented at the Hemophilia Symposium: "Full Steam

Ahead," Memphis, July 9–10, 1971. See van Eys, "Home Transfusion for Hemophilia," p. 198. Halden also gave brief testimony to the U.S. Congress about home transfusion care on the November 15, 1973, hearings in support of the Hemophilia Act of 1973.

43. Oscar Ratnoff in "Discussion Following Dr. Telfer's Chapter [on "Home Transfusion Programs"], in David Green, ed., *Hemophilia: A Manual of Outpatient Management* (Springfield, IL: Charles C. Thomas, 1973), pp. 61–62.

44. Louis Aledort, *The Treatment of Hemophilia: Current Management; A Physician's Manual* (New York: National Hemophilia Foundation, 1978), 9 pp.

45. Richard A. Rettig, "Origins of the Medicare Kidney Disease Entitlement: The Social Security Amendments of 1972," in Kathi E. Hanna, ed., *Biomedical Politics: Institute of Medicine Report of the Committee to Study Biomedical Decision Making* (Washington, DC: National Academy Press, 1991), pp. 176–208. See also David J. Rothman, *Beginnings Count: The Technological Imperative in American Health Care* (New York: Oxford University Press, 1997), pp. 87–110, and Steven J. Peitzman, "From Bright's Disease to End-Stage Renal Disease," in Charles Rosenberg and Janet Golden, eds., *Framing Disease: Studies in Cultural History* (New Brunswick, NJ: Rutgers University, 1992), pp. 4–19.

46. Rettig, "Origins of the Medicare Kidney Disease Entitlement," pp. 195–96.

47. Ibid., p. 189, and *National Health Insurance Proposals. Hearing before the Committee on Ways and Means, House of Representatives, 92nd Congress, First Session on the Subject of National Health Insurance Proposals, Part 7 of 13 Parts, November 3 and 4, 1971* (Washington, DC: U.S. Government Printing Office, 1972), pp. 1524–47.

48. *Hemophilia Act of 1973*, pp. 3–4.

49. Ibid., p. 1.

50. The NHF appointed two popular professional football players as honorary chairmen in the early 1970s, George Blanda and Roger Staubach. See ibid., p. 18.

51. Ibid., pp. 19–22.

52. Ibid., pp. 31–32.

53. Ibid., pp. 38–39.

54. Ibid., pp. 40–41.

55. Ibid., p. 41.

56. See Arlene Silberman, "No Wheelchair for Steven," *Good Housekeeping* 173 (November 1971): 99, 206–11; Edwin Kiester Jr., "Lifeblood for Young Cliff Watson, Hemophiliac," *Today's Health* 51 (December 1973): 42–47, 60–63; and John Marsh, "Magic in a Shoebox," *Seventeen Magazine* 37 (April 1978): 223.

57. See, e.g., Robert M. Smith, "President Vetoes Health Care Bill; Senate Overrides," *New York Times*, July 27, 1975, pp. A1, A19.

58. For further details on the legislative history on the hemophilia act, see Resnick, *Blood Saga*, pp. 73–89.

59. Peter Levine and Anthony Britten, "Supervised Patient-Management of Hemophilia: A Study of 45 Patients with Hemophilia A and B," *Annals of Internal Medicine* 78 (1973): 195–201; and Peter Levine, "Efficacy of Self-Therapy in Hemophilia, A Study of 72 Patients with Hemophilia A and B," *New England Journal of Medicine* 291 (1974): 1381. See also NHLI, *Pilot Study*, and Resnick, *Blood Saga*, pp. 70–89.

60. Carol Kasper, Shelby Dietrich, and Samuel Rapaport, "Hemophilia Prophylaxis with Factor VIII Concentrate," *Archives of Internal Medicine* 125 (June 1970): 1004–9. See also Smith, "Economic Implications," pp. 70–76.

61. *The Journey and the Dream: The History of the American Diabetes Association* (Alexandria, VA: American Diabetes Association, 1990), p. 51. Also quoted by Resnick, *Blood Saga*, p. 82.

62. Massie and Massie, *Journey*. Portions of the book first appeared in 1973 in *Family Health* and *Ladies Home Journal*. In 1975 excerpts of *Journey* were also published in various U.S. newspapers.

63. See Robert K. Massie, *Nicholas and Alexandra* (New York: Atheneum Press, 1967).

64. Robert Kirsch, "U.S. Neglect of the Chronically Ill," *Los Angeles Times*, July 28, 1975, p. D1.

65. See, e.g., Kirsch as well as Christopher Lehmann-Haupt, "Books of The Times; It Was Awful and Wonderful," *New York Times*, May 9, 1975, p. A33.

66. Jill Smolowe, "Hemophiliac Finds Key to an Active Campus Life," *New York Times*, November 27, 1977, p. NJ22.

67. Kirsch. "U.S. Neglect of the Chronically Ill."

68. Joseph Fratantoni and David Aronson, eds., *Unsolved Therapeutic Problems in Hemophilia*, DHEW Publication No. NIH 77-1089 (Washington, DC: U.S. Government Printing Office, 1976), p. 1.

69. See Jessica H. Lewis, "Hemophilia, Hepatitis, and HAA," *Vox Sang* 19 (1970): 406–9; Robert H. Wagner, "Hepatitis in Hemophilia," *Thrombosis and Diathesis Haemorrhagica Suppl.* 40 (1970): 377; Harry S. Kingdon, "Hepatitis after Konyne," *Annals of Internal Medicine* 73 (1971): 656–57; B. F. Boklan, "Factor IX Concentrate and Viral Hepatitis," *Annals of Internal Medicine* 74 (1971): 298; L. K. Hellerstein and D. Deykin, "Hepatitis after Konyne Administration," *New England Journal of Medicine* 284 (1971): 1039–40; R. Faria and N. J. Finamara, "Hepatitis B Associated with Konyne," *New England Journal of Medicine* 287 (1972): 358–59; Carol L. Kasper and S. A. Kipnis, "Hepatitis and Clotting-factor Concentrates," *Journal of the American Medical Association* 221 (1972): 510;

M. M. Oken, L. Hostkin, and R. L. De Jager, "Hepatitis after Konyne Administration," *American Journal of Digestive Disorders* 17 (1972): 271–74; S. G. Sandler, C. E. Rath, and A. Juder, "Prothrombin Complex Concentrates in Acquired Hypoprothrombinemia," *Annals of Internal Medicine* 79 (1973): 485–91; J. H. Lewis, N. G. Maxwell, and J. M. Brandon, "Jaundice and Hepatitis B Antigen/Antibody in Hemophilia," *Transfusion* 14 (1974): 203–11; and overviews, circa 1976, found in Fratantoni and Aronson, *Unsolved Therapeutic Problems in Hemophilia*, especially Leonard B. Seeff and Jay Hoofnagle, "Acute and Chronic Liver Disease in Hemophilia," pp. 61–72, and H. R. Lesesne et al., "Liver Biopsy in Hemophilia A," pp. 73–76. Quote from W. P. Webster et al., "Liver Function Tests in Hemophiliacs," p. 48.

70. NHLI, *Pilot Study*, 142.

71. Seeff and Hoofnagle, "Acute and Chronic Liver Disease in Hemophilia," pp. 61–72, quotes on pp. 61, 69. The earliest reports of the rise in post-transfusion hepatitis in hemophilia patients that Seeff and Hoofnagle could find dated from 1970, which suggested to them that hemophilia experts were relatively late in acknowledging that hepatitis rates among recipients of pooled products were a problem.

In fact, Seeff had already entered the debate on the risks of post-transfusion hepatitis in March 1975 by explaining to readers of the *New England Journal of Medicine* that rates of post-transfusion hepatitis dropped dramatically (62 percent) at one Veteran Administration Hospital in Illinois after the state of Illinois instituted its Blood Labeling Act on October 1, 1972. That law had dramatically reduced the use of paid blood donors in the state by 40–50 percent according to Dr. J. Garrott Allen. Veterans Administration hospitals outside of Illinois, which continued to use blood from paid donors, did not experience reductions in rates of post-transfusion hepatitis. See L. B. Seeff, H. J. Zimmerman, E. C. Wright, and H. B. Greenlee, "Rates of Post-Transfusion Hepatitis," *New England Journal of Medicine* 292 (March 6, 1975): 532–33, and J. Garrott Allen, "Advantages of Volunteer Blood Donors," *New England Journal of Medicine* 291 (December 19, 1974): 1365–66.

On the discovery of hepatitis B surface antigen, see Baruch S. Blumberg and Harvey J. Alter, "A 'New' Antigen in Leukemia Sera," *Journal of the American Medical Association* 191 (1965): 101–6, and Baruch S. Blumberg, *Hepatitis B: The Hunt for a Killer Virus* (Princeton, NJ: Princeton University Press, 19), p. 81.

72. Louis Aledort, "The Cause of Death in Hemophiliacs," in Fratantoni and Aronson, *Unsolved Therapeutic Problems in Hemophilia*, pp. 9–14, quote on p. 13.

73. NHLI, *Pilot Study*, p. 142.

74. Resnick, *Blood Saga*, p. 66.

75. See Goldsmith, "Brief of the National Hemophilia Foundation as *Amicus Curiae*," p. 18, in folder "NHF Medical Advisory Council, 1970," Brinkhous Papers.

76. Letter from J. Garrott Allen to Ian A. Mitchell, April 15, 1975, MSC 393, folder 16-11, U.S. Dept. of Health, Education, and Welfare, National Blood Policy Papers, 1969–81, Gift of Dr. Ian Mitchell, History of Medicine Division, National Library of Medicine, Bethesda, MD.

77. Ibid.

78. Draft, "Policy Statement by the National Hemophilia Foundation on the National Blood Policy and the American Blood Commission," p. 1 of 2, which was circulated by George J. Theobald Jr., National Executive Director of the NHF to Trustees of the NHF on December 30, 1975, box 49: "Professional Organizations, N–P," folder 5: "National Hemophilia Foundation, Memoranda," Maxwell Myer Wintrobe Papers, Accn. #954, Manuscript Division, J. Willard Marriott Library, University of Utah, Salt Lake City, Utah.

79. Allen's concern about Konyne was prompted by his reading of Lewis et al., "Jaundice and Hepatitis B Antigen/Antibody in Hemophilia." Quote from J. Garrott Allen's letter to Dr. W. D'A. Maycock, Blood Products Laboratory, Lister Institute, Elstree, Herts., England, December 20, 1974, MSC 393, folder 16-9, National Blood Policy Papers.

80. Letter from J. Garrott Allen to Ian A. Mitchell, November 18, 1974, MSC 393, folder 16-9, National Blood Policy Papers.

81. Letter from J. Garrott Allen to Ian A. Mitchell, April 15, 1975, MSC 393, folder 16-11, National Blood Policy Papers. As detailed in his letter to Mitchell, Allen's distrust of the "Private Sector" was confirmed by *Journey*'s account of the efforts by Hyland/Baxter and other concentrate manufacturers to put the American Red Cross out of the business of concentrate development and production. See Massie and Massie, *Journey*, pp. 280–81.

82. Starr, *Blood*, p. 257.

Chapter 7: The Mismanagement of Hemophilia and AIDS

1. During the 1990s, as these events were being investigated, everyone agreed that there were at least sixteen thousand hemophilia patients in the United States, and at least half contracted HIV through their treatments. The figures, which are now recognized to be low, came from the CDC and hemophilia treatment centers in 1992–94. Despite being contested, these numbers were employed, for instance, by the Institute of Medicine's Committee to Study HIV Transmission through Blood and Blood Products and widely used in the policy discussions and court disputes of the 1990s. See the "Executive Summary of the

Institute of Medicine's Committee to Study HIV Transmission through Blood and Blood Products," in Lauren B. Leveton, Harold C. Sox Jr., and Michael A. Stoto, eds., *HIV and the Blood Supply: An Analysis of Crisis Decisionmaking* (Washington, DC: National Academy Press, 1995), p. 1, and the Rand Institute for Civil Justice study, "Blood Clotting Products for Hemophiliacs: In Re Factor VIII or IX Concentrate Blood Products," in Deborah Hensler et al., *Class Action Dilemmas: Pursuing Public Goals for Private Gain* (Santa Monica, CA: RAND, 2000), pp. 293–317.

Ronald Bayer's historical analysis on the "epidemiological toll" of transfusion-related AIDS on hemophiliacs from 1978 to 1985 provides a good summary. Bayer notes that rates of infections were estimated in 1994 to be 96% among "high-dose factor VIII recipients, 92% of moderate-dose recipients, and 56% of low-dose recipients." He cites "75% to 85%" infection rates among hemophiliacs treated between 1978 and 1985, and emphasizes that "62% to 89% of hemophilia A patients who would be infected had already become so" by January 1983, the date of the CDC's first public meeting on transfusion-related AIDS. Bayer, "Blood and AIDS in America: The Making of an Iatrogenic Catastrophe," in Eric Feldman and Ronald Bayer, eds., *Blood Feuds: AIDS, Blood, and the Politics of Medical Disaster* (New York: Oxford University Press, 1999), pp. 33–35.

Beyond Bayer's account, see Terence Chorba, Robert Holman, Tara Strine, Matthew Clarke, and Bruce Evatt, "Changes in Longevity and Causes of Death among Persons with Hemophilia A," *American Journal of Hematology* 45 (February 1994): 112–21; and, more recently, J. Michael Soucie, Rachelle Nuss, Bruce Evatt, et al., "Mortality among Males with Hemophilia: Relations with Source of Medical Care," *Blood* 96 (July 15, 2000): 437–42, and Terence Chorba, Robert Holman, Matthew Clarke, and Bruce Evatt, "Effects of HIV on Age and Cause of Death for Persons with Hemophilia A in the United States," *American Journal of Hematology* 66 (2001): 229–40.

2. Louis Aledort, "HIV and Hemophilia," *Journal of Thrombosis and Haemostasis* 5 (2007): 607–10, quotes on p. 607. Aledort's piece responds to Bruce Evatt, "The Tragic History of AIDS in the Hemophilia Population, 1982–1984," *Journal of Thrombosis and Haemostasis* 4 (2006): 2295–2301.

3. The best historical writing and scholarship on the intersection of hemophilia and AIDS in the United States begins with David Kirp, "Look Back in Anger: Hemophilia, Rights, and AIDS," *Dissent* 44 (Summer 1997): 65–70; Douglas Starr, *Blood: An Epic History of Medicine and Commerce* (New York: Alfred Knopf, 1998); Susan Resnick, *Blood Saga: Hemophilia, AIDS, and the Survival of a Community* (Berkeley: University of California Press, 1999); Michael Davidson, "Strange Blood: Homophobia and the Unexplored Boundaries of Queer

Nation," in Timothy Powell, ed., *Beyond the Binary: Reconstructing Cultural Identity in a Multicultural Context* (New Brunswick, NJ: Rutgers University Press, 1999), pp. 39–60; Salmaan Keshavjee, Sheri Weiser, and Arthur Kleinmann, "Medicine Betrayed: Hemophilia Patients and HIV in the US," *Social Science and Medicine* 53 (2001): 1081–94; Patricia Siplon, "Blood Policy in the Age of AIDS," in Patricia Siplon, *AIDS and the Policy Struggle in the United States* (Washington, DC: Georgetown University Press, 2002), pp. 42–66.

For the U.S. situation in comparative perspective with other nations, see Feldman and Bayer, *Blood Feuds*; André Picard, *The Gift of Death: Confronting Canada's Tainted-Blood Tragedy* (Toronto: HarperCollins Publishers, 1995); and Rosemary Daly and Paul Cunningham, *A Case of Bad Blood: The Human Story behind the Public Tragedy* (Dublin: Poolbeg, 2003).

These participant histories are also critical sources: Corey Dubin, "Hemophilia: A Story of Success—Disaster and the Perseverance of the Human Spirit, Parts I & II," *Journal of the Association of Nurses in AIDS Care* 10 (May–June 1999): 90–93, and 10 (July–August): 88–92; Charles Kozak, "Hemophilia Holocaust Litigation Related to Blood Factor VIII and IX Products and AIDS Transmission," in James O'Donnell, ed., *Drug Injury: Liability, Analysis, and Prevention*, 2nd ed. (Tucson, AZ: Lawyers and Judges Publishing, 2005), pp. 633–48; and Evatt, "The Tragic History of AIDS."

Essential memoirs and firsthand accounts include Peter Brandon Bayer, "A Life in Limbo," *New York Times Magazine*, April 2, 1989, pp. 48–55; Nancy Shaw, *Blood Brothers: Ryan, Chris, and Hemophilia* (Wilson, NC: Star Books, 1989); Ryan White and Ann Marie Cunningham, *Ryan White: My Own Story* (New York: Dial Books, 1991); Abraham Verghese, *My Own Country: A Doctor's Story* (New York: Vintage Books, 1994); Elaine DePrince, *Cry Blood Murder: A Tale of Tainted Blood* (New York: Random House, 1997); Tom Andrews, *Codeine Diary: A Memoir* (Boston: Little, Brown, 1998); Kathy Seward MacKay and Stacy Milbouer, *Dying in Vein: Blood, Deception . . . Justice* (Hollis, NH: Hollis Publishing, 2002); Ogden M. Forbes and M. Jane Forbes, *Surviving the American Medical System in the 21st Century: Stories of American Citizens with Hemophilia* (San Marino, CA: Forbes Research International, 2003); Shawn Decker, *My Pet Virus: The True Story of a Rebel without a Cure* (New York: Tarcher-Penguin, 2006); Laura Gray and Christine Chamberlain, *The Gift of Experience: Conversations about Hemophilia* (Boston: Boston Hemophilia Center, 2007); Henry J. Nichols, *Henry for President* (Seattle: Create Space, 2008).

4. Keshavjee, Weiser, and Kleinmann, "Medicine Betrayed," p. 1081.

5. On "canaries in the mine shaft," see Resnick, *Blood Saga*, pp. x, 2–3, 225.

6. Starr, *Blood*, pp. 250–65.

7. Dubin, "Hemophilia: A Story of Success—Disaster and the Perseverance of the Human Spirit, Part I," p. 91.

8. Author's interview with Harvey Alter, M.D., associate director for research and chief of Infectious Disease Section, Department of Transfusion Medicine, NIH Clinical Center, Bethesda, MD, July 30, 1998.

9. See Evatt, "Tragic History."

10. Elizabeth Fee and Theodore Brown, "Michael S. Gottlieb and the Identification of AIDS," *American Journal of Public Health* 96 (June 2006): 982–83.

11. The very idea that AIDS "spread" from the gay community is problematic from the standpoint that it presumes that AIDS was principally a disease of male homosexuals, which it never was. There was, for instance, a silent epidemic of AIDS among intravenous drug users in New York City in the era. Yet, I use the word because it reveals how prominent investigators conceptualized AIDS as a local problem at the earliest stages of the epidemic.

12. On controversies related to the consensus surrounding the HIV-equals-AIDS hypothesis, see Steven Epstein, *Impure Science: AIDS, Activism, and the Politics of Knowledge* (Berkeley: University of California Press, 1994), pp. 45–178.

13. See Evatt, "Tragic History"; Randy Shilts, *And the Band Played On: Politics, People, and the AIDS Epidemic* (New York: St. Martin's Press, 1987), pp. 160–61; and Starr, *Blood*, pp. 266–73.

14. Evatt, "Tragic History," p. 2296; Shilts, *And the Band Played On*, pp. 160–61; and Bruce Evatt, M.D., phone interviews by Stephen Pemberton, August 21–22, 2008.

15. Dale Lawrence, M.D., interview by Stephen Pemberton, Historical Office of the National Institutes of Health, Bethesda, MD, October 15, 1998. Also Evatt, "The Tragic History;" Shilts, *And the Band Played On*, p. 161; and Starr, *Blood*, p. 267.

16. Siplon, "Blood Policy in the Age of AIDS," p. 47.

17. CDC, "Epidemiological Notes and Reports Pneumocystis carinii Pneumonia among Persons with Hemophilia A," *Morbidity and Mortality Weekly Report* 31 (July 16, 1982): 365–67.

18. Also present were representatives from the New York City Health Department and the New York Inter-Hospital Study Group on AIDS and KS. See William H. Foege, "Summary Report on Open Meeting of PHS Committee on Opportunistic Infections in Patients with Hemophilia, August 6, 1982," reprinted in Leveton et al., *HIV and the Blood Supply*, pp. 266–68.

19. Evatt, "Tragic History," p. 2296.

20. National Hemophilia Foundation, *Hemophilia Newsnotes: Hemophilia Patient Alert #1*, July 14, 1982, reprinted in Leveton et al., *HIV and the Blood*

Supply, p. 265. See also Robert K. Massie, "Blood Feud: A Mother Takes the Hemophilia Tragedy to Court," *New Yorker* 73 (June 16, 1997): 100.

21. CDC investigators identified the first cases of AIDS among Haitians in the spring of 1982, leading them to categorize Haitians as a high-risk group. The stereotyping of Haitians was particularly pernicious given the history of U.S.-Haitian relations and the broader history of scapegoating immigrants as "disease carriers" in American history. See Shilts, *And the Band Played On*, pp. 135–36; Paul Farmer, *AIDS and Accusation: Haiti and the Geography of Blame* (Berkeley: University of California Press, 1992); and Alan Kraut, *Silent Travelers: Germs, Genes, and the "Immigrant Menace"* (New York: Basic Books, 1994).

22. Evatt, "Tragic History," and Evatt, phone interviews.

23. Ibid.

24. Shilts, *And the Band Played On*, p. 171.

25. Starr, *Blood*, pp. 273, 281, and Evatt, phone interviews.

26. CDC, "Epidemiologic Notes and Reports Possible Transfusion-Associated Acquired Immune Deficiency Syndrome (AIDS)—California," *Morbidity and Mortality Weekly Report* 31 (December 10, 1982): 652–54. See also Evatt, "Tragic History," p. 2297, and Shilts, *And the Band Played On*, pp. 195, 199, 220–24.

27. Evatt, phone interviews, and Starr, *Blood*, pp. 272–76.

28. Leveton et al., *HIV and the Blood Supply*, pp. 175–79.

29. See Public Health Service Committee on Opportunistic Infections in Patients with Hemophilia, *Summary Report on Open Meeting of PHS Committee on Opportunistic Infections in Patients with Hemophilia* (Washington, DC: U.S. Public Health Service, 1982); Shilts, *And the Band Played On*, pp. 169–71; and Siplon, *AIDS and the Policy Struggle in the United States*, p. 48.

30. Resnick, *Blood Saga*, p. 122.

31. Leveton et al., *HIV and the Blood Supply*, pp. 172–81.

32. Starr, *Blood*, quotes on pp. 269, 399.

33. Ibid., p. 272.

34. There was diversity of opinion among gay advocacy groups on questions of blood policy, yet the vast majority resisted a universal ban on gay donors. See John-Manuel Andriote, *Victory Deferred: How AIDS Changed Gay Life in America* (Chicago: University of Chicago Press, 1999), pp. 59–65.

35. Shilts, *And the Band Played On*, p. 222; Starr, *Blood*, pp. 271–72.

36. Starr, *Blood*, p. 271.

37. Bayer, "Blood and AIDS in America," p. 24.

38. Shilts wrote that hemophilia care advocates exclaimed, "What about the hemophiliac's right to life?" in *And the Band Played On*, p. 222, but did not attribute the quote. Starr, *Blood*, p. 272, quotes Louis Aledort as articulating this

position: Aledort said, "I disagree vehemently with the National Gay Task Force. They may want to protect their rights, but what about the hemophiliacs' right to life." Douglas Starr's documentation of the January 4 meeting is detailed on p. 399.

39. Ronald Bayer has effectively explained the debate over "surrogate testing" of blood using the hepatitis B core antibody test. No one knew for certain if this test would work. To this day, it remains contested: some experts saying it would have cut tremendously into the rates of transfusion-related HIV; others saying that it has been demonstrated that it would not work. See Bayer, "Blood and AIDS in America," pp. 27–29.

40. David J. Gury, vice president, Plasma Supply, Alpha Therapeutic Corporation, Letter to all source affiliates, December 17, 1982, in Leveton et al., *HIV and the Blood Supply*, quotes on pp. 269, 272. See also Starr, *Blood*, pp. 269–72.

41. See Donald P. Francis, interview by Sally Smith Hughes, in Regional Oral History Office of the Bancroft Library, *The AIDS Epidemic in San Francisco: The Medical Response, 1981–1984*, vol. 4 (Berkeley: University of California, 1997), pp. 60–66, quote on p. 62.

42. On "blood shield laws," see Leveton et al., *HIV and the Blood Supply*, pp. 2, 48–49, 139, 223–24, and Starr, *Blood*, pp. 206, 323.

43. See Donald Francis, interview by Hughes, *The AIDS Epidemic in San Francisco*, 4:60–66, quotes on pp. 64–65. Herbert Perkins reportedly made this or a similar statement at the December 1983 meeting of the Blood Products Advisory Committee. For Perkins's account, see Hughes's interview of him in Regional Oral History Office of the Bancroft Library, *The AIDS Epidemic in San Francisco: The Medical Response, 1981*, vol. 5 (Berkeley: University of California, 1997), 212 pp.

44. At the January 4, 1983 meeting, the CDC's Thomas Spira presented the option of investigating five tests as candidates for a "surrogate" AIDS test. These included the test for the antibody to hepatitis B core antigen, the test for the antibody to hepatitis B surface antigen, a test for the T-cell helper-suppressor ratio, a test for the absolute lymphocyte count, and a fifth for measuring immune complexes. In December 1983 the FDA Blood Products Advisory Committee decided to implement a three-month study of the issue, which proved inconclusive. Throughout the dispute, blood bankers remained resistant to using any surrogate AIDS test, and the efforts of the few blood banks that initiated surrogate testing were denounced as "hysteria mongering," according to Ronald Bayer. See Bayer, "Blood and AIDS in America," p. 28, and Sally Smith Hughes's interview of Herbert Perkins in *The AIDS Epidemic in San Francisco*, 5:29.

45. Starr, *Blood*, pp. 250–65.

46. See Herbert Perkins, interview by Hughes, section on "'One-in-a-million' Risk of Transfusion AIDS," in *The AIDS Epidemic in San Francisco*, 5:22–25.

47. The uneasy alliance between blood bankers and gay advocates had a history. For many gay activists of the era, blood donation was viewed as a meaningful expression of their civic identity, a gesture toward building the gay community into a respected minority within American society, and a symbol of solidarity between gay culture and the nation's majority culture. Gay Americans reportedly gave blood in disproportionately higher numbers than other groups in some U.S. cities, which prompted blood bankers to worry not only about the cost of the hepatitis B tests but also about the danger that the test would drive these valued donors away. (Sources: Evatt, phone interviews by Pemberton, and Perkins, interview by Hughes, in *The AIDS Epidemic in San Francisco*, vol. 5.)

48. David Kirp, "The Politics of Blood: Hemophilia Activism in the AIDS Crisis," in Feldman and Bayer, *Blood Feuds*, pp. 293–321. See also Davidson, "Strange Blood: Hemophobia and the Unexplored Boundaries of Queer Nation."

49. Starr, *Blood*, p. 272, and Oscar Ratnoff, telephone interview by Susan Resnick, November 5, 1991. Courtesy of Susan Resnick.

50. The unpublished "Reporter Notes" of B. D. Colon (*Newsday* journalist) as quoted in Starr, *Blood*, p. 273.

51. Quotes from Shilts, *And the Band Played On*, p. 220. See also Starr, *Blood*, p. 273, based on his interview with Donald Francis, and Hughes's interview with Francis, *The AIDS Epidemic in San Francisco*, 4:60–66.

52. American Red Cross National Headquarters, Memorandum to Mr. de-Beufort from Dr. Cumming, February 5, 1983, reproduced in Leveton et al., *HIV and the Blood Supply*, p. 287.

53. Starr, *Blood*, p. 300.

54. The processes included detergent solvents as well as heat treatments to destroy the lipid coating on hepatitis viruses. Accounts of this history are available in Leveton et al., *HIV and the Blood Supply*, pp. 83–96, and more provocatively in DePrince, *Cry Bloody Murder*, pp. 51–53, 58–61.

55. Bayer, "Blood and AIDS in America," p. 31, and Leveton et al., *HIV and the Blood Supply*, p. 92.

56. Leveton et al., *HIV and the Blood Supply*, p. 177.

57. Author's interview with Harvey Alter; interview with Leon Hoyer, M.D., director, Holland Laboratories, American Red Cross, Rockville, MD, October 13, 1998; and interview with Dale Lawrence, National Institutes of Health, Bethesda, MD, October 15, 1998. See also Bayer, "Blood and AIDS in America," p. 31, and Walt Bodanich and Eric Koli, "Tainted Exports: Two Paths of Bayer Drug in 80's: Riskier Type Went Overseas," *New York Times*, May 22, 2005, p. A1.

58. Andrews, *Codeine Diary*, pp. 22–23.

59. David Whitman, "To a Poster Child, Dying Young," *U.S. News & World Report* 108 (April 16, 1990): 8. See also Doris Zames Fleischer and Frieda Zames, "'Wheelchair Bound' and the 'Poster Child,'" in the *Disability Rights Movement: From Charity to Confrontation* (Philadelphia: Temple University Press, 2001), pp. 1–13.

60. Charles Rosenberg, "Disease and Social Order in America: Perceptions and Expectations," in Elizabeth Fee and Daniel Fox, eds., *AIDS: The Burdens of History* (Berkeley: University of California Press, 1988), pp. 12–32, quote on p. 13.

61. Davidson, "Strange Blood: Hemophobia and the Unexplored Boundaries of Queer Nation," especially p. 44. See also Dennis Altman, *AIDS in the Mind of America: The Social, Political, and Psychological Impact of a New Epidemic* (New York: Anchor Press/Doubleday, 1986).

62. Kenneth Orr, "Hemophiliacs and AIDS: Contracting a Killer," *Christian Century* 105 (March 9, 1988): 247–48.

63. Quotes in "Remembering Ryan White," *Newsweek* 115 (April 23, 1990): 24, and Whitman, "To a Poster Child, Dying Young," p. 8.

64. The *Ryan White Comprehensive AIDS Resources Emergency (CARE) Act*, Pub. L. 101-381, 104 Stat. 576, was enacted on August 18, 1990. See Andriote, *Victory Deferred*, pp. 211–89, and Siplon, *AIDS and the Policy Struggle in the United States*, pp. 93–100, on the history and politics surrounding the CARE Act, including how Ryan White's image helped the U.S. Congress frame their support of AIDS prevention and treatment as a benefit for majority Americans (not gay Americans and other minority groups).

65. David Kirp, *Learning by Heart: AIDS and Schoolchildren in America's Communities* (New Brunswick, NJ: Rutgers University Press, 1989).

66. Michael Doan, "The Little Hostage to a Killer in the Blood," *U.S. News & World Report* 101 (September 8, 1986): 10.

67. Jennet Conant, "AIDS in the Classroom," *Newsweek* 107 (March 3, 1986): 6.

68. Jack Friedman and Bill Shaw, "The Quiet Victories of Ryan White," *People Weekly* 29 (May 30, 1988): 88–96.

69. The cover of *People Weekly* 29 (May 30, 1988) pictures Ryan White alone with the lede: "Amazing Grace: In the shadow of death from AIDS, hemophiliac Ryan White, 16, has found a great gift for living. This is a boy you'll never forget."

70. Ryan White and Anne Marie Cunningham, *Ryan White: My Own Story* (New York: Dial Books, 1991), p. 5.

71. Nadine Brozan, "Chronicle: On the Talk-Show Circuit with Ryan White's Mother," *New York Times*, April 22 1991, p. B8.

72. Whitman, "To a Poster Child, Dying Young."

73. James Barron, "AIDS Sufferer's Return to Classes Is Cut Short," *New York Times*, February 22, 1986, p. A6.

74. Dirk Johnson, "Ryan White Dies of AIDS at 18; His Struggle Helped Pierce Myths," *New York Times*, April 9, 1990, p. D10.

75. White and Cunningham, *Ryan White: My Own Story*, p. 11.

76. Quoted in Sander Gilman, *Disease and Representation: Images of Illness from Madness to AIDS* (Ithaca: Cornell University Press, 1988), p. 268. See also Dorothy Nelkin and Stephen Hilgartner, "Disputed Dimensions of Risk: A Public School Controversy over AIDS," *Milbank Quarterly* 64, suppl. 1 (1986): 118–42.

77. Gilman, *Disease and Representation*, pp. 267–68.

78. "Brothers with AIDS Virus Return to Florida Classes under Guard," *New York Times*, August 25, 1987, p. A12; "Fire Damages Home of Boys Ordered Admitted to School," *New York Times*, August 29, 1987, p. A32; "Family in AIDS Case Quits Florida Town after House Burns," *New York Times*, August 30, 1987, p. A1; Jon Norheimer, "To Neighbors of Shunned Family, AIDS Fear Outweighs Sympathy," *New York Times*, August 31, 1987, p. A1; Paula Chin and Meg Grant, "Seize the Day: AIDS Victim Ricky Ray, 14, Plans His Marriage," *People* 35 (June 17, 1991): 39; "Ricky Ray, 15, Dies: Known for AIDS Cause," *New York Times*, December 13, 1992, p. B8; Stephen Buckley, "AIDS in America: Twenty Years Later, Slow Change of Heart," *St. Petersburg Times*, September 2, 2001, p. A1.

79. Interview with Andrew Flagg, in Laura Gray and Christine Chamberlain, eds., *The Gift of Experience*, pp. 159–66, quote on p. 163.

80. Bayer, "A Life in Limbo," p. 48.

81. Cindy Patton, *Sex and Germs: The Politics of AIDS* (Boston: South End Press, 1985), p. 23.

82. Bayer, "A Life in Limbo," p. 55.

83. Oscar Ratnoff, telephone interview by Susan Resnick, November 5, 1991, courtesy of Susan Resnick. See also Resnick, *Blood Saga*, pp. 122–32, and Jacalyn Duffin, *Lovers and Livers: Disease Concepts in History* (Toronto: University of Toronto Press, 2005), pp. 98–100.

84. Dale Lawrence, interview by Pemberton, and Ratnoff, interview by Resnick.

85. Robert Simon, "The Family and Hemophilia," in Margaret Hilgartner and Carl Pochedy, eds., *Hemophilia in the Child and Adult*, 3rd ed. (New York: Raven Press, 1989), p. 214.

86. Andrews, *Codeine Diary*, p. 23.

87. Resnick, *Blood Saga*. See also Starr, *Blood*, pp.241–42 and 281–82, where he discusses Dietrich's dilemmas.

88. *Hemophilia Newsnotes, NHF Medical Bulletin #7, Chapter Advisor #8,* May 11, 1983, reprinted in Leveton et al., *HIV and the Blood Supply,* pp. 295–96.

89. Profilate ad, *Hemophilia Letter: A Quarterly Newsletter Devoted to Hemophilia* (Alpha Therapeutic Corporation, Los Angeles) 3, no. 2 (Summer 1981): 5. See also Louis M. Aledort, "Methods of Care, Products Available, Complications of Therapy," and Judith Best, "Lesson Plan for Self-Treatment in Hemophilia," *Mount Sinai Journal of Medicine* 44 (1977): 332–38, 470–76, which are each referenced in the ad, pp. 4–5.

90. "Alpha Moves to Protect Hemophiliacs against Risk of AIDS," *Hemophilia Letter: A Quarterly Newsletter Devoted to Hemophilia* (Alpha Therapeutic Corporation, Los Angeles) 4, no. 2 (Winter 1982): 1. "It Takes a Team," Profilate ad in same newsletter, p. 5. Quotes from pp. 1, 5. See Starr, *Blood,* p. 270.

91. Ronald Bayer and Gerald Oppenheimer, *AIDS Doctors: Voices from the Epidemic* (New York: Oxford University Press, 2000), p. 22.

92. Bayer, "A Life in Limbo."

93. Dubin, "Hemophilia: A Story of Success—Disaster and the Perseverance of the Human Spirit."

94. Siplon, "Blood Policy in the Age of AIDS."

95. Charles Bosk, *Forgive and Remember: Managing Medical Failure,* 2nd ed. (Chicago: University of Chicago Press, 2003). See also recent debates surrounding medical mistakes in organ transplantation in Keith Wailoo, Julie Livingston, and Peter Guranaccia, eds., *A Death Retold: Jesica Santillan, the Bungled Transplant, and Paradoxes of Medical Citizenship* (Chapel Hill: University of North Carolina Press, 2006).

96. Aledort, "HIV and Hemophilia." See also Evatt, "Tragic History."

97. For very different strategies to telling this history, one might compare Keshavjee, Weiser, and Kleinmann, "Medicine Betrayed," with the documentary films of Alexander Marengo, Nick Read, and Gino Del Guercio, *Red Gold: The Epic Story of Blood* (PBS/Educational Broadcasting Corporation, 2002); Kelly Duda, *Factor 8: The Arkansas Prison Blood Scandal* (Concrete Films USA, 2005); and Marilyn Ness, *Bad Blood: A Cautionary Tale* (Necessary Films, 2010).

Conclusion

1. Charles Rosenberg, "Pathologies of Progress: The Idea of Civilization as Risk," *Bulletin of the History of Medicine* 72 (1998): 714–30, quote on p. 726. See also Rosenberg, *Our Present Complaint: American Medicine, Then and Now* (Baltimore: Johns Hopkins University Press, 2007), especially pp. 77–112.

2. "By 1982, 73% of persons with hemophilia A treated at U.S. hemophilia

treatment centers received lyophilized concentrates, with the majority receiving their therapy almost exclusively at home." Terence Chorba, Robert Holman, Matthew Clarke, and Bruce Evatt, "Effects of HIV Infection on Age and Cause of Death for Persons with Hemophilia A in the United States," *American Journal of Hematology* 66 (2001): 230.

3. Originally, there were 22 federally funded HTCs. Each included a coagulation laboratory, a blood bank, and a multidisciplinary hemophilia treatment team. Individual states also began funding their own HTCs according to this model. In 1975 there were an additional 21 HTCs funded at the state level. By 2005 there were more than 130 HTCs in the United States that received federal funding through the Health Resources and Services Administration and CDC. They provide comprehensive care, preventive services, and disease surveillance to more than fifteen thousand people with hemophilia and more than ten thousand patients with other types of bleeding disorders. Scott D. Grosse, Michael S. Schecter, Roshni Kulkarni, et al., "Models of Comprehensive Multidisciplinary Care for Individuals in the United States with Genetic Disorders," *Pediatrics* 123 (January 2009): 409.

4. On Dana Kuhn, see Susan Resnick, *Blood Saga: Hemophilia, AIDS, and the Survival of a Community* (Berkeley: University of California Press, 1999), pp. 93, 162–63; Douglas Starr, *Blood: An Epic History of Medicine and Commerce* (New York: Alfred Knopf, 1998), pp. 278, 321, 326; and Patricia Siplon, *AIDS and the Policy Struggle in the United States* (Washington, DC: Georgetown University Press, 2002), p. 55.

5. Resnick, *Blood Saga*, and David Kirp, "The Politics of Blood: Hemophilia Activism in the AIDS Crisis," in Eric Feldman and Ronald Bayer, eds., *Blood Feuds: AIDS, Blood, and the Politics of Medical Disaster* (New York: Oxford University Press, 1999), pp. 293–322.

6. Resnick, *Blood Saga*, and Siplon, *AIDS and the Policy Struggle in the United States*.

7. Ronald Bayer, "Blood and AIDS in America: The Making of a Catastrophe," in Feldman and Bayer, *Blood Feuds*, p. 39, and Siplon, *AIDS and the Policy Struggle in the United States*, p. 58.

8. Steven Epstein, *Impure Science: AIDS, Activism, and the Politics of Knowledge* (Berkeley: University of California Press, 1994).

9. Resnick, *Blood Saga*, pp. 174–82, and Barry Meier, "Blood, Money, and AIDS: Hemophiliacs are Split," *New York Times*, June 11, 1996, p. D1.

10. Siplon, *AIDS and the Policy Struggle in the United States*.

11. In 2004 the *Lancet* published the first scientific report to claim that vCJD was transmissible by blood. A. H. Peden, M. W. Head, D. L. Ritchie, J. E. Bell, and

J. W. Ironside, "Preclinical vCJD after Blood Transfusion in a PRNP Codon 129 Hetereozygous Patient," *Lancet* 354 (August 7–13, 2004): 527–29.

12. "Prodigal Dad," season 1, episode 15, of *Gideon's Crossing* aired on the American Broadcasting Company network on February 12, 2001. Leslie Libman, director. Andre Braugher played Dr. Gideon.

13. Robert Massie and Suzanne Massie, *Journey* (New York: Alfred Knopf, 1975), p. 269.

14. See again Brinkhous's remarks, ibid.

15. Jeremy Laurance, "800 Haemophiliacs Given Tainted Blood at Risk of vCJD," *Independent* (London, England), May 20, 2009.

16. Walt Bogdanich and Eric Koli, "Tainted Exports: Two Paths of Bayer Drug in 80's: Riskier Type Went Overseas," *New York Times*, May 22, 2005, p. A1.

17. Ibid.

18. Eric Feldman, "HIV and Blood in Japan: Transforming Private Conflict into Public Scandal," in Feldman and Bayer, *Blood Feuds*, pp. 60–93.

19. Ian Fischer, "The Struggle for Iraq: Public Health; Iraqi AIDS Patients Faced Confinement as Well as Pain and Death," *New York Times*, October 24, 2003, Health Section, p. A12.

20. Brian O'Mahony, "WFH: Back to the Future," *Haemophilia* 10 (2004): 1–8.

21. See, e.g., K. M. Brinkhous, "Gene Transfer in the Hemophilias: Retrospect and Prospect," *Thrombosis Research* 67 (1992): 329–38.

22. Keith Wailoo and Stephen Pemberton, *The Troubled Dream of Genetic Medicine: Ethnicity and Innovation in Tay-Sachs, Cystic Fibrosis, and Sickle Cell Disease* (Baltimore: Johns Hopkins University Press, 2006), pp. 103–10.

23. See, e.g., M. A. Kay, S. Rothenberg, C. N. Landen, D. A. Bellinger, F. Leland, C. Toman, M. Finegold, A. R. Thompson, M. S. Read, K. M. Brinkhous, and S. L. C. Woo, "In Vivo Gene Therapy of Hemophilia B: Sustained Partial Correction in Factor IX-deficient Dogs," *Science* 262 (1993): 117–19; M. A. Kay, C. N. Landen, S. Rothenberg, L. A. Taylor, F. Leland, S. Wiehle, F. Bingliang, D. Bellinger, M. Finegold, A. R. Thompson, M. S. Read, K. M. Brinkhous, and S. L. C. Woo, "In Vivo Hepatic Gene Therapy: Complete Albeit Transient Correction of Factor IX Deficiency in Hemophilia B Dogs," *Proceedings of the National Academy of Sciences USA* 91 (1994): 2353–57; and J. N. Lozier and K. M. Brinkhous, "Gene Therapy and the Hemophilias," *Journal of the American Medical Association* 271 (1994): 47–51.

24. J. H. Lewis, F. A. Bontempo, J. A. Spiro, M. V. Ragni, and T. E. Starzl, "Liver Transplantation in a Hemophiliac [Letter]," *New England Journal of Medicine* 312 (1985): 1189, and F. A. Bontempo, J. H. Lewis, T. J. Gorenc, J. A. Spero,

M. V. Ragni, J. P. Scott, and T. E. Starzl, "Liver Transplantation in Hemophilia A," *Blood* 69 (1987): 1721–24.

25. See Stephen Pemberton, "Canine Technologies, Model Patients: The Historical Production of Hemophiliac Dogs in American Biomedicine," in Susan Schrepfer and Philip Scranton, eds., *Industrializing Organisms: Introducing Evolutionary History* (New York: Routledge, 2004), pp. 191–213.

26. Robert Massie Jr.'s Web site, http://bobmassie.org/ accessed February 23, 2010, and November 2, 2010.

INDEX

Abilgaard, Charles, 215
Abbott Laboratories, 158, 178–79, 260
ACT-UP (AIDS Coalition to Unleash
    Power), 288
"Adam H.," 176
Addis, Thomas, 55–58, 60, 62–65, 68,
    74–75, 318n35
advocacy, disease, 127, 134, 218,
    226–27
Aggeler, Paul, 98, 100–101, 112, 330n54
AIDS (acquired immunodeficiency
    syndrome), 4, 10, 16, 237, 242–79,
    288, 303; as blood borne, 118,
    245–49, 259, 270, 277; and blood
    supply, 238, 246, 250–62; causation,
    243, 259; denial, 247–48, 250,
    253, 259, 280; as disease of "sex
    and drug abuse," 243, 245–46,
    254–55, 263, 267–70, 295–98; era
    of, 7, 242, 262, 289, 294–96; as "gay
    disease," 243, 264, 267, 354n11; and
    "high-risk groups," 246, 254–55,
    355n21; naming of, 243, 251–52; as
    sexually transmitted, 243, 245, 247;
    skepticism, 247–48, 250, 253, 259,
    280; and stigma, 250, 263–65,
    267–70, 295. See also HIV; HIV/
    AIDS; people with AIDS; post-
    transfusion infections; transfusion-
    related HIV/AIDS
Albert, Prince Consort (husband of
    Queen Victoria), 33
Albucasis, 20
Aledort, Louis, 217, 220, 231, 245–46,
    274, 288, 355–56n38; on clotting
    factor concentrates, 248, 253, 259;
    on history, 237–38, 282, 352n2
Alexander, Benjamin, 130

Allen, J. Garrott, 234–35, 350n71,
    351n81
Alpha Therapeutics, 255–56, 261,
    275–78
Alter, Harvey, 230
American Association of Blood Banks
    (AABB), 204, 257, 260
American Red Cross (ARC), 121, 124,
    127, 163, 166, 170, 204, 287; and
    AIDS, 257, 259–60; and clotting
    factor concentrates, 175, 351n81
Andrews, Tom, 262, 274
anemia, 55; pernicious, 62–63, 68;
    sickle cell, 197, 200
Appleton, Oliver, 40
Archer inquiry, 293
Armour Laboratories, 94–95, 171, 261,
    327n32
Armstrong, Donald, 254
autonomy, 9–11, 16, 160, 195, 239, 258,
    286–87, 289–90; and clotting factor
    concentrates, 172, 209, 279. See also
    people with hemophilia

Backer, Frank, 223
Backer, Frank, Jr., 223
Bassen, Frank, 130
Baxter (pharmaceutical co.), 157–58,
    177–78, 180–81, 215, 261, 342n43,
    351n81
Bayer (pharmaceutical co.), 294–95
Bayer, Peter Brandon, 269–70, 280
Behringwerke Corp., 260
Beth Israel Hospital (Brooklyn, NY), 90
Bias, Val, 288
Biggs, Rosemary, 92, 98–99
Binder, David, 162, 166
Birch, Carroll LaFleur, 86–90

bleeder patients, 20, 22, 26, 29–30, 42, 47, 93, 114; and advocacy, 111, 122–23, 136; and AIDS, 262; as "experiments of nature," 79–80; female, 38–41, 81–91, 100, 104–10, 112, 335n36; and marriage, 41, 43; as normal people, 190–91; and specialists, 106–9. *See also* patients; people with bleeding disorders; people with hemophilia

bleeding disorders, ix–x, 2–3, 15, 76–77, 91, 99–102, 173, 292; diagnosis of, 86, 93, 108–9

blood, 237, 299; and AIDS screening, 249–50, 254–56; as "borrowed," 161, 165; as commodity, 10, 107, 120, 197, 257, 327n36; donor as "paid," 235, 241, 350n71; as "foreign," 296; as gift, 172, 197; as national resource, 16, 197–98, 203; vs. plasma delivery systems, 172–76, 207–8; of questionable quality, 164–65, 202; as "unavoidably unsafe," 233. *See also* blood products; plasma; plasma fractions

blood bankers, 120–21, 163, 169–70, 175–76, 202, 299; in AIDS era, 244, 246–47, 250, 255–68, 356n44, 357n47

blood banks, xiii, 119, 124, 165–66, 171, 180, 203, 287; commercial, 162–64, 168; and cryoprecipitate, 174–77; founding of, 16; and HIV testing, 260. *See also* blood industry

blood clotting nomenclature, 75, 87, 101, 103–4, 113

blood clotting research, x, 19, 50, 55–63, 68–73, 74, 330n50; cascade or waterfall hypothesis, 113–14; classic theory of Morawitz, 57, 62, 70, 96, 317n19; confusion about, 75, 99–104, 331n70; golden age of, 58, 91–92, 114; Howell's theories, 59, 61–62, 317n25

blood credits, 165–66, 170

blood donation, 1–3, 79, 81, 128, 172; in AIDS era, 252, 254, 256–58; as burden, 120–24, 165–67, 181–83; as civic duty, 120, 122, 127–28, 161, 167–68; as "gift exchange," 170, 191–92; as voluntary, 120–22, 152–54,

161–64, 167–68, 180–82, 202, 208, 233

blood donors, 3, 111, 120–21, 124, 153; ban on gay, 246, 250, 254–55, 257–58, 260, 355n34; as "family," 122; high-risk, 232–33, 235, 250, 252, 255, 260; paid, 162–64, 170, 175, 202, 235, 241; and plasma donors, 170–71; screening of, 237, 246–47, 254–56, 260; voluntary, 161, 175, 177

blood economy, 9, 160, 162–63, 166, 181–83, 255, 257, 294–96

blood industry, 1, 202, 238–39, 252, 277, 287. *See also* blood banks; plasma banks; plasma fractionation industry

blood products, ix; and post-transfusion infections, 244, 275, 293, 350n71. *See also* plasma products

Blood Products Advisory Committee (FDA), 289, 356nn43–44

blood profiteering, 163–64, 172, 202

blood resources in the U.S., 3, 16, 197–98, 202–4, 208, 224

blood safety, 232–35, 248, 250–62

blood services, 119–20, 124, 137–38, 292; access to, 160–61, 183, 233; delivery system, 198, 207–8, 241, 244; reform of, 202, 233, 241–42

blood shield laws, 256

blood shortages, 160–72, 177, 194, 240

blood transfusions, ix, 2, 49, 51, 79, 81, 182; for hemophilia generally, 81, 94, 118, 318n38; for hemophilia in 1800s, 52–54, 318n9; for hemophilia in 1910s, 57, 60–61, 63–65, 67–68; for hemophilia in 1930s, 71, 73–74; for hemophilia in post–WWII America, 118–19; rise of transfusion medicine, 63–67. *See also* plasma transfusions

Blumberg, Baruch, 230

Blundell, James, 52–53

Bogdanich, Walt, 294–95

Boone, Donna, 7

Bosk, Charles, 281

Brinkhous, Kenneth Merle, x–xii, 147–48, 292, 301, 331n70; and clotting factor concentrates, xi, 158, 177; and factor VIII discovery, xi, 76, 322n77; in Iowa, 68–74, 76; and NHF

Foundation for Bleeders (Omaha, NE), 123–24
Francis, Donald, 256, 259
Friedland, Eric, 195, 219–22, 226
Friedland, Louis, 219–22, 226
Friedrich William of Hesse and by Rhine, Prince (grandson of Queen Victoria), 33, 36
Furnas, Helen, 81–83, 90, 104, 105–12, 125

Garner, Jim, 153–54, 347n40
Gaughenbaugh, Don, 123
gay community, 8, 246, 354n11, 358n64; activism, 247, 250, 254–55, 288, 355n34; and blood donation, 258, 357n47; and hemophilia community, 255, 258
Gelsinger, Jesse, 299
gender, attitudes toward, 8, 110, 258
gene therapy research, 291, 299–301
Giamona, Angelo, 121
Gideon's Crossing (TV series), 291, 362n12
Gilbert, Marvin, 222
Gilman, Sander, 268
Glazer, Shep, 219, 222
globalization, disease risks of, 293–98
Goffman, Erving, 12
Gottlieb, Michael, 242
governance, and hemophilia management, 8–9, 16, 84, 198, 283–84, 298
government (U.S. federal), 3, 193–94, 238, 287–88; accountability of, 279, 281; and blood supply safety, 208, 239, 241, 299; delayed response of, to AIDS, 251–52; and funding for hemophilia care, 196–203, 209, 227; presumed incompetence of, xiii, 4, 218–19, 241, 250, 267
Graham, John B., 90
Grandidier, Ludwig, 29–30, 39, 44
Green, Mrs. J., 215–16
Green Cross (Japan), 296
Groves, Ernest W. Hey, 55, 57

Haas, Greg, 288
Haitians, 246, 254, 255, 355n21

Haldane, J. B. S., 35–36, 44–46, 311n37
Halden, Richard, Jr., 216
"Harry B.," 187
Harvard University, 59–60, 75, 77–78, 93–95, 97, 130, 238, 318n35, 322n77
Hassan, Muhanid, 297
Hay, John, 40, 309n19, 313n54
health care, 10, 16, 238, 274; access to, 160, 183, 196, 198–200; affordability of, 1, 8–9, 163; cost of, 198–200, 202, 292
health insurance, 166, 182, 193, 198–200, 207, 209, 232, 273
heart disease, 2, 201, 228–29, 232
Heavner, Roy, 220
hematologists, x, 15, 55–62, 81–87, 129–30; and blood coagulation specialists, 68–80, 90–114, 173; and hemophilia community, 192, 205; and patients, 106–12, 120, 126
hematology, 1, 15, 48–49, 116, 323n5; promises of, 127–28, 136; specialty of, 91, 102–3, 108, 134
hemodialysis, 178, 215, 219, 285
hemophilia, ix–x, 5, 16, 46, 227, 283–85; among African Americans, 38; as Anglo-Germanic disease, 31–38; as bleeding disorder, 49, 76–78, 81, 284; and blood clotting, 2, 48–50, 54–63, 76; as blood disease, 14, 18, 49–51, 78; and blood supply debates, 162, 202–9, 232–35; characteristics of, 2, 10, 13–14; and class, 14, 18–19, 21, 34–36, 47; concept of, 14, 18–31, 38, 47, 105, 284–86; as constitutional, 32, 50, 78; crippling in, 10–12, 125, 140, 146, 186, 211–12, 220–22, 225; cure for, 290–91, 299–302; definition of, 8; as "democratic" disease, 1, 111, 185, 226; *de novo* cases of, 31–32, 35, 45, 86; diagnosis of, 8, 38, 81, 86, 91, 104, 108, 290; and ethnicity, 14, 18–19, 21, 32, 38, 47, 187; in females, 38–44, 81–91, 100, 104–10; and gender, 7–9, 14, 18–19, 21, 37, 47, 285, 303; and gendered identities, 83, 110–11, 150–51, 224, 258; and German medicine, 19, 25–32, 34, 50, 56, 295; as hereditary disease, 18,

hemophilia (*cont.*)
31–36, 39–47, 81, 284; historical interpretation of, 6–7, 10–13, 18–21, 238–40, 284–86, 302–3; history of, ix, xiii, 2, 8–9, 14; and identity, 18, 47; in Jews, 20–21, 37, 91; joint bleeding in, 2, 211–12, 222; as "lonesome" disease, 81–84, 110–12, 119; as "male" disease, 7, 39, 44, 81, 84–86, 89, 108–11; as manageable, 10–11, 15, 49, 158, 236, 264; in nonhuman animals, xii, 20, 73, 90, 301; and pain, ix, 2, 10–11, 124, 150–51, 211, 213; as personal challenge, 81, 117, 294; and progress, 6, 14, 44, 47, 227, 283–86; psychosocial perspectives on, 185–89; and race, 14, 18–19, 21, 37–38, 46–47, 188; as "royal" disease, 1–2, 21–22, 32–36, 44–45, 111, 143, 226; and sex hormones, 86–88; as sex-linked, 7, 18–19, 41, 81, 85–86, 309n19; and sexual identity, 38–39; stereotyped portraits of, 143–46, 187; transformation of, into chronic manageable disease, ix–x, 1–4, 19, 49–50, 118, 191, 239, 303; visibility of, 1–2, 13, 18–19, 44, 47, 124, 138, 262; word *hemophilia*, 1, 28–29, 31, 33, 38, 86. *See also* hemophilia A; hemophilia B; hemophilia C; hemophilia management; people with hemophilia
hemophilia A, 26, 92, 101, 104–5, 110, 113, 173. *See also* factor VIII deficiency
hemophilia advocacy, 176, 191–92, 194, 197–98, 224, 236; in AIDS era, 286–90, 296. *See also* hemophilia associations; hemophilia community; people with hemophilia
"hemophilia AIDS holocaust," 288
hemophilia associations, 5, 110, 120–21, 123, 126–27, 135, 155, 296; in AIDS era, 280–81; as "corrupt," 234; as "sob sisters," 189. *See also* Canadian Hemophilia Society; Committee of Ten Thousand; Foundation for Bleeders; Hemophilia/HIV Peer Association; National Hemophilia

Foundation; U.K. Haemophilia Society; World Federation of Hemophilia
hemophilia B, 92, 101, 104, 113, 206, 229. *See also* factor IX deficiency
hemophilia C, 81, 91, 101, 105. *See also* factor IX deficiency
hemophilia community, 3–4, 8–9, 15–16, 83, 122, 160, 203, 286; and adult patients, 190–91; as "blood brotherhood," 151, 155–56; as "categorical illness group," 201, 292; and clotting factor concentrates, 172, 180–82, 190–91, 196, 219, 258–59, 272; as "community of fate," 127; demands for justice from, 238, 281–82; emergence of, 117–37; as "fractional population," 292; and gay community, 255; and gender anxiety, 8, 306–7n15; and home care, 212, 215–16; and isolation, 124, 127, 137, 187; and knowledge of AIDS, 250, 252, 262, 267, 278, 279, 288; and NHLI *Blood Resources Study*, 204–9; overcoming mistakes, 279–82; political advocacy by, 3–4, 198, 201–2, 205; and specialists, 111–12, 126, 128–37, 192. *See also* hemophilia advocacy; hemophilia associations
Hemophilia/HIV Peer Association (H/HIV Peer), 280, 288
hemophilia management, ix–x, xii, 1, 3, 49–50, 73, 107, 289; access to, 198–201, 226; as "back to the future" enterprise, 298, 301; as benign, 7; cost of, 160, 191, 206; definition of, 284; experience of, 285; failures in AIDS era, 238, 268, 279–80; goals of, 7, 16, 116–18, 290; globalization of, 293–98; historical analysis of, 6, 9, 78–80, 83, 117, 209, 281–82, 284–85; ironies of, 302–3; promises of, 16, 92, 120, 172, 235; and prophylactic use of plasma products, 211–12, 214, 292; prophylactic vs. episodic care, 206; revolution in, 181; risks of, 16; as technological enterprise, 5; "total care" vs. home care, 209, 217. *See also* complications of hemophilia

treatment; comprehensive care for hemophilia; home transfusion care; therapeutic revolution
hemophilia treatment centers (HTCs), 16, 201, 210, 224–25, 232–33, 287, 346n21, 361n3; in AIDS era, 249, 253, 256, 271, 274, 351n1, 360–61n2
hemophilia treatment specialists, 172, 176, 202, 204–6, 209–10, 217, 227–28, 231–32; blame of, 5, 280; and comprehensive care, 183–90, 253; as patient advocates, 224, 276–78; and post-transfusion hepatitis, 208, 229, 231–32, 350n71; responses of, to AIDS, 237, 252–53, 258, 262, 270, 274; supply vs. safety, 232, 234, 258
hemophobia, 269
Henry, Betty Jane, 124–25
Henry, Lee, 82, 125
Henry, Robert Lee, 124–25, 129, 131–12, 134–35, 143, 331n70, 335n36
Henry family, 125–27, 129, 155
hepatitis, 6, 179, 208, 229–30, 260–61, 299; and paid donors, 164, 202, 241, 350n71; in people with hemophilia, 208, 229–32, 241, 277, 279
hepatitis B virus, 229–30, 232, 240, 242, 245, 259–60, 277, 299; testing for, 249–50, 254–57, 260, 278, 356n39, 356n44, 357n47
hepatitis C virus (HCV), ix, 5, 231, 240, 242, 291, 293, 301
hereditary conditions, 1, 22, 27, 44–46
Hexter, Margaret, 132–33, 335n39
Hilgartner, Margaret, 277
Hitler, Adolf, 46
HIV (human immunodeficiency virus), 4, 237, 240, 267, 293, 301; discovery of, 260–62
HIV/AIDS, 4, 7, 242, 267, 270, 274, 280, 297; among people with hemophilia, ix, 240, 351n1; and blood test, 237, 260, 262; in Iraq, 299; as manageable, 283, 301
Holmstrom, Kenny, 123
home transfusion care, 209–17, 225–26, 287, 347n31, 361n2. See also self-administration of blood products

homosexuality, 8, 258, 264, 267
Hoofnagle, Jay, 230–31, 350n71
Hooper Foundation, 68
Hopff, Freidrich, 28
Howard County Hemophilia Society, 266
Howell, William Henry, 55, 58–62, 68, 74, 317n25, 318n35
Hudson, Rock, 264
Huff, Sam, 220
Hussein, Saddam, 297
Hyland Division, 177–78, 180–81, 215, 339n4, 342n43, 351n81. See also Baxter

Immerman, Hermann, 37, 41, 43, 51
Ingram, G. Isley, 20
inhibitors, 228, 231–32
Institute of Medicine (IOM) of the U.S. National Academy of Sciences (NAS), 238, 288, 351n1
insulin, 2, 285; insulin-like treatment, 112, 177–78
insurance companies, 182, 194, 273, 287. See also health insurance
International Committee on Blood Clotting Factors, 103–5
intravenous drug users, 243, 246, 254–55
Iowa Group, 68–75
Iowa test, 69–70
Irwin Memorial Blood Bank, 249, 256

Jabbar, Khalid Ali, 297–98
Jaffe, Harold, 249
James, Chris, 293
Javits, Jacob, 219
Jewett, Warren, 223, 226
Jewish Hospital (Cincinnati, OH), 90
John, Elton, 265
Johns Hopkins University School of Medicine (Baltimore, MD), 59
Jordan, Henry, 82, 130, 152
Journey (book), 226, 234–35, 290, 302, 351n81
justice, 16, 281–82, 286–87, 289–90, 296

Kansas City Hospital Association, 164
Kapp, Christian Erhard, 26

National Heart and Lung Institute
(NHLI), 203–4, 206–10, 228, 232–34
National Hemophilia Foundation
(NHF), 110, 112, 176, 193–94,
228, 280, 287–88; and access to
hemophilia care, 199–201, 233–34;
and AIDS, 245–46, 249–58, 261–62,
271, 274–75, 279; blame of, 5, 279;
and blood credits, 162, 164–65;
and blood safety, 233–34; board
of trustees, 133–35; and CDC,
245–46, 248–49, 252–55, 257, 277;
chapters, 131–33, 165, 335n36; as
"consumer's union," 196; direct loan
programs, 132, 162, 165–66; early
years as Hemophilia Foundation,
Inc. (1948–55), 124–27, 129–30,
335n36; endorsements of clotting
factor concentrate use, 244, 253, 275,
277; exclusionary focus on males,
306–7n15; failures of, 238, 262, 267;
and first commercial clotting factor
concentrate, 180–81; and football
players, 220, 348n50; founding of,
3, 124; *Home Care of the Hemophilic
Child* (treatment guide), 147–49;
Man's Advocacy Network (MANN),
287; Medical Advisory Council (MAC)
or Medical and Scientific Advisory
Council (MASAC), 110, 130–31, 134,
136, 252, 261; Metropolitan New York
chapter (New York, NY), 111, 135, 162,
165, 167; Midwest chapter (Chicago,
IL), 133, 135, 143; Montreal chapter
(Canada), 131, 155; name change,
131, 133; New England chapter
(Boston, MA), 213; New York chapter
(Rochester, NY), 131, 135, 147, 185,
187; and "normality within limits,"
147–49; political advocacy, 3, 16, 197,
201–2, 209, 217–27; publicity efforts,
126, 139–40, 143–45, 195–96, 198,
222, 344n1; research investments,
133–37; Southern California chapter
(Los Angeles, CA), 133, 144, 184
National Institutes of Health (NIH),
232, 247, 251, 261, 287
Nesbit, Robert, 38

New York Blood Center (New York,
NY), 176
Nicholas and Alexandra (book/movie),
226
Nixon, Richard, 199–201, 203–4, 208,
218, 345n5
Nobel Prize in Medicine or Physiology,
62, 68, 230
normality/normalcy, 4, 7, 141, 172, 209,
288; and AIDS, 16, 237, 239, 262,
271–72, 288–91; and clotting factor
concentrates, 258, 275–76, 278–79;
and experts, 83, 127, 137–38, 185;
and gay community, 258; hemophilia
patients' aspirations for, 168, 188–
89, 191–92, 198, 236, 266, 286;
interpretations of, 10–12, 116–17, 138,
160; "normality within limits," 115,
148–51, 156; promise vs. reality, 139,
190, 192–93; words *normality* and
normalcy, 116
normalization, ix, 4, 7–10, 187–88, 286,
303; of blood clotting defects, 95,
106, 138; in orthopedics, 138, 152,
222; technological means of, 4, 200,
290
"normal lives" (for people with hemophilia), 3, 16, 116, 147, 197, 201,
286, 290–91; in AIDS era, 268; and
hemophilia advocacy movement, 11,
15, 117–18, 129, 138, 140, 145, 240;
public testimonies of, 220–21; and
therapeutic technologies, 112, 160–61,
172, 177–79, 206, 227
normal people/"normals," 12–13, 15,
128, 185, 197, 266
Northwestern University, 301

O'Brien, Mrs., 215
O'Mahony, Brian, 298, 301
O'Neil, Jack, 265
organ transplantation, 6, 300–302
Orthopaedic Hospital (Los Angeles,
CA), 184, 216
orthopedic braces, 125, 132, 152, 212,
220–23
Osler, Sir William, 32, 51, 54–55
Ottenberg, Reuben, 64–65

Otto, John Conrad, 22–25, 38, 284, 309nn11 and 19
Owen, Charles, 68
Owren, Paul, 95–97, 99
Oxford University, 92–93, 98–99, 104, 114, 322n77

Patek, Arthur J., 75–78, 93, 97
paternalism, 239, 277, 279, 289
patients, ix, 16, 290, 292; adolescent hemophilia, 192, 223, 227; adult hemophilia, 185–89, 192, 213, 223, 227–28, 232, 273, 300; and doctor-patient relation, 78–79, 107; pediatric hemophilia, 3, 7, 109, 111, 116, 141, 184, 213, 291; pediatric hemophilia/AIDS, 263, 267–68; treatment among younger vs. older, 206–7. *See also* bleeder patients; people with hemophilia
Pavlovsky, Alfredo, 96–98, 328n39
PCP *(Pneumocystis pneumonia)*, 242–45, 248
Pearson, Karl, 40, 84
Peitzman, Steven, 218
Penrose, Lionel, 45
people with AIDS, 263–64, 267–70, 288, 294–97. *See also* HIV; HIV/AIDS
people with bleeding disorders, 207, 236, 267, 297. *See also* bleeder patients; patients
people with hemophilia, ix, 5–6, 10, 15, 138–51, 153, 155, 201; as activists, 176, 286–90; as adolescents, 160, 187, 190–93, 291; as adults, 185–89, 223; and AIDS, xiii, 4–5, 118, 238, 251, 263, 267–79, 281, 288, 353n3; asymptomatic females, 7, 27, 41; and autonomy, 9, 16, 158, 160, 167, 180, 195–96, 200–201, 227, 236, 271–72; as blood consumers, 120–24, 152–54, 161–62, 166–68, 182, 204, 207–8, 241, 346n18; as boys, 117–18, 124–25, 138–42, 145–51, 160, 184–85, 187–93, 223; burdens on, 5, 121, 161, 165–66, 224; characterizations of, 12, 145–46, 148, 150–51, 166, 190, 223, 271–73; as children, 139–40, 221, 291; in China, 294–96; as consumers of plasma

products, 178, 182, 202; as creditable individuals, 12–13, 15, 124, 127–28, 138, 144, 168, 190, 196–99, 209; and cryoprecipitate, 176; and dependency, 10, 15, 128, 139, 186–87, 192; and disability, 9, 228; in early American republic, 22–25; as financial risk, 166, 182; and hepatitis, 300–302; and hospitals, 119; and iatrogenic infections, 4, 229–31, 237, 351n1; identity of, 3, 158; in Iraq, 296–98; as invalids, 128, 138, 141, 146, 186–87, 272; isolation of, 2, 11, 81–83, 111–12, 119, 124, 146; in Japan, 296; life expectancy of, 3–4, 140–41, 173, 185, 206, 306n5; as men, 116, 138, 145, 147, 150, 184–93; and military service, 168; as "normal" people, 121, 141, 144, 168, 189–92, 222–23, 267, 271–72; and parents, 150; population in the U.S., 173, 183, 198, 205–6, 345n23, 346n21; as "poster child(ren)," 223, 262–63, 266–67; as research subjects, 15, 48–50, 55–57, 71–74, 77–80, 208, 230–31; and rights, 196–98, 233, 258, 273; and risky behaviors, 185, 190–93, 273; and "safe sex," 273; "special needs" of, 124, 189, 192, 209; and sports, 149, 222; and stigma, 121, 124, 146, 187–89, 263–65, 267–70; and surgery, 44, 52–53, 64, 73, 124–25, 174; as test of national blood resources, 203, 240–42; and trust, 262, 279–82; as victim, 4, 143–44, 168, 263, 267–70, 280; vulnerabilities of, 13, 120–23, 241–42, 287. *See also* bleeder patients; carriers of hemophilia; hemophilia advocacy; "normal lives"; patients
Perkins, Herbert, 256, 356n43
pharmaceutical industry, xiii, 4, 194, 203, 224, 234, 287, 295–96; and plasma as profitable commodity, 94–95, 169, 171–72, 175. *See also* plasma fractionation industry
Physicians for Human Rights, 254
Pierce, Glenn, 288
plasma, 3, 172–76, 179–80, 207–8, 299; and AIDS screening, 254–55;

as commodity, 160, 172–73, 183, 294; fresh or fresh-frozen, 124, 157, 161, 215; as gift, 172; as "industrial affair," 171, 183; as national resource, 197–98, 203; and "paid" donors, 235, 241; and pooling, 175, 180, 229–30, 253, 259, 261, 270. *See also* blood; plasma fractions; plasma products
plasma banks, 171–76, 180–81
plasma fractionation, 94–95, 169, 223, 230, 327n36
plasma fractionation industry, 160, 169–71, 180, 235, 275, 287–88, 294–96, 327n32; and AIDS, 244, 246, 255–56, 260–61, 277–79; and hepatitis B, 299; legal settlement with people infected with HIV, 281, 289, 296
plasma fractions, xi, 77, 93–94, 136, 169–71, 173, 177; Cohn fraction I, 94–95, 97–98, 143, 153, 170, 174. *See also* clotting factor concentrates; cryoprecipitate
plasmapheresis, 169–73, 175, 180
plasma products, 16, 160, 207; and AIDS or hepatitis transmission, 235, 237, 253, 256, 277, 350n71; as pooled products, 4, 208–9, 229. *See also* blood products; clotting factor concentrates; cryoprecipitate; plasma; plasma fractions
plasma thromboplastin antecedent (PTA) deficiency, 82–83, 105, 108, 110, 114. *See also* factor XI deficiency
plasma thromboplastin component (PTC) deficiency, 98, 100, 104, 110, 114. *See also* factor IX deficiency
plasma transfusions, 94, 124, 157, 161, 215
polio, 123, 134
Pool, Judith Graham, 173–76
poster child/children, 223, 262–63, 266–67
post-transfusion infections, ix, 232–33, 279, 289, 291; and pooling of blood plasma, 229–30, 253, 259; as iatrogenic catastrophe, xiii, 4, 16, 239–40, 280; management of, 300–302; as "natural disaster," 16, 281; as revenge

effect, 6, 230; risks for, 203, 229–30, 242, 250, 277, 279, 299. *See also* hepatitis; tranfusion-related HIV/AIDS
President's Commission on AIDS, 265–66
Protein Foundation, Inc., 135
prothrombin tests, 79, 92; one-stage prothrombin assay (PT or Quick test), 69–70, 93, 95–96, 102, 105; two-stage prothrombin assay (Iowa test), 69–70
PTA-type hemophiliod, 82, 107–9
Public Citizen Health Research Group, 295
Puckett, Pearl, 123–24

Quick, Armand, 69–70, 75, 130
Quick test, 69–70, 93, 95–96, 102, 105

Rabiner, Fred, 213–15
Rackermann, Francis, 77
Rasputin, 184
Ratnoff, Oscar, 78, 114, 185, 216–17, 258, 271–73
Ray, Ricky, 268, 272
Ray family, 268
Reagan, Ronald, 247, 251, 263, 272, 274
Resnick, Susan, 126–27, 176, 201, 216, 232, 272
revenge effects, 5–6, 285
Rice, Terry, 289
Richmond, Julius, 38
Ricky Ray Hemophilia Relief Act, 281, 289
rights, 8–9, 16, 158, 209, 303. *See also* people with hemophilia
Romanov family, 226
Rosenberg, Charles, 285
Rosenberg, Michael, 288
Rosenthal, Martin, 130–31, 136–37, 147–48, 181, 190, 193
Rosenthal, Nathan, 90
Rosenthal, Robert, 90–91, 93
Rush, Benjamin, 22
Ryan White Comprehensive AIDS Resources Emergence (CARE) Act, 263, 358n64

Scheinfeld, Amram, 42, 44–46
Schnabel, Frank, 117–18, 138, 151, 153, 155
Schönlein, Johann Lukas, 27–31
Seeff, Leonard, 230, 350n71
Seegers, Walter, 68, 72
Segal, Bernard, 165, 167
self-administration of blood products, 176, 178–79, 193, 210–11, 214–15, 221–23, 347n40. *See also* home transfusion care
sex (biological), 83–91, 105–6, 237, 267. *See also* sex-linked inheritance
sex hormones, 87–88
sex-limited disease, 86–87
sex-linked inheritance, 1, 22, 31, 41–42, 44, 84–91, 104–6, 284
Sharp and Dohme (pharmaceutical co.), 95, 327n32
Shilts, Randy, 251, 355n38
Shulman, Irving, 98
Siplon, Patricia, 288
Sloan-Kettering Memorial Cancer Center (New York, NY), 254
Smith, Edward, 146
Smith, Harry Pratt, 68–69, 71–72
Smith, Nathan, 196
Spaet, Theodore, 85, 100, 112, 153
Spielberg, Steven, 190
Spira, Thomas, 249, 356n44
Spock, Benjamin, 149
Squibb (pharmaceutical co.), 95, 327n32
Stanford University, 58, 85, 94, 100, 112, 173, 212, 234
Starr, Douglas, 163, 171, 235, 241, 253–54, 356n38
Stetson, Richard, 75–77, 93
stigma, 9–13, 121, 124, 146, 187–89, 263–65, 267–70
Sullivan, Robert, 267
Surgenor, Douglas, 203–4
surgery, 5–6; and hemophilia, 44, 52–53, 64, 73, 124–25, 174

tainted blood scandals, 1, 202–3, 208, 240, 292, 296
Takehido, Kawano, 296
Taylor, Elizabeth, 265

Taylor, F. H. Laskey, 75–77, 93, 95, 97
technological ethos, 14, 49–50, 79, 83
technological innovation, 15, 91, 183
technological ways of being, xi, 2, 4–5, 10, 92, 284–85, 299
technology, 3–11, 15, 53, 55, 68, 83, 182, 284; laboratory, 49, 70, 92–93, 97–99, 284; technical fixes, 4, 290, 300
Telfer, Margaret, 213–16
Tenner, Edward, 5
therapeutic revolution, ix, 15, 158, 172, 183, 194, 209
tests. *See* prothrombin tests
Thomas, Henry Bascom, 87–88
Thorndike Memorial Laboratory (Boston, MA), 75, 77–78, 318n35
thromboplastic assays, 79, 92–93, 102
Tiddrick, Robert, 72
Titmuss, Richard, 208
Tocantins, Leandro, 130
"total care," 217, 253, 279, 286
transfusion-related HIV/AIDS, 249–50, 259–60, 262, 351n1, 356n39; as agent of change, 16–17, 286, 289; and clotting factor concentrates, 243–45, 248–49, 360–61n2; as failure of management, 237–39, 251; perceived risk of, 250, 257, 262, 271, 277, 279; secondary epidemic among wives, 272–73
Tufts–New England Medical Center (Boston, MA), 213, 225

U.K. Haemophilia Society, 293
University Hospital (Cleveland, OH), 185, 306n5
University of California at Los Angeles (UCLA), 187, 242
University of Colorado Medical Center, (Denver, CO), 244
University of Illinois, Chicago, 86–87
University of Iowa, x, 68, 71–72
University of North Carolina at Chapel Hill, x–xi, 76, 90
University of Pittsburgh, 79, 300–301
University of Rochester, 68, 70, 126, 147
U.S. Congress, 16, 164, 197, 217–20, 223–25, 227, 238, 263, 281